C0-AKF-409

PULMONARY DEVELOPMENT

LUNG BIOLOGY IN HEALTH AND DISEASE

Executive Editor: **Claude Lenfant**

Director, National Heart, Lung, and Blood Institute
National Institutes of Health
Bethesda, Maryland

Volume 1 IMMUNOLOGIC AND INFECTIOUS REACTIONS IN THE LUNG, *edited by Charles H. Kirkpatrick and Herbert Y. Reynolds*

Volume 2 THE BIOCHEMICAL BASIS OF PULMONARY FUNCTION, *edited by Ronald G. Crystal*

Volume 3 BIOENGINEERING ASPECTS OF THE LUNG, *edited by John B. West*

Volume 4 METABOLIC FUNCTIONS OF THE LUNG, *edited by Y. S. Bakhle and John R. Vane*

Volume 5 RESPIRATORY DEFENSE MECHANISMS (in two parts), *edited by Joseph D. Brain, Donald F. Proctor, and Lynne M. Reid*

Volume 6 DEVELOPMENT OF THE LUNG, *edited by W. Alan Hodson*

Volume 7 LUNG WATER AND SOLUTE EXCHANGE, *edited by Norman C. Staub*

Volume 8 EXTRAPULMONARY MANIFESTATIONS OF RESPIRATORY DISEASE, *edited by Eugene Debs Robin*

Volume 9 CHRONIC OBSTRUCTIVE PULMONARY DISEASE, *edited by Thomas L. Petty*

Volume 10 PATHOGENESIS AND THERAPY OF LUNG CANCER, *edited by Curtis C. Harris*

Volume 11 GENETIC DETERMINANTS OF PULMONARY DISEASE, *edited by Stephen D. Litwin*

Volume 12 THE LUNG IN THE TRANSITION BETWEEN HEALTH AND DISEASE, *edited by Peter T. Macklem and Solbert Permutt*

Volume 13 EVOLUTION OF RESPIRATORY PROCESSES: A COMPARATIVE APPROACH, *edited by Stephen C. Wood and Claude Lenfant*

Volume 14 PULMONARY VASCULAR DISEASES,
edited by Kenneth M. Moser

Volume 15 PHYSIOLOGY AND PHARMACOLOGY OF THE AIRWAYS,
edited by Jay A. Nadel

Volume 16 DIAGNOSTIC TECHNIQUES IN PULMONARY DISEASE (in two parts),
edited by Marvin A. Sackner

Volume 17 REGULATION OF BREATHING (in two parts),
edited by Thomas F. Hornbein

Volume 18 OCCUPATIONAL LUNG DISEASES:
RESEARCH APPROACHES AND METHODS,
edited by Hans Weill and Margaret Turner-Warwick

Volume 19 IMMUNOPHARMACOLOGY OF THE LUNG,
edited by Harold H. Newball

Volume 20 SARCOIDOSIS AND OTHER GRANULOMATOUS
DISEASES OF THE LUNG,
edited by Barry L. Fanburg

Volume 21 SLEEP AND BREATHING,
edited by Nicholas A. Saunders and Colin E. Sullivan

Volume 22 *PNEUMOCYSTIS CARINII* PNEUMONIA:
PATHOGENESIS, DIAGNOSIS, AND TREATMENT,
edited by Lowell S. Young

Volume 23 PULMONARY NUCLEAR MEDICINE:
TECHNIQUES IN DIAGNOSIS OF LUNG DISEASE,
edited by Harold L. Atkins

Volume 24 ACUTE RESPIRATORY FAILURE,
edited by Warren M. Zapol and Konrad J. Falke

Volume 25 GAS MIXING AND DISTRIBUTION IN THE LUNG,
edited by Ludwig A. Engel and Manuel Paiva

Volume 26 HIGH-FREQUENCY VENTILATION IN INTENSIVE CARE
AND DURING SURGERY,
edited by Graziano Carlon and William S. Howland

Volume 27 PULMONARY DEVELOPMENT: TRANSITION
FROM INTRAUTERINE TO EXTRAUTERINE LIFE,
edited by George H. Nelson

Volume 28 CHRONIC OBSTRUCTIVE PULMONARY DISEASE, second edition, revised and expanded
edited by Thomas L. Petty

Volume 29 THE THORAX (in two parts),
edited by Charis Roussos and Peter T. Macklem

Other volumes in preparation

THE PLEURA IN HEALTH AND DISEASE,
edited by Jacques Chrétien, Jean Bignon, Albert Hirsch, and Gerard Huchon

PULMONARY DEVELOPMENT

TRANSITION FROM INTRAUTERINE TO EXTRAUTERINE LIFE

Edited by
George H. Nelson
Medical College of Georgia
Augusta, Georgia

MARCEL DEKKER, INC. New York • Basel

Library of Congress Cataloging in Publication Data

Main entry under title:

Pulmonary development.

(Lung biology in health and disease ; v. 27)
Includes indexes.
1. Respiratory distress syndrome. 2. Hyaline membrane disease. 3. Lungs–Growth. 4. Fetus–Growth. I. Nelson, George H. II. Series. [DNLM: 1. Fetal Organ Maturity. 2. Fetus–physiology. 3. Lung–embryology. 4. Respiratory Distress Syndrome. W1 LU62 v.27 / WS 410 P982]
RJ274.P85 1985 618.3'26 85-7047
ISBN 0-8247-7316-0

Marcel Dekker, Inc.
270 Madison Avenue, New York, New York 10016

Current printing (last digit):
10 9 8 7 6 5 4 3 2 1

Printed in the United States of America

To
Anne, Martha, Elizabeth,
Rose, and Caroline,
and
Rosemary Nelson Hutto

CONTRIBUTORS

John E. Bleasdale, Ph.D. Assistant Professor, Departments of Biochemistry and Obstetrics-Gynecology, University of Texas Health Science Center at Dallas, Dallas, Texas

Geoffrey S. Dawes, C.B.E., D.M., F.R.S. Director, The Nuffield Institute for Medical Research, University of Oxford, Oxford, England

Goran Enhorning, M.D. Professor, Department of Obstetrics and Gynaecology, University of Toronto, Toronto, Ontario, Canada

John F. Evans, M.D. Associate Professor, Department of Obstetrics and Gynecology, and Assistant Professor, Department of Pediatrics, University of Kansas School of Medicine–Wichita, and Wesley Medical Center, Wichita, Kansas

Hossam E. Fadel, M.D., D.G.O., D.S., M.S. Professor, Maternal-Fetal Medicine Section, Department of Obstetrics and Gynecology, Medical College of Georgia, Augusta, Georgia

Robert O. Fisch, M.D. Professor, Department of Pediatrics, University of Minnesota Hospitals, Minneapolis, Minnesota

Fritz Fuchs, M.D. Professor, Department of Obstetrics and Gynecology, Cornell University Medical College, New York, New York

Gary R. Gutcher, M.D. Associate Professor, Department of Pediatrics, University of Wisconsin School of Medicine, Madison, Wisconsin

John M. Johnston, Ph.D. Professor, Department of Biochemistry, University of Texas Health Science Center at Dallas, Dallas, Texas

William P. Kanto, Jr., M.D. Chief, Section of Pediatric Neonatology, and Professor, Department of Pediatrics, Medical College of Georgia, Augusta, Georgia

Donald L. Levy, M.D. Associate Professor and Director, Division of Maternal-Fetal Medicine, Department of Obstetrics and Gynecology, Eastern Virginia Medical School, Norfolk, Virginia

James C. McPherson, Jr., M.D. Associate Professor, Departments of Surgery and Cell and Molecular Biology, Medical College of Georgia, Augusta, Georgia

Carole R. Mendelson, Ph.D. Assistant Professor, Departments of Biochemistry and Obstetrics-Gynecology, University of Texas Health Science Center at Dallas, Dallas, Texas

John C. Morrison, M.D. Professor, Department of Obstetrics and Gynecology, University of Mississippi Medical Center, Jackson, Mississippi

George H. Nelson, Ph.D., M.D. Professor, Department of Obstetrics and Gynecology, Medical College of Georgia, Augusta, Georgia

Ronan O'Rahilly, M.D. Director, Carnegie Laboratories of Embryology, California Primate Research Center, and Professor, Human Anatomy and Neurology, University of California at Davis, Davis, California

John E. Patrick, M.D., F.R.C.S.(C) Professor, Department of Obstetrics and Gynecology and Department of Physiology, Medical Research Council Group in Reproductive Biology, St. Joseph's Hospital Research Institute, University of Western Ontario, London, Ontario, Canada

Robert H. Perelman, M.D. Associate Professor, Department of Pediatrics, University of Wisconsin School of Medicine, Madison, Wisconsin

Lynne M. Reid, M.D. Pathologist-in-Chief, The Children's Hospital, and Wolbach Professor of Pathology, Harvard Medical School, Boston, Massachusetts

Daniel K. Roberts, M.D., Ph.D. Professor and Chairman, Department of Obstetrics and Gynecology, and Professor, Department of Pathology, University of Kansas School of Medicine–Wichita; Chief, Obstetrics and Gynecology Service, Wesley Medical Center, Wichita, Kansas

William E. Roberts, M.D. Fellow, Maternal-Fetal Medicine, Department of Obstetrics and Gynecology, University of Mississippi Medical Center, Jackson, Mississippi

Alex. F. Robertson, III, M.D. Professor, Department of Pediatrics, Medical College of Georgia, Augusta, Georgia

Jeanne M. Snyder, Ph.D. Research Assistant Professor, Departments of Cell Biology and Obstetrics-Gynecology, University of Texas Health Science Center at Dallas, Dallas, Texas

Joseph F. Tomashefski, Jr., M.D.* Research Fellow, Department of Pathology, The Children's Hospital, and Harvard Medical School, Boston, Massachusetts

Gordon F. Vawter, M.D. Associate Pathologist-in-Chief, The Children's Hospital, and Professor, Department of Pathology, Harvard Medical School, Boston, Massachusetts

Preston Lea Wilds, M.D.[†] Professor, Division of Maternal-Fetal Medicine, Department of Obstetrics and Gynecology, Eastern Virginia Medical School, Norfolk, Virginia

Present affiliation:
*Assistant Professor, Department of Pathology, Case Western Reserve University School of Medicine, and Cleveland Metropolitan General Hospital, Cleveland, Ohio
†Consultant, Maternal and Child Health, Community Health Services—Eastern Virginia Regional Office, Virginia Department of Health, Virginia Beach, Virginia

PREFACE

Abnormal pulmonary function is by far the most critical problem encountered by genetically normal premature newborns. This potentially lethal condition serves as the general theme for this book, which has been organized to present in a temporal fashion pulmonary maturation from early lung development in utero to long-term follow-up of survivors of respiratory distress syndrome. Between these end points in time, the attempt has been made to discuss critical points of development and important events that might alter the ultimate outcome.

The 19 chapters herein are grouped into eight parts. Chapters 1 through 4 make up the first part. The embryology (Chapter 1), anatomy (Chapter 2), and biochemistry (Chapter 3) of early human lung development are covered in these chapters. In Chapter 4 Dawes and Patrick review the physiology of fetal breathing activity and discuss the importance of fetal breathing movements in lung development.

The second part (Chapters 5 through 7) covers the methods available to the obstetrician for gestational age estimation and fetal maturity evaluation. The principal ways of doing this utilize ultrasonography and amniotic fluid analysis. In addition, Chapter 7 presents a historical review of evaluation of fetal lung maturity at the Medical College of Georgia.

Part 3 comprises Chapters 8 through 10. These chapters present some factors that may influence fetal lung maturation during gestation. A possible role of diet in fetal lung maturation is proposed and, in addition, the effects of various maternal drugs and maternal-fetal disorders are reviewed.

Part 4 discusses important events that occur just prior to delivery. Chapter 11 presents the Kansas experience in maternal transport. I think everyone would agree with the concept that the uterus is the best transport incubator and maternal transport should be utilized, whenever possible, when premature delivery is threatening. Chapter 12 discusses prevention of premature deliveries and presents appropriate precautions should delivery be imminent.

The events in Chapters 13 and 14 (Part 5) occur in the delivery room. Enhorning updates the reader on the possible future use of surfactant administration in the delivery room. In addition, immediate resuscitation of the newborn is considered in Chapter 14.

In Part 6 the scene shifts to the neonatal intensive care unit (NICU). Special problems encountered in the unit, as well as perinatal regionalization, are discussed by Gutcher and Perelman, who describe their experience in Wisconsin (Chapter 15). In addition, the differential diagnosis of the various respiratory distress syndromes encountered in the NICU are presented with special emphasis on hyaline membrane disease (Chapter 16).

Infants who suffer from respiratory distress syndrome either succumb to their disease or recover only to have potential long-term consequences. Part 7 (Chapters 17 and 18) discusses these two outcomes. Tomashefski, Vawter, and Reid present the pathological picture of infants who do not survive, while Fisch discusses the potential future problems to be encountered by the survivors.

The final part—Chapter 19—was written to allow chapter contributors to express their opinions with regard to areas of future research and development in the broad context of pulmonary maturation. In addition, a few select authorities in perinatal medicine were asked to contribute their thoughts.

It is quite apparent that considerable progress has been made in recent years in understanding, preventing, and treating neonatal pulmonary immaturity; nevertheless, it still remains a formidable threat to medical personnel interested in the newborn infant. This book was written with those individuals in mind. Obviously the prime audience that this book was designed for are those physicians and nurses who are directly responsible for the care and welfare of pregnant women and newborn infants. However, hospital and state administrators, emergency medical technicians, medical technologists, respiratory therapists, students of medicine, nursing, and graduate studies, epidemiologists, basic scientists, pathologists, and others might find this material interesting reading.

George H. Nelson

INTRODUCTION

Ontogeny, the key to structure.

These were the first words of E. A. Boyden's final publication, which appeared in the sixth monograph of the series "Lung Biology in Health and Disease." The title of the monograph was *Development of the Lung*, and W. A. Hodson was the editor.

If ontogeny is the key to structure, then structure is the key to function. Thus, it should surprise no one that this series, which is devoted to the understanding of lung biology, i.e., function, again includes a volume concerned with pulmonary maturation.

At the time of birth, the lung undergoes dramatic changes of major functional significance and potential clinical importance. Of course, the degree of lung maturation at birth determines how the lung will respond to its first contact with air, but the attendant care given by obstetricians and pediatricians also contributes to the success of this event. In fact, subsequent respiratory health may very well depend on the course of lung maturation in utero and on whether the infant's entry into the world is with a healthy or a diseased lung.

The field of neonatology is advancing at a rapid pace and remarkable progress has been made during the last few years, especially with regard to lung biology. Dr. Nelson's volume not only is a treatise on the history of the lung from its embryonic stage to its response to birth, but is all novel in concept and in content. Dr. Nelson selected authors who are new to the series but experts in their fields. Each of them brings a point of view that adds considerably to the entire series. From my own vantage point, the last chapter, entitled "Areas of Future Research and Development," is of special interest because it shows how many questions remain unanswered, even though so much new knowledge has been gained. It reminds us that research pursuits in the area of lung maturation will continue to challenge us in the years ahead.

Dr. Nelson and the authors of his volume have provided the series with a major contribution for which we are very grateful.

Claude Lenfant, M.D.
Bethesda, Maryland

CONTENTS

Part Two METHODS OF EVALUATION

Part Three INFLUENCING FACTORS

Part Four PREDELIVERY

Part Five THE DELIVERY ROOM

Part Seven THE NONSURVIVORS AND THE SURVIVORS

Part Eight THE FUTURE

PULMONARY DEVELOPMENT

Part One

BASIC SCIENCE

1

The Early Prenatal Development of the Human Respiratory System

RONAN O'RAHILLY

California Primate Research Center
University of California at Davis
Davis, California

I. Introduction

It is almost 100 years since Wilhelm His investigated the development of the human lungs. A number of studies of embryonic development have appeared in the intervening years, culminating in the description of the origin of the bronchopulmonary segments by Wells and Boyden in 1954 [1].

The most precise account of early respiratory development is that by O'Rahilly and Boyden [2], in which only data based on staged human embryos were included. In the Carnegie system of staging, as promulgated by O'Rahilly [3,4], the embryonic period proper, i.e., the first 8 post-ovulatory weeks of development, is subdivided into 23 stages based on morphological criteria (Table 1). The fetal period, i.e., from 8 weeks to birth, has not yet been staged.

Supported by research grant HD-16702, Institute of Child Health and Human Development, National Institutes of Health.

Table 1 Developmental Stages in Human Embryos

Carnegie stage	Pairs of somites	Length (mm)	Age (days)	Features
1				Fertilization
2			1½–3	From 2 to about 16 cells
3			4	Free blastocyst
4			5–6	Attaching blastocyst
5		0.1–0.2	7–12	Implanted although previllous
5a		0.1	7–8	Solid trophoblast
5b		0.1	9	Trophoblastic lacunae
5c		0.15–0.2	11–12	Lacunar vascular circle
6		0.2	13	Chorionic villi; primitive streak may appear
6a				Chorionic villi
6b				Primitive streak
7		0.4	16	Notochordal process
8		1.0–1.5	18	Primitive pit; notochordal and neurenteric canals
9	1–3	1.5–2.5	20	Somites first appear
10	4–12	2–3.5	22	Neural folds begin to fuse; 2 pharyngeal bars; optic sulcus
11	13–20	2.5–4.5	24	Rostral neuropore closes; optic vesicle
12	21–29	3–5	26	Caudal neuropore closes; 3 pharyngeal bars; upper limb buds appearing

13	30–?	4–6	28	Four limb buds; lens disc; optic vesicle
14		5–7	32	Lens pit and optic cup; endolymphatic appendage distinct
15		7–9	33	Lens vesicle; nasal pit; antitragus beginning; hand plate; trunk relatively wider; cerebral vesicles distinct
16		8–11	37	Nasal pit faces ventrally; retinal pigment visible in intact embryo; auricular hillocks beginning; foot plate
17		11–14	41	Head relatively larger; trunk straighter; nasofrontal groove distinct; auricular hillocks distinct; finger rays
18		13–17	44	Body more cuboidal; elbow region and toe rays appearing; eyelids beginning; tip of nose distinct; nipples appear; ossification may begin
19		16–18	47½	Trunk elongating and straightening
20		18–22	50½	Upper limbs longer and bent at elbows
21		22–24	52	Fingers longer; hands approach each other, feet likewise
22		23–28	54	Eyelids and external ear more developed
23		27–31	56½	Head more rounded; limbs longer and more developed

Source: Ref. 3. Courtesy of the Carnegie Institution of Washington.

II. Sequence of Events

The sequence of the chief developmental events will now be presented chronologically. Only the lower part of the respiratory system (from the larynx downward) will be considered here.

A. Second Week

In the chick embryo, it has been possible by means of radioautographic mapping to delineate areas of pulmogenic endoderm and mesoderm [5]. These early stages probably correspond to human embryos of 2 weeks (stages 6 and 7). However, no morphological evidence of the respiratory apparatus is found for another week.

B. Third Week

The foregut is established by 20 postovulatory days (stage 9), and it includes the embryonic pharynx with its median groove and keel. By 22 days (stage 10), when the embryo is about 3 mm in length, the median pharyngeal groove is seen to include a slightly more defined laryngotracheal sulcus, the caudal end of which is enlarged to form the respiratory primordium [6].

According to Puiggrós-Sala [7], what may be termed the respiratory field (*Lungenfeld*) includes not only the ventral border (*Vorderdarmkante*) but also portions of both lateral walls of the foregut.

C. Fourth Week

At 24 days (stage 11) the respiratory primordium (Fig. 1) is more evident and appears as a thickened elevation immediately rostral to the hepatic primordium [7,8]. There is some evidence that the respiratory primordium is bilateral in origin [8]. Unilateral failure of development would be expected to result in agenesis of the lung.

The mesenchyme around the respiratory primordium is believed to determine the pattern of growth and branching of the endodermal component. Subsequently the mesenchyme will give rise to the connective tissue, muscle, and cartilage of the bronchial tree.

At 26 days (stage 12) the respiratory primordium assumes the form of a rounded bud (Fig. 1). The part of the foregut immediately caudal to the bud may now be termed the esophagus [9]. However, the existence of an epithelial tracheo-esophageal septum as usually described [10] has recently been denied as a result of a careful reassessment of early human embryos [11]. It is now suggested that what was formerly interpreted as

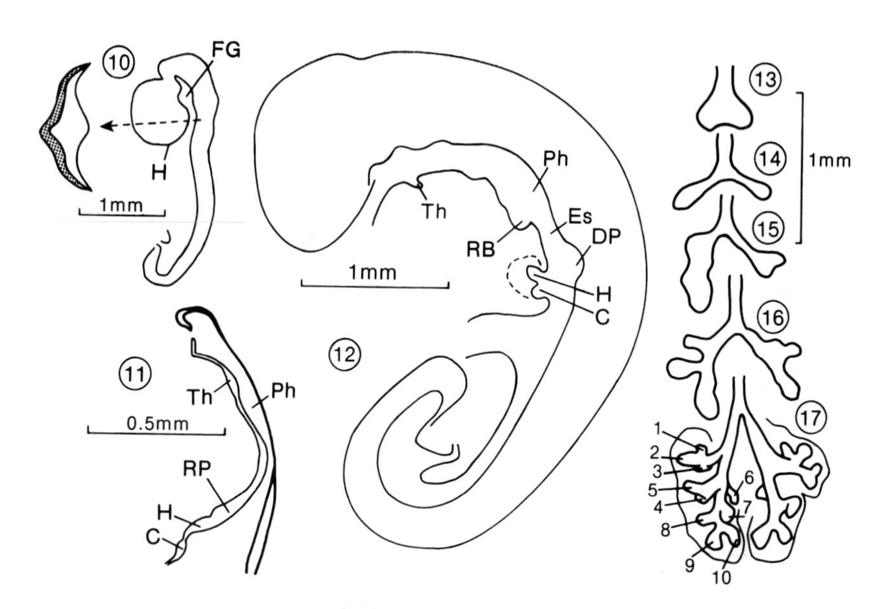

Figure 1 The embryonic respiratory system from 3 to 6 weeks. A transverse section (arrow) at stage 10 shows the embryonic pharynx with its laryngotracheal sulcus. The close relationship of the respiratory primordium (RP) to the hepatic (H) and cystic (C) primordia is well seen at stage 11. The respiratory primordium has formed a bud (RB) at stage 12, and the esophagus (Es) is distinguishable from the pharynx (Ph), although a trachea is not yet delineated. The respiratory tree is shown in ventral view on the right-hand side of the drawing. The primary bronchi of stages 13 and 14 give rise to lobar bronchi at stages 15 and 16, and to segmental buds (1–10) at stage 17. Additional abbreviations: FG, foregut; DP, dorsal pancreas; Th, thyroid gland.

a tracheoesophageal septum is actually the curved floor of the pharynx between the pharynx (not esophagus) behind and the respiratory bud (not the trachea) in front (Fig. 2). Nevertheless, a mesenchymal partition separates the trachea from the esophagus, and the term tracheoesophageal septum can still be used [12].

At 28 days (stage 13) the main bronchi are represented by right and left lung buds [7]. The point of division is opposite approximately the sixth pair of somites, which would correspond to the mid-cervical region. Later during this stage the elongating stalk that gives rise to the lung buds forms the trachea. The pulmonary arteries and veins are now evident [13] and a common pulmonary vein is recognizable [14]. The embryo is about 5 mm in length.

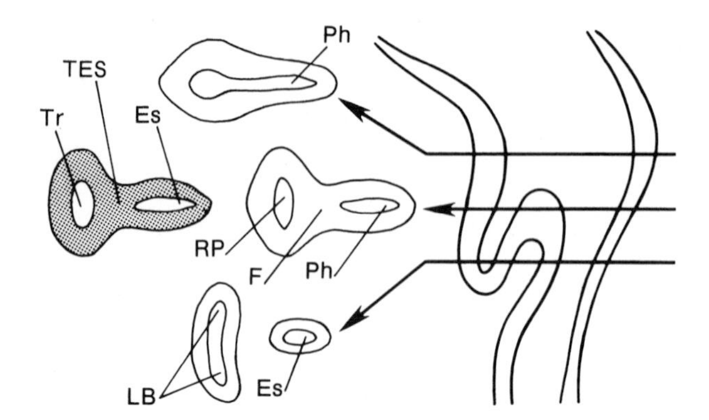

Figure 2 Median section and transverse sections of the foregut at 4 weeks (stage 13). According to the usual account–e.g., that of Smith in 1957 [10] – a tracheoesophageal septum (TES) is postulated between the trachea (Tr) and esophagus (Es) (stippled section). To the right, Zaw-Tun's 1982 interpretation [11] is illustrated. According to this, the trachea has not yet differentiated, and the cavity of the respiratory primordium is separated from that of the pharynx by the curved pharyngeal floor (F). Additional abbreviations: F, floor of embryonic pharynx; LB, lung buds.

D. Fifth Week

At 32 days (stage 14) the larynx is taking form [15]. The paired lung buds are elongating to become lung sacs; the right one usually longer and directed caudally, the left one generally shorter and more transverse. The main bronchi are beginning to curve dorsally to embrace the esophagus. By 33 days (stage 15) the lung sacs are giving rise to lobar buds: three on the right and two on the left. Angiogenesis is occurring around the primary bronchi.

E. Sixth Week

By 37 days (stage 16) the lobar buds have elongated and become more definite (Figs. 1 and 3). The embryo is now about 10 mm in length. Instances of atresia of the esophagus and tracheoesophageal fistula have been recorded from stage 16 to stage 19 [10]. At 41 days (stage 17), when the embryo is about 11-14 mm in length, the bronchopulmonary segments arise as segmental buds on the bronchial tree [1]. The surface of the developing lung is lobulated and the elevations represent at first the underlying bronchopulmonary segments. Segmental anomalies, caused by the displaced origin of buds, may develop at this time. The lobar fissures are present by this stage.

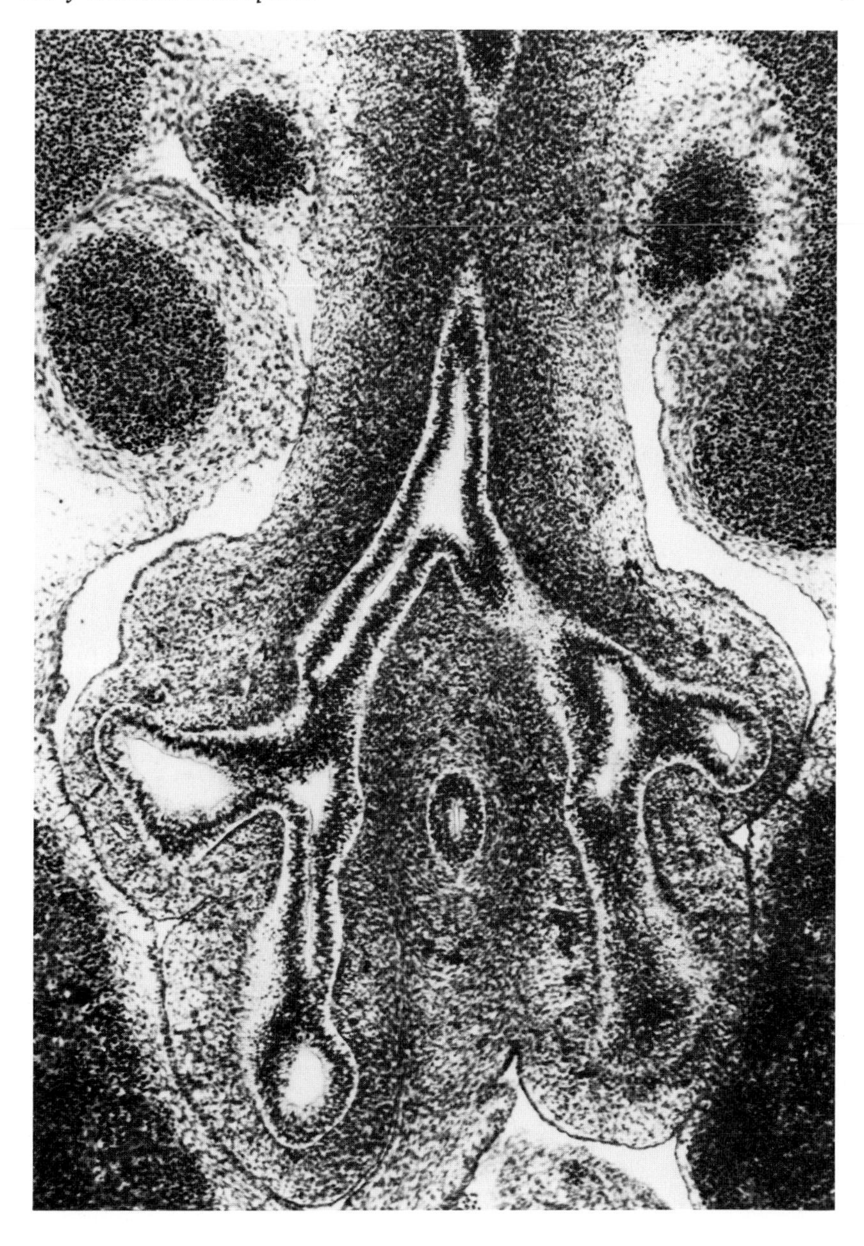

Figure 3 Coronal section through the trachea and lobar buds at 37 days (stage 16), 11 mm. Below the carina, the lower end of the esophagus is visible in cross section. The parietal and visceral layers of the pleura are evident.

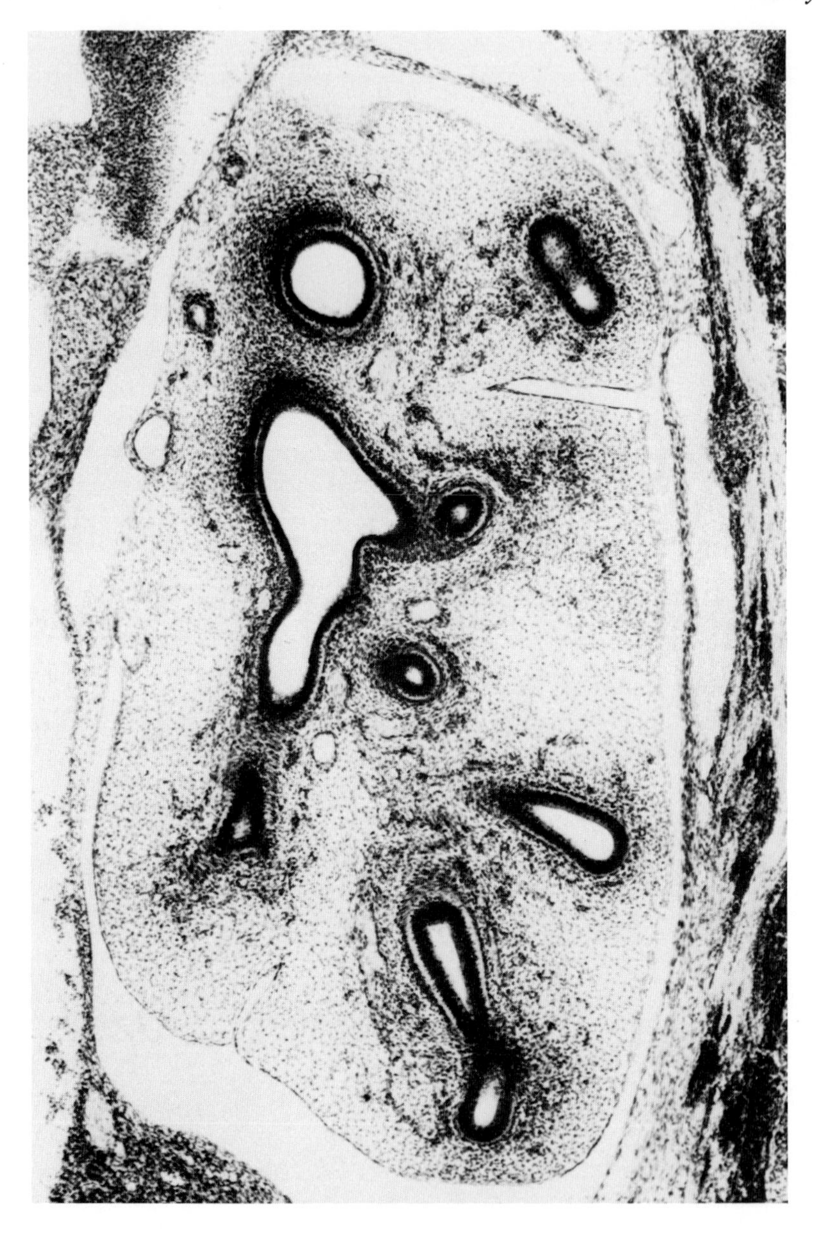

Figure 4 Sagittal section through a lung at 48 days (stage 19), 18 mm. Several large bronchi can be seen in section, surrounded by condensations of the mesenchyme. The lung does not fill the pleural cavity completely. Indications of interlobar fissures can be discerned.

F. Seventh Week

By 44 days (stage 18) a few subsegmental buds begin to appear. The left lung lags behind the right lung in size and degree of development until the end of the embryonic period proper [16]. By 48 days (stage 19; Fig. 4) the first generation of subsegmental bronchi is complete [1]. The elevations on the surface of the lung represent mostly the underlying subsegments and give the lung the appearance of a mulberry. The lungs have grown laterally but have not yet curved ventrally, so that they are wedged between the heart and the vertebral column. The lungs lie between the second and the sixth to ninth ribs [1], and hence will later grow both rostrally and caudally, but primarily caudally. The main developmental events during the first 7 weeks are summarized in Figure 5.

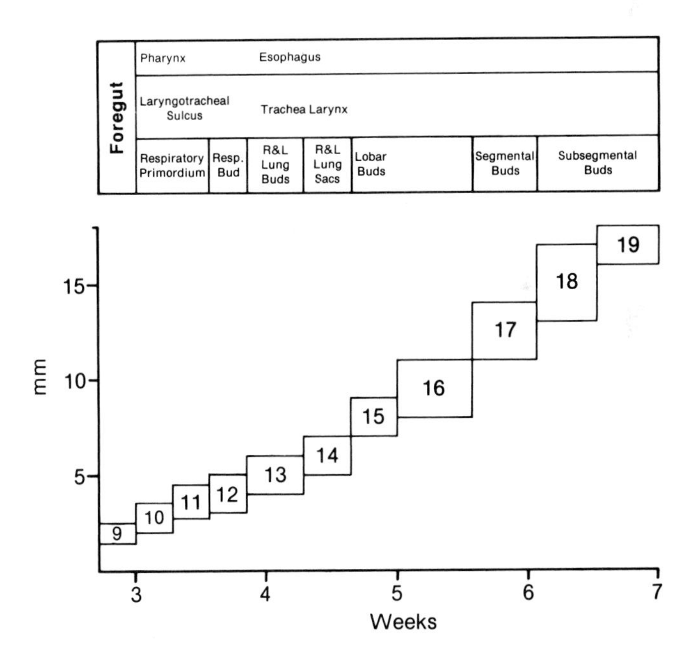

Figure 5 Scheme of the development of the respiratory system. The rectangles represent stages (from 9 to 19) above which the appropriate developmental features are indicated. The ordinate represents embryonic length in millimeters and the abscissa shows embryonic age in weeks and days.

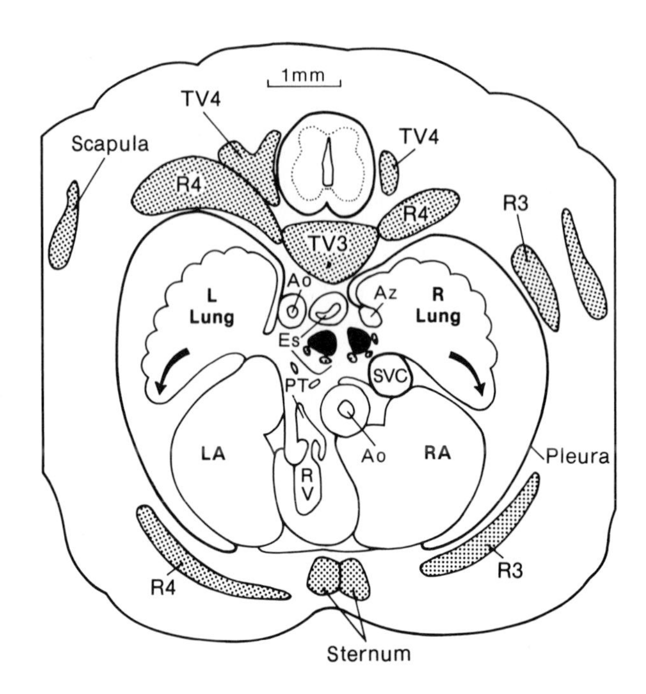

Figure 6 Horizontal section through an embryo of 8 weeks (stage 23) immediately below the tracheal bifurcation. Parts of the third and fourth thoracic vertebrae (TV3, TV4) and ribs (R3, R4) are visible. The primary bronchi are indicated in black, each surrounded by several pieces of cartilage. The lungs extend laterally into the pleural cavities, which they do not fill, and they are now beginning to grow ventrally as well (arrows). Other features shown include the sternum (of bilateral origin), the scapulae (very high at this stage), and the aorta (Ao, sectioned twice), azygos vein (Az), esophagus (Es), left atrium (LA), pulmonary trunk (PT) and pulmonary valve, right atrium (RA), right ventricle (RV), and superior vena cava (SVC).

G. Eighth Week

By 51 days (stage 20) the second generation of subsegmental bronchi is forming. The formation of new bronchi appears to occur only at the growing tips of the tree, especially where the basement membrane is incomplete [17]. The lungs appear to occupy only half of the pleural cavity. The pleuroperitoneal canals are closing [18]. The embryo is about 20 mm in length. By 52 days (stage 21) the pleural sacs are closed and they extend between the first and twelfth ribs [18].

The conclusion of the embryonic period proper is at 8 postovulatory weeks (stage 23), when the embryo is about 30 mm in length (Figs.

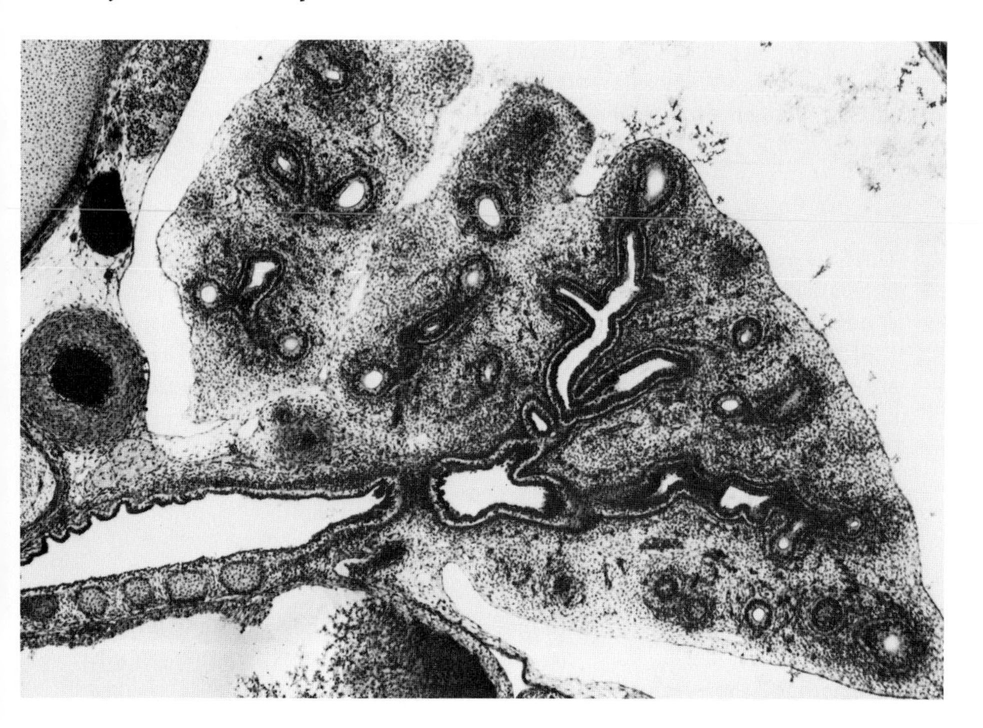

Figure 7 Horizontal section through the left lung at 57 days (stage 23), 31 mm. The left main bronchus, the cartilaginous plates of which are visible in section, can be traced toward the periphery, where the lung is in its pseudoglandular phase. The bronchial tubules are embedded in mesenchyme, which is condensed around them. The pleural cavity is wide. Dorsal to the left main bronchus, the descending aorta, filled with blood, is visible in corss section.

6 and 7); the lungs are in the pseudoglandular phase. The various bronchial tubules are embedded in loose mesenchyme, which constitutes the bulk of the lungs. We have observed that most of the tubules contain a relatively large lumen and are lined by a thick pseudostratified columnar epithelium, which is covered by a well-marked basement membrane. The tubules are surrounded by mesenchymal condensations. The lung is limited peripherally by a layer of pleural mesothelium. The pleural cavity, at least in histological sections, is wide. (According to Wells and Boyden [1], "in both fresh and fixed specimens the lungs do not fill the pleural sacs.") The trachea is approximately 3 mm in length. In three embryos at this stage the tracheal bifurcation occurred at the level of the third thoracic vertebra. Cartilage is present in the trachea and in the primary bronchi.

A detailed histological account and a reconstruction of the bronchial tree at this important stage would be a valuable contribution to our knowledge of pulmonary development. Considerable information concerning the larynx at this stage is being accumulated [19].

H. Early Fetal Period

The fetal period of development begins with the ninth week. The pseudoglandular phase persists until about 14-16 weeks. Cartilage develops in more peripheral tubules, particularly during the first half of prenatal life, as do also glands [20]. Glands may be found in the trachea as early as 57 mm [21]. The pulmonary epithelium in most of the peripheral bronchial tubules diminishes from columnar to cuboidal early in the fetal period, and cytoplasmic glycogen increases in amount [22].

III. Discussion

Although staging has been mentioned only briefly in this account, it should be stressed that the use of a recognized staging system is essential in order to determine the precise sequence of developmental events. Most systems of the body have now been investigated developmentally in reference to the Carnegie system of stages, and data are readily available [4].

It should also be emphasized that the structure of the lungs shows marked species differences, and hence "the physiologist who neglects the study of the anatomy of human lungs during development" does so at his peril [23].

The respiratory apparatus is a derivative of the embryonic pharynx. The pharynx served originally as a strainer for food but later it became subserviant to respiration and also participated in the formation of an assortment of nonrespiratory structures, such as the thyroid gland. These developmental deviations are well exemplified by the pharyngeal pouches, which in fish are elaborated into gill-slits, whereas in reptiles, birds, and mammals they are converted into an array of other structures. Such instances "have been used erroneously to support the biogenetic law" [24], whereby it was claimed that ontogeny recapitulated phylogeny. In point of fact, the pharyngeal pouches of embryonic reptiles, birds, and mammals "bear little resemblance to the gill-slits of the adult fish" [24]. Moreover, it is half a century since in a discussion of "fishy nomenclature" it was recommended that the word branchial be dropped from mammalian embryology [25].

Puiggrós-Sala [7], who made and illustrated careful reconstructions from embryos of stages 10-13, subdivided the early development of the respiratory apparatus into five phases. It was stressed that variations do occur and that the events do not always follow precisely the same sequence. The phases are:

1. The respiratory field (*Lungenfeld*) arises as a thickening of both the ventral and lateral walls of the foregut between the pharyngeal pouches rostrally and the hepatic anlage caudally (stage 10).
2. Two lateral protrusions arise from the respiratory field and meet at the ventral border of the foregut (*Vorderdarmkante*) (stages 11 and 12). The foregut grows in length, so that the respiratory primordium becomes further separated from the pharyngeal pouches and from the hepatic primordium.
3. Differential growth results in caudoventral rotation of the lateral protrusions (stage 12).
4. Lateral grooves begin to separate the respiratory bud (*Lungenanlage*) from the esophagus (stages 12 and 13).
5. The right and left lung buds (*primäre Lungensäckchen*) are formed (stage 13).

Although such terms as pulmonary primordium are frequently used (2), Puiggrós-Sala (7) has pointed out that the *Lungenanlage* includes the future larynx, trachea, bronchi, and lungs.

It is reasonable to assume, in the absence of evidence to the contrary, that the respiratory apparatus develops (as do the limb buds) in rostrocaudal sequence, so that the first portion to be formed is laryngeal rather than pulmonary [15]. The various segments, such as the trachea, however, cannot at first be distinguished from each other.

In the development of the respiratory system, "observations of organ cultures of human foetal lung show that the morphogenesis of the bronchial tree is brought about by mitosis, cell death and cell migration" [26]. Recently it has been suggested that, as a bronchial tip grows, "resistance to its further advance increases progressively as a result of compression by the mesenchymal tissues at the tip, approach to the pleural surface, or approach to neighboring bronchi" [17]. Division and further growth of the bronchus take place in areas of lower resistance. This is correlated with an increase in the proportion of tracheobronchial tissue and a decrease in the proportion of mesenchyme within the developing lungs.

It is interesting to reflect that embryonically the lungs begin as thick-walled buds that project into a dense mass of connective tissue, "a condition having no counterpart in any adult. The respiratory epithelium is a later-developing product of this preliminary condition" [27]. This is one of many illustrations of the principle that present developmental changes in the embryo or fetus anticipate future requirements for the survival and welfare of the organism [28].

Although the pseudoglandular period is concerned with the establishment of air-conducting tubules, it has recently been proposed (on the basis of studies of the mouse) that it must include the beginning of the development of the respiratory portion of the lung early in fetal life, perhaps at 11-12 weeks [29].

IV. Summary

The beginning of the respiratory system awaits the appearance of the foregut, which is established by 20 days. The respiratory primordium develops within the next few days, and right and left lung buds can be distinguished by 4 weeks. Each lung bud gives rise to lobar buds at 5 weeks. Segmental buds are present by 6 weeks and subsegmental buds by 7 weeks. The surrounding mesenchyme is essential to these events. The respiratory system develops as a ventral outgrowth of the foregut but the existence of an epithelial tracheoesophageal septum has recently been denied. Much further work remains to be done and it is pointed out, for example, that no detailed account of the respiratory system at the end of the embryonic period proper is available.

References

1. Wells, L. J., and E. A. Boyden, The development of the bronchopulmonary segments in human embryos of horizons XVII to XIX, *Am. J. Anat.*, **95**:163-201 (1945).
2. O'Rahilly, R., and E. A. Boyden, The timing and sequence of events in the development of the human respiratory system during the embryonic period proper, *Z. Anat. Entw.*, **141**:237-250 (1973).
3. O'Rahilly, R., *Developmental Stages in Human Embryos, Including a Survey of the Carnegie Collection. Part A: Embryos of the First Three Weeks (Stages 1 to 9).* Carnegie Institution of Washington, Washington, D.C. (1973).
4. O'Rahilly, R., Early human development and the chief sources of information on staged human embryos, *Europ. J. Obstet. Gynec. Reprod. Biol.*, **9**:273-280 (1979).
5. Rosenquist, G. C., The origin and movement of prelung cells in the chick embryo as determined by radioautographic mapping, *J. Embryol. Exp. Morphol.*, **24**:497-509 (1970).

6. Corner, G. W., A well-preserved human embryo of 10 somites, *Contr. Embryol. Carneg. Instn.,* **20**:81–101 (1929).
7. Puiggrós Sala, J., Über die Entwicklung der Lungenanlage des Menschen, *Z. Anat. Entw.,* **106**:209–225 (1937).
8. Davis, C. L., Description of a human embryo having twenty paired somites, *Contr. Embryol. Carneg. Instn.,* **15**:1–51 (1923).
9. Bejdl, W., and G. Politzer, Über die Frühentwicklung des telobranchialen Körpes beim Menschen, *Z. Anat. Entw.,* **117**:136–152 (1953).
10. Smith, E. I., The early development of the trachea and esophagus in relation to atresia of the esophagus and tracheoesophageal fistula, *Contr. Embryol. Carneg. Instn.,* **36**:41–57 (1957).
11. Zaw-Tun, H. A., The tracheo-esophageal septum—fact or fantasy? The origin and development of the respiratory primordium and esophagus, *Acta Anat.,* **114**:1-21 (1982).
12. O'Rahilly, R., and Müller, F., Respiratory and alimentary relations in staged human embryos. New embryological data and congenital anomalies, *Ann. Otol. Rhinol. Laryngol.,* **93**:421–429 (1984).
13. Congdon, E. D., Transformation of the aortic-arch system during the development of the human embryo, *Contr. Embryol. Carneg. Instn.,* **14**:47–110 (1922).
14. Neill, C. A., Development of the pulmonary veins, *Pediatrics,* **18**:880–887 (1956).
15. O'Rahilly, R., and J. A. Tucker, The early development of the larynx in staged human embryos, *Ann. Otol. Rhinol. Laryngol.,* **82**(Suppl. 7):1–27 (1973).
16. D. M. Palmer, The lung of a human foetus of 170 mm. C.R. length, *Am. J. Anat.,* **58**:59–72 (1936).
17. Hutchins, G., H. M. Haupt, and G. W. Moore, A proposed mechanism for the early development of the human tracheobronchial tree, *Anat. Rec.,* **201**:635–640 (1981).
18. Wells, L. J., Development of the human diaphragm and pleural sacs, *Contr. Embryol. Carneg. Instn.,* **35**:107–134 (1954).
19. Müller, F., R. O'Rahilly, and J. A. Tucker, The human larynx at the end of the embryonic period proper. 1. The laryngeal and infrahyoid muscles and their innervation, *Acta Otolaryngol.,* **91**:323–336 (1981).
20. Bucher, U., and L. Reid, Development of the intrasegmental bronchial tree: The pattern of branching and development of cartilage at various stages of intra-uterine life, *Thorax,* **16**:201–218 (1961).
21. Tos, M., Development of the tracheal glands in man, *Acta Pathol. Microbiol. Scand.,* **68**(Suppl. 185):1–128 (1966).

22. E. Hage, The morphological development of the pulmonary epithelium of human foetuses studied by light and electron microscopy, *Z. Anat. Entw.*, **140**:271–279 (1973).
23. Emery, J., *The Anatomy of the Developing Lung.* London, Heinemann (1969).
24. DeBeer, G., *Embryos and Ancestors,* 3rd ed. London, Oxford University Press, 1958.
25. Frazer, J. E., The nomenclature of diseased states caused by certain vestigial structures in the neck, *Br. J. Surg.,* **11**:131–136 (1923).
26. Glücksmann, A., Mitosis and degeneration in the morphogenesis of the human foetal lung *in vitro, Z. Zellforsch.,* **64**:101–110 (1964).
27. Torrey, T. W., and A. Feduccia, *Morphogenesis of the Vertebrates,* 4th ed., New York, Wiley, 1979.
28. Reynolds, S. R. M., Developmental changes and future requirements, *Cold Spring Harbor. Symp. Quant. Biol.,* **19**:1–2 (1954).
29. Ten Have-Opbroek, A. A. W., The development of the lung in mammals: An analysis of concepts and findings, *Am. J. Anat.,* **162**:201–219 (1981).

2

The Morphology of Lung Development in the Human Fetus

JEANNE M. SNYDER, CAROLE R. MENDELSON, and JOHN M. JOHNSTON

University of Texas Health Science Center at Dallas
Dallas, Texas

I. Introduction

The human fetal lung at birth mediates gas exchange between blood and air. An inability to assume this function properly has life-threatening consequences. Respiratory distress syndrome (RDS) of the newborn, the leading cause of death in premature human newborns [1], is caused by an inadequate production of surfactant by the fetal type II pneumonocyte [2]. Lung surfactant is a lipoprotein substance that lines the alveolus and by reducing its surface tension overcomes the tendency of the alveoli to collapse during expiration [3].

A goal of many investigators is to determine methods for stimulating normal lung maturation either in utero or after birth so as to prevent the development of RDS. In order to understand and interpret data concerning the therapeutic manipulation of human fetal lung maturation, it is necessary first to understand the normal process of human fetal lung differentiation. The morphology of developing fetal lung is described in detail in several review papers [4-7]. However, few reports are concerned specifically with the morphological

---

Supported by USPHS grant HD13912.

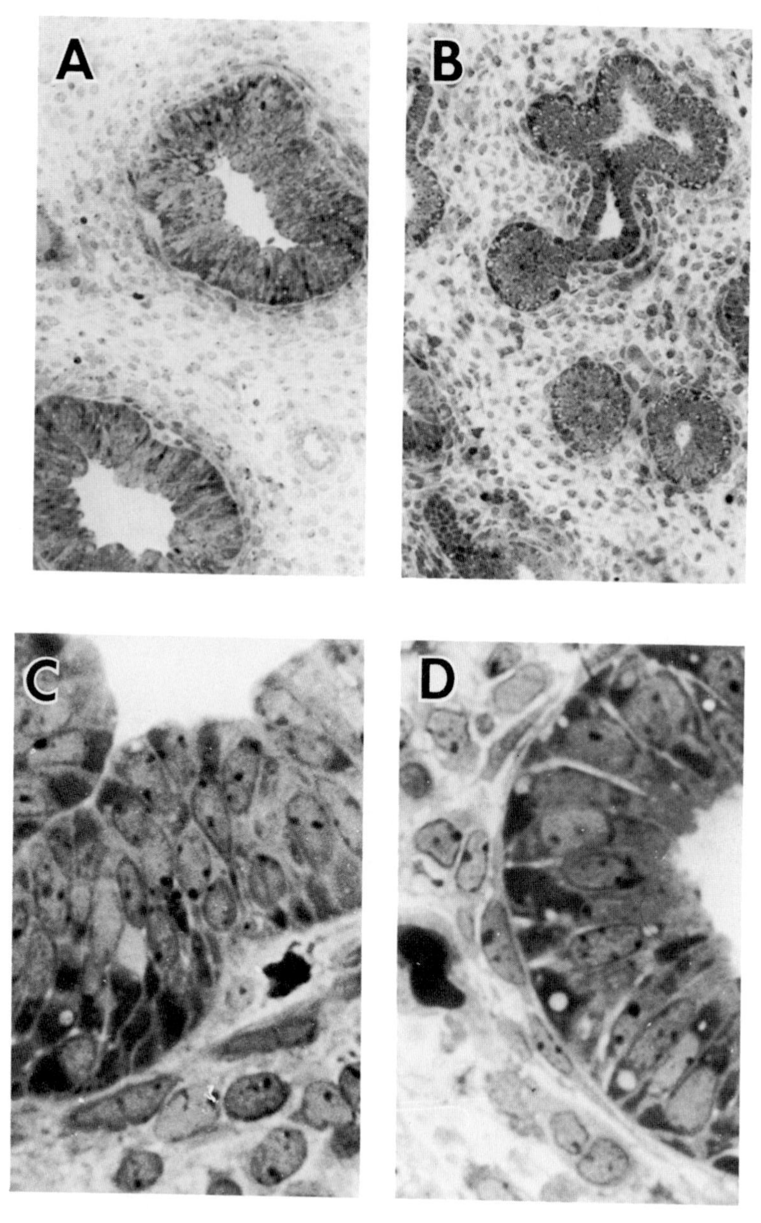

Figure 1 Morphology of human fetal lung at the pseudoglandular stage of development. A. Lung tissue from an 8-week gestational age human embryo. Gestational ages were estimated from foot length data. Ducts are lined by a pseudostratified columnar epithelium and are surrounded by abundant connective tissue (160X). B. Lung tissue from a 16-week gestational age human fetus. The

and biochemical differentiation of human fetal lung. Therefore, information concerning human fetal lung development is emphasized in this chapter. In addition, where pertinent, the reader is referred to biochemical studies which confirm or expand morphological observations concerning human fetal lung maturation.

II. Embryonic Lung Development

The human fetal lung originates as a ventral diverticulum that arises from the caudal end of the laryngotracheal groove of the foregut of the 3-week-old embryo [8]. The diverticulum grows caudally to form the primitive trachea and then, by 4 weeks, the end of the diverticulum divides into the two sacs, the lung buds. The two lung buds then develop lobar buds which correspond to the mature lung lobes, i.e., three on the right and two on the left. By about 6 weeks, the lobar buds have further subdivided and formed the bronchopulmonary segments.

The primitive lung bud is lined by an endodermally derived epithelium which differentiates into both the respiratory epithelium lining the airways [9] and the specialized epithelium that lines the alveoli and permits gas exchange [10]. The lung bud grows into a rounded mass of mesodermal cells from which the blood vessels, smooth muscle, cartilage, and other connective tissues that form the framework of the lung differentiate [11]. Ectoderm contributes to the innervation of the lung [12].

The cells lining the ducts of the very early lung (i.e., <8 weeks) form a tall, pseudostratified, columnar epithelium (Fig. 1a and c). The epithelial cells contain large glycogen pools and sit on a thick continuous basement membrane to which a layer of flattened connective tissue cells is tightly apposed. Beneath the cuff formed by the basement membrane and fibroblasts are found connective tissue cells with many branching processes. A small number of capillaries are dispersed in the connective tissue.

---

ducts have branched extensively and are now lined by a columnar epithelium. The tissue contains very few blood vessels (160X). C. Higher magnification photograph of the epithelium lining the ducts shown in A. The pseudostratified columnar cells contain dark-staining pools of glycogen. A prominent basement membrane underlines the epithelium and beneath this a cuff of connective tissue cells surrounds the duct (800X). D. Higher magnification photograph of the epithelium lining the ducts shown in B. The columnar cells have a basally situated nucleus and contain large pools of glycogen above and below the nucleus. The basement membrane beneath the epithelium is adjacent to a layer of connective tissue cells oriented at right angles to the epithelium (800X)

III. The Pseudoglandular Phase of Lung Development

From the seventh to the sixteenth week of gestation the embryonic bronchial tree undergoes repeated dichotomous branching, resulting in 16-25 generations of presumptive airways [8]. The branching ducts of the primitive bronchial tree are surrounded by abundant mesenchyme, and in cross section the tissue resembles glandular tissues; therefore, this has been termed the pseudoglandular phase of lung development [11]. By 16 weeks of gestation all of the bronchial airways have been formed and further growth of the airways occurs by elongation and widening of existing airways and not by further branching of existing airways [8]. Toward the end of the glandular phase of lung development the bronchiolar tree ends in structures designated as terminal bronchi from which three or four orders of respiratory bronchioles originate [8]. The respiratory bronchioles in turn end in terminal sacs which are the presumptive alveolar ducts.

The cells lining the presumptive alveolar ducts of fetal lung at the glandular phase of development form a columnar epithelium (Fig. 1b and d). A layer of fibroblasts is apposed to the prominent, continuous basement membrane. There are wide empty spaces between connective tissue cell processes. Ultrastructurally, the epithelial cells contain large pools of glycogen and few cytoplasmic organelles (Fig. 2). The cells are joined by junctions at their upper lateral surfaces. Wide intercellular gaps are frequently observed.

Starting at about 7 weeks cilia appear on some of the cells lining the upper airways (Fig. 3). Goblet cells are detected as early as the tenth week of gestation. A detailed review of the differentiation of fetal lung airways appears in Ref. 13.

Mesenchymal-epithelial interactions are necessary for normal lung airway morphogenesis [14]. Spooner and Wessels [15] have shown that endodermal lung buds will undergo normal bronchiolar branching in vitro only if exposed to bronchial mesoderm (no other mesoderm, including tracheal, would substitute). Other investigators have shown that the rate and extent of bronchial branching is directly proportional to the amount of mesenchyme present [14]. It has been reported that close cell contacts between epithelial and mesenchymal cells are found in mouse lung at the glandular stage of development [16]. In addition, collagen synthesis seems to be necessary for the branching of airways during morphogenesis of the lung [17].

In order for bronchial cytodifferentiation to occur a minimal amount of mesenchyme is necessary [14]. In fact, with increasing amounts of mesenchyme, epithelial differentiation is shifted from bronchial (i.e., ciliated columnar cells and goblet cells) to alveolar (primarily type II pneumonocytes) [14]. Lung

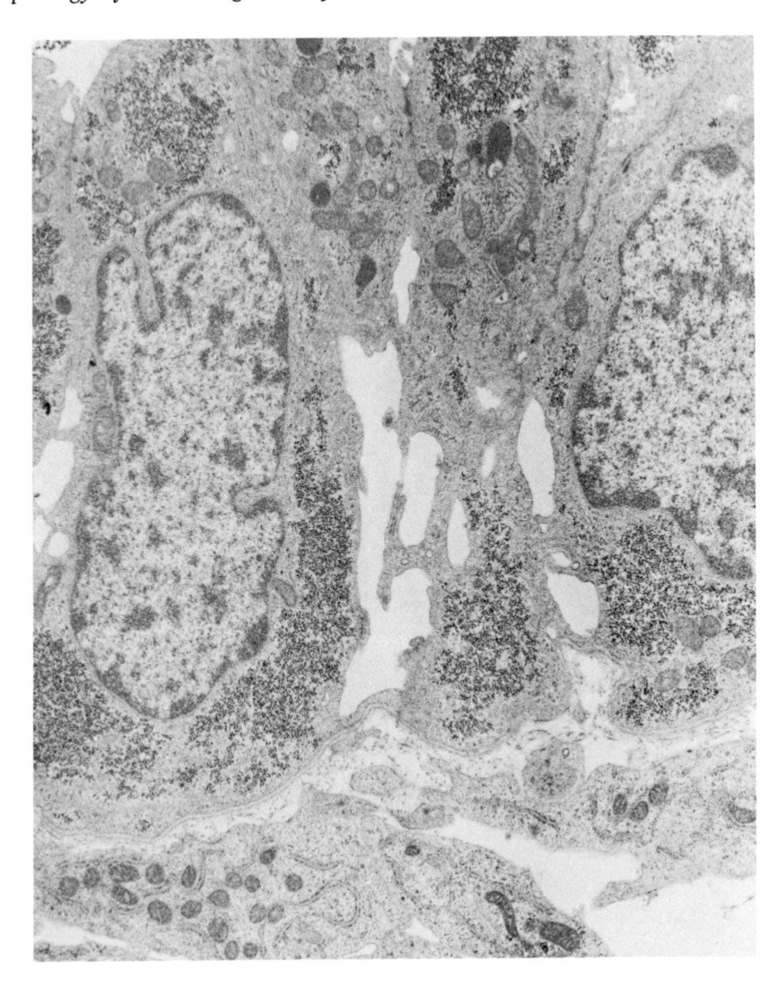

Figure 2 Electron micrograph of the cells lining the ducts of lung tissue from a 16-week gestational age human fetus. The columnar cells contain large pools of glycogen. The cells are separated by wide intracellular spaces at their lower lateral borders and are joined by tight junctions at their apex. The cells contain mitochondria, a few lysosomes, and very small amounts of rough endoplasmic reticulum. A prominent basement membrane underlies the epithelium and beneath this are scattered collagen fibrils. Connective tissue cells beneath the epithelium are oriented at right angles to the epithelium. The connective tissue cells also contain large pools of glycogen (12.250X).

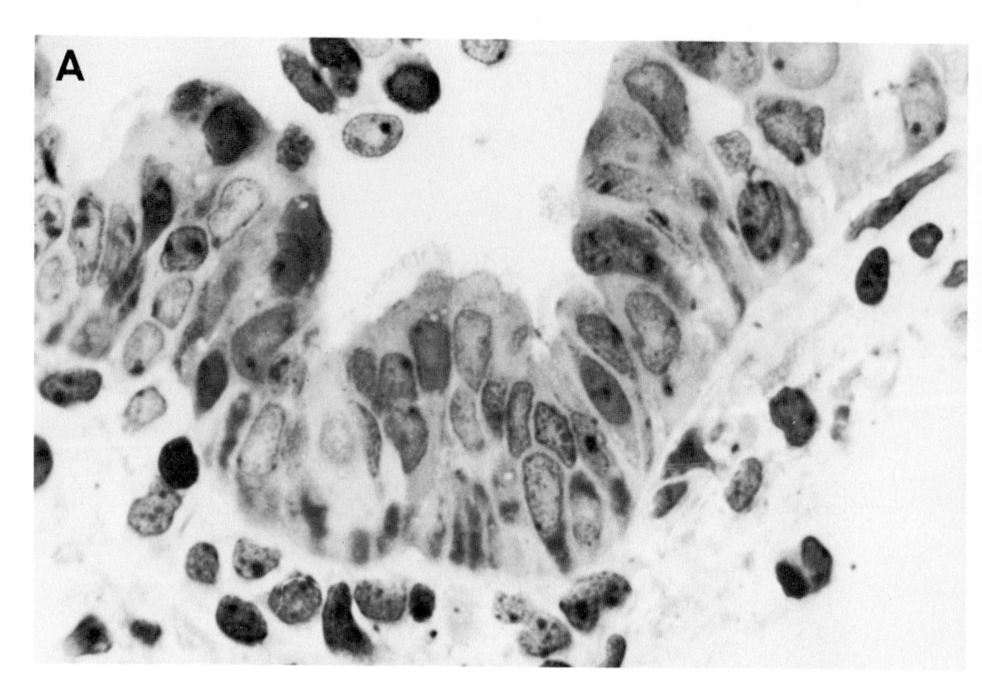

Figure 3 Differentiated airway in lung tissue from a 13–14-week gestational age human fetus. A. Light micrograph of a portion of a differentiated airway. Some of the tall pseudostratified columnar cells lining the airway are ciliated (1630X). B. Electron micrograph of cells from the same tissue as shown in A. Some of the cells lining the airway have many cilia on their apical surface. Nonciliated cells are interspersed with the ciliated cells. The cells lining the airway are joined by tight junctions at their apical borders (9750X). (Courtesy of M. T. Stahlman and M. E. Gray.)

mesenchymal cytodifferentiation (into smooth muscle, blood vessels, cartilage, etc.) will occur only when lung epithelium and lung mesenchyme are cocultivated [18]. In addition, a morphological difference between the connective tissue surrounding the trachea and that surrounding the bronchial buds has been described [19].

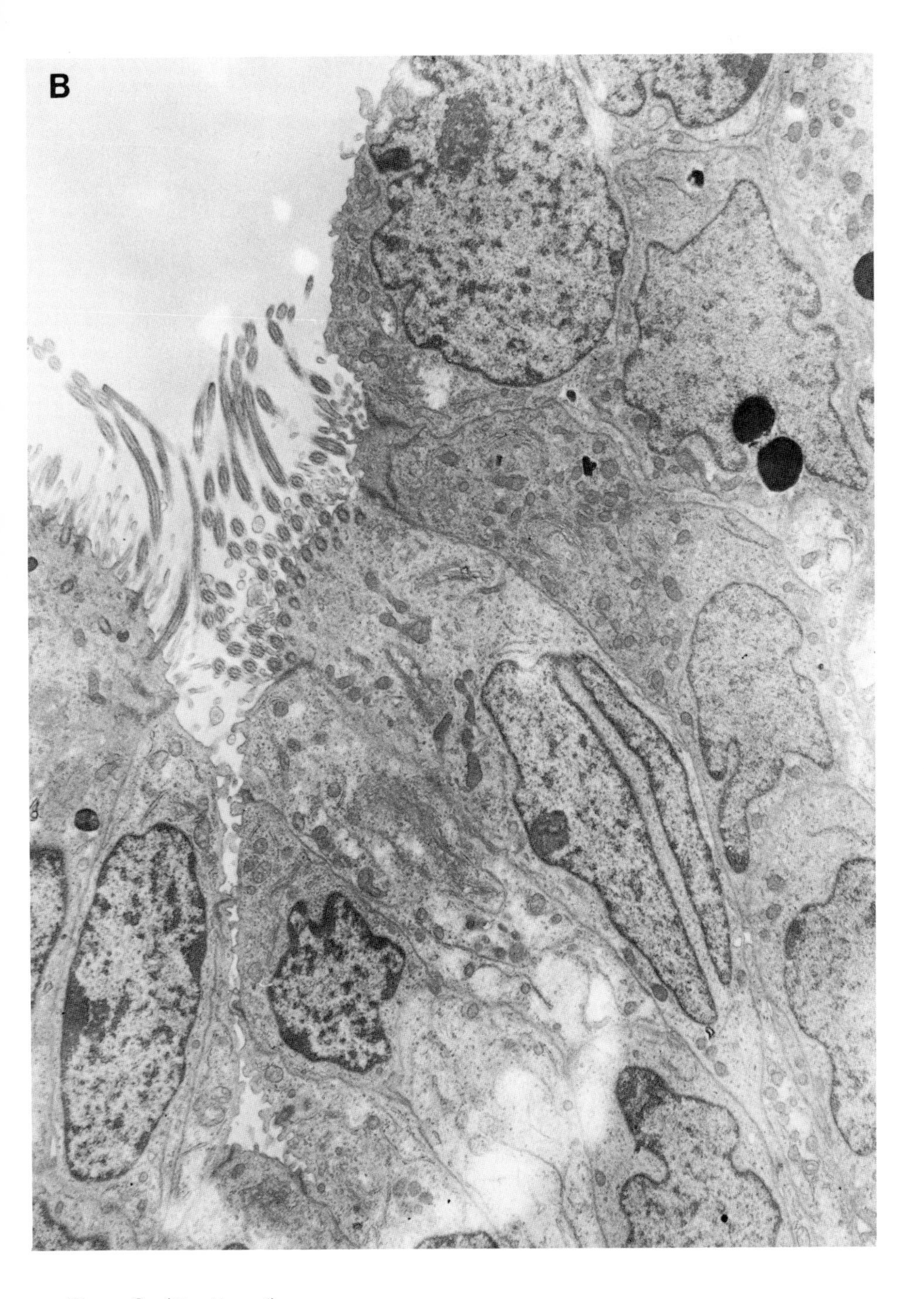

Figure 3 (Continued)

IV. The Canalicular Phase of Lung Development

The canalicular or second phase of lung development takes place from the sixteenth to the twenty-fourth week of gestation. It is characterized by the differentiation of the alveolar epithelium, a decrease in the relative amount of connective tissue in the lung, and an increase in the number of blood vessels. The first morphological evidence of this new phase of lung differentiation is the growth and movement of capillaries close to the tubule wall (Fig. 4A). The signal for the increase in capillary growth is not known. However, the growth of capillaries close to the lumen of the duct has the effect of thinning the cytoplasm of the overlying epithelial cells, the type I pneumonocytes (Fig. 4B). Simultaneously, the first appearance of differentiated (i.e., lamellar body-containing) type II

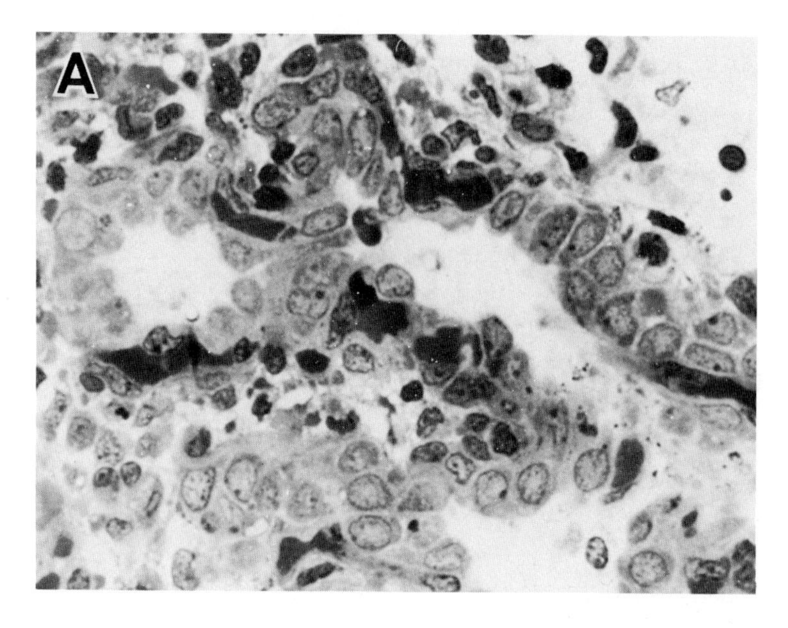

Figure 4 Human fetal lung at the canalicular stage of development (20 weeks gestational age). A. Light micrograph of a duct surrounded by connective tissue. The duct is lined by cuboidal epithelium. Beneath many of the epithelial cells are capillaries filled with red blood cells. The epithelial cells overlying the capillaries are flattened when compared to adjacent cells (500X). B. Electron micrograph of the same tissue shown in A. The cuboidal epithelial cells are filled with glycogen and have many apical cytoplasmic projections. A capillary extends into the epithelium. The underlying connective tissue cells have many long, thin processes which lie directly beneath the basement membrane and ramify within the connective tissue (5500X).

pneumocytes occurs (Fig. 5A). The first unstructural changes that are observed within the presumptive type II pneumonocytes lining the terminal ducts are increased rough endoplasmic reticulum, Golgi apparatus, and multivesicular bodies (Fig. 5C). Dense organelles resembling primary lysosomes are also frequently observed (Fig. 5B). As the cells mature, the junctions between adjacent cells are formed at the base of the cell, so that the cell bulges into the lumen of the duct or alveoli. Initially, the cells are filled with glycogen and as differentiation proceeds, the amount of glycogen in the cells decreases. This loss of glycogen appears to occur concurrently with the increase in surfactant lipid synthesis [20].

The differentiated type II pneumonocyte has many cytological specializations which are indicative of an uptake mechanism occurring in these cells. The apical surface of the type II pneumonocyte is covered with microvilli which increase its surface area. Coated pits and coated vesicles are frequently observed in the apical cytoplasm. Multivesicular bodies and lysosomes are also abundant in differentiated type II pneumonocytes. All of these organelles may be involved in the reuptake of surfactant from the lumen and its reutilization in lamellar bodies [21].

Many investigators have shown that the type I and II pneumonocytes are related developmentally and that in the adult lung the type I pneumonocyte

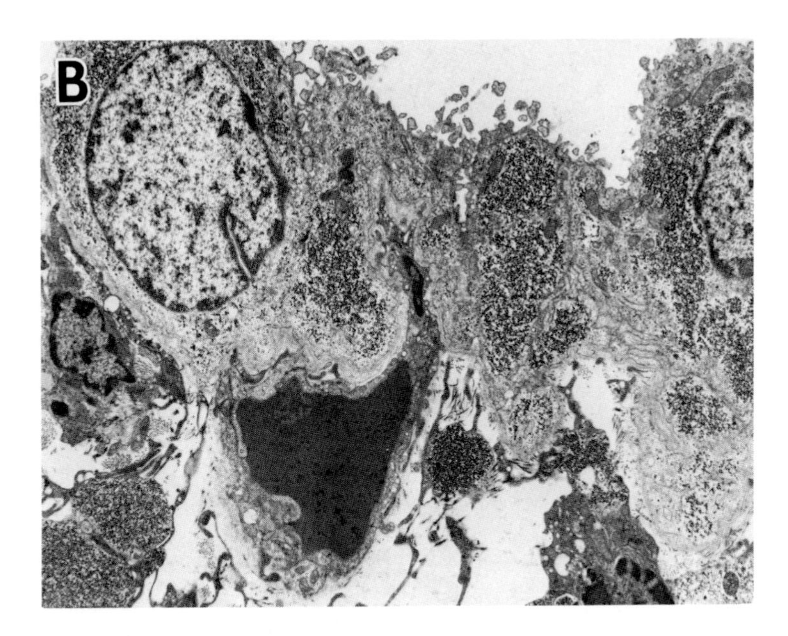

Figure 4 (Continued)

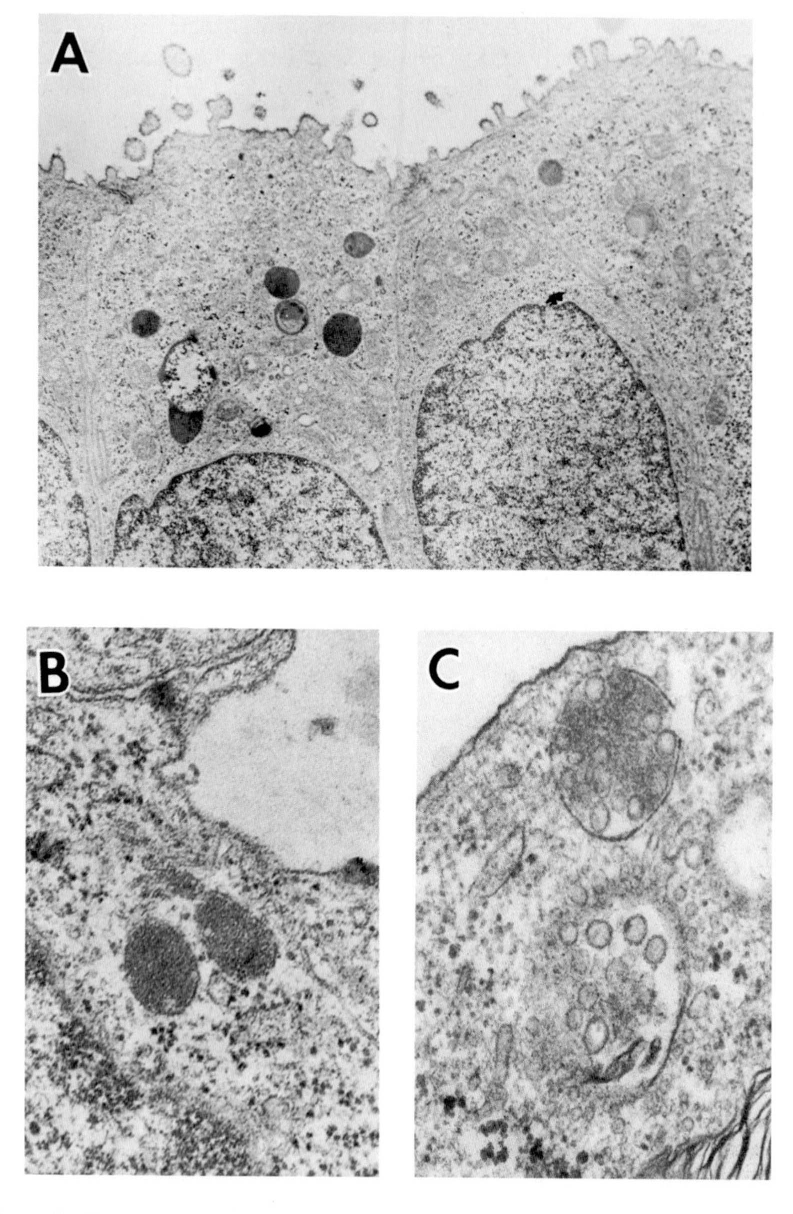

Figure 5 Electron micrographs of lung ductal epithelial cells from a 21-week gestational age human fetus. A. The ductal epithelial cells have reduced amounts of intracellular glycogen when compared to earlier stages of development. A prominent Golgi apparatus and dense membrane-bound organelles resembling

is probably derived from the type II pneumonocyte [22,23]. Injury to the alveolar epithelium of adult lung tissue results in first a proliferation of type II pneumonocytes and then the differentiation of type I pneumonocytes. Most investigators have described fetal lung type I pneumonocyte differentiation occurring via the proliferation of capillaries under an epithelium comprised of undifferentiated cells. The cells directly above a capillary subsequently thin and become type I pneumonocytes. Adamson and Bowden, however, have observed that type I pneumonocytes develop from differentiated type II pneumonocytes during lung development in the fetal rat [24]. Whether this is a normal phenomenon in all species is not known. Stahlman and Gray [6] observed human fetal type II pneumonocytes, which contain lamellar bodies, being invaded and "thinned" by a capillary. It seems certain that a direct interaction between the capillary and an epithelial cell (either undifferentiated or type II) is necessary for type I cell differentiation.

In some specimens of human fetal lung between the twentieth and the twenty-second weeks of gestation, the entire epithelium of the terminal sacs is composed of type II pneumonocytes which contain lamellar bodies (J. Snyder, unpublished observations) [25]. The proliferation of capillaries beneath the epithelium has not yet occurred at this time in development. Presumably, in this lung tissue the type I cell would be derived from a morphologically identifiable type II cell, i.e., the same differentiation pattern shown to exist in adult lung and in fetal rat lung. It is also pertinent to point out that explants of undifferentiated fetal lung tissue of 12–18 weeks' gestational age (i.e., epithelium plus adjacent mesenchymal tissues) maintained in vitro develop an epithelium comprised entirely of type II pneumonocytes [26] (Fig. 6). Blood vessels are not maintained in these explants and type I pneumonocyte differentiation is not observed. Since the differentiation of type II pneumonocytes can occur precociously in human fetal lung maintained in vitro, it is possible that type II pneumonocyte differentiation in vivo may be under an inhibitory influence.

---

lysosomes are observed in the apical cytoplasm. Short, blunt microvilli project from the apical surface of the cells (9700X). B. High-magnification electron micrograph of dense lysosomelike organelles observed in presumptive type II pneumonocytes (43,500X). C. Multivesicular bodies are also frequently seen in differentiating fetal lung type II cells. These structures are membrane bound and contain many small vesicles with a variable amount of dense material in the area between the small vesicles. These structures are usually observed in the apical cytoplasm directly beneath the plasma membrane. They are more frequently observed in cells which contain mature lamellar bodies (34,000X).

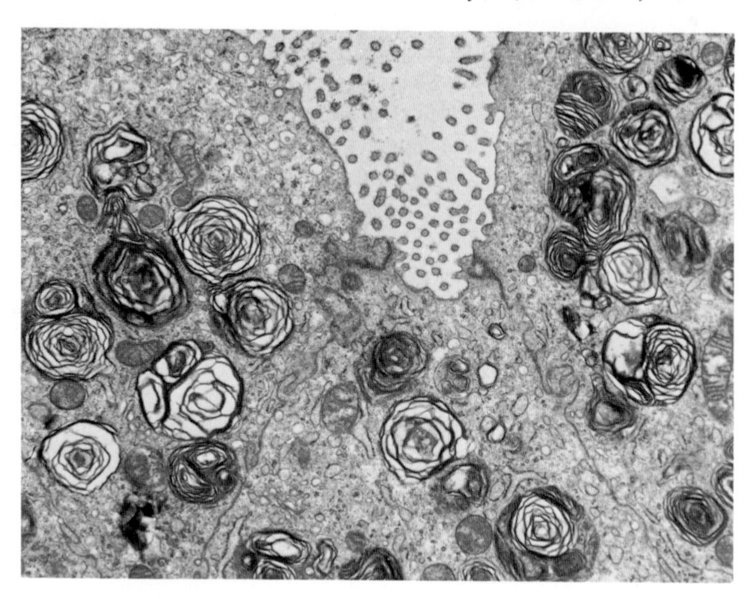

Figure 6 Electron micrograph of ductal epithelial cells in an explant of a 16-week gestational age human fetal lung tissue which had been maintained in vitro for 5 days. The apical cytoplasm of the cells is filled with many large lamellar bodies. The glycogen content of the cells is reduced. The amounts of Golgi apparatus and rough endoplasmic reticulum are increased in these cells. Microvilli line the apical surface of the cells (10,000X).

Smith [27] has reported that a factor derived from cultures of lung fibroblasts promotes the differentiation of lung type II cells. This finding is interesting in view of the well-documented requirement for interactions between lung mesenchyme and epithelium during lung development [14,15,19]. It has been reported that purified type II pneumonocytes cannot be maintained for long periods in vitro [28], perhaps because in order to maintain differentiation type II pneumonocytes require interaction with the connective tissue matrix which forms part of their normal environment in vivo [29]. Vaccaro and Brody [30] have reported that direct contacts between the type II cells and connective tissue cells exist in adult lung. This direct contact is mediated via foot processes of the type II cell that protrude through the basement membrane and come into close contact with fibroblasts beneath the basement membrane. Similar processes are not found on type I cells.

The role of the basement membrane in the differentiation of type I and II pneumonocytes is not known, but interactions of cells with basement membranes have been shown to be a requisite for cell differentiation in other tissues [29]. Vaccaro and Brody have reported that the basement membranes underlying the types I and II pneumonocytes in adult lung are different, by both morphological and biochemical criteria [30]. Using ultrastructural histochemical techniques, they observed that the basement membrane underlying the type II cell is enriched in the glycosaminoglycan, heparan sulfate. We have reported that the synthesis of heparan sulfate is increased greatly during type II pneumonocyte differentiation in cultured explants of human fetal lung tissue [31]. Vaccaro and Brody also described ultrastructural differences between the basement membranes of type I and II pneumonocytes [30]. We have observed similar differences in human fetal lung tissues (Fig. 7A and B).

Several sulfated, glycosylated proteins associated with basement membrane have been isolated and characterized [32-34]. Fibronectin, a 220,000 molecular weight glycoprotein, is found in the basement membranes of several embryonic tissues. Laminin has been detected in basement membranes of adult lung tissue [33]. Both of these structural proteins are probably involved in the attachment of epithelial cells to the basement membrane and/or to collagen. Using immunohistochemical techniques we have observed the binding of antibodies to fibronectin and laminin to human fetal lung tissues at the glandular phase of development (Fig. 7C and D). Both proteins are present in the basement membranes underlying all of the primitive ducts at this stage of development. We observed some discontinuities in the basement membrane similar to those reported by Bernfield and Banerjee [35] in an investigation of the salivary gland. Fibronectin and laminin immunofluorescence was also detected in some cells within the connective tissue compartment. The role of these proteins in fetal lung differentiation has not been investigated. In fetal kidney tissue laminin synthesis has been shown to precede tubule formation [36].

Hyaline membranes are characteristic of the lungs of infants who die from RDS. These membranes are formed as a result of transudation from the alveolar capillaries [25] and the sloughing of the alveolar epithelium. The intercellular junctions between the sloughed off epithelial cells remain intact. The basement membranes also are intact but still adherent to the alveolar wall [37]. It would seem pertinent to investigate the presence or absence of substances such as laminin, entactin, fibronectin, type IV collagen, and glycosaminoglycans (especially heparan sulfate) in fetal lungs during development, particularly in the lungs of infants who die from the complications of RDS. These substances are either components of the basement membrane or may be involved in the adherence of epithelial cells to the basement membrane.

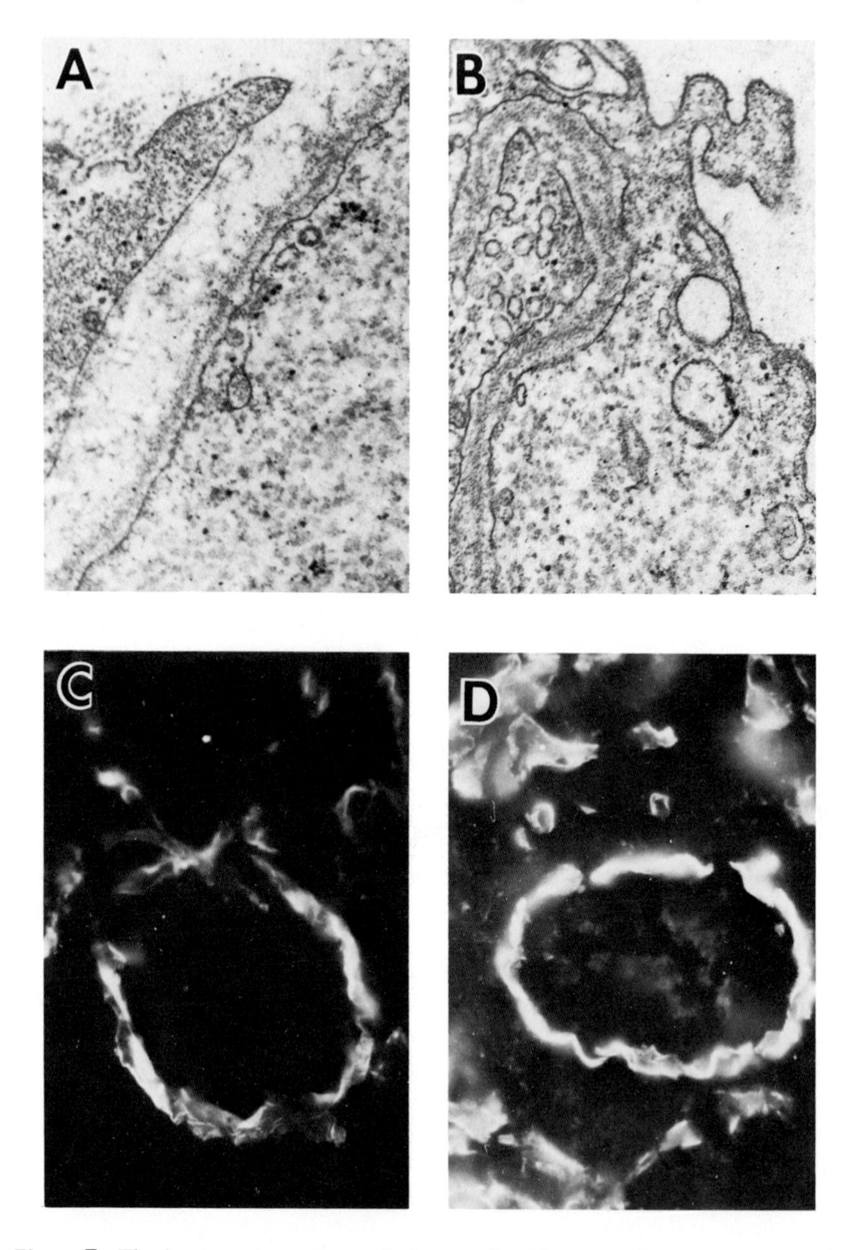

Figure 7 The basement membrane in human fetal lung. A. Electron micrograph of the basement membrane beneath an undifferentiated epithelial cell. The basement membrane is composed of an electron lucent lamina rara externa directly beneath the cell, a dense lamina densa, and a layer of filamentous

V. The Terminal Saccular Phase of Lung Development

From the twenty-fourth week of gestation until term the lung undergoes a third morphological differentiation period, the terminal saccular phase of lung development. During this period the distal lung tissue is remodeled into structures more closely resembling adult lung tissue parenchyma. The amount of connective tissue relative to the amount of epithelium is further reduced (Fig. 8A and B). The capillary bed hypertrophies, thus increasing steadily the surface area available for gas exchange in the distal parts of the lung.

The cells lining the saccules of human fetal lung at this stage of development are recognizable type I and II pneumonocytes. Morphologically they are indistinguishable from the corresponding cells described in neonatal or adult human lung tissue. Biochemically, however, the surfactant produced by the fetal lung differs from that produced later in gestation [38]. Immature lungs produce surfactant enriched in phosphatidylinositol, while lungs late in gestation produce surfactant enriched in phosphatidylglycerol. No changes in lamellar body morphology during gestation have been described. However, we have observed that lamellar bodies produced by human fetal lung explants treated with hormones and shown to be enriched in phosphatidylglycerol are larger than the phosphatidylinositol-containing lamellar bodies produced in control explants [39].

Lamellar bodies are first observed in the cytoplasm of human fetal lung epithelial cells at about the twentieth to twenty-fourth week of gestation. Since the phosphatidylcholine content of amniotic fluid does not increase

---

material extending from the lamina densa to the region of connective tissue cells (30,500X). B. Electron micrograph of the basement membrane beneath a presumptive type I pneumonocyte. The basement membrane appears to be a fusion of the basement membrane associated with the capillary and with the epithelial cell. It is thicker and more amorphous than the basement membrane of the presumptive type II cell (30,500X). C. Immunofluorescent localization of laminin in 14-week gestational age human fetal lung. The laminin is located primarily in the basement membrane beneath the epithelial ducts. The basement membrane is not continuous. Some cells in the connective tissue also are positively stained for laminin. There appears to be no cytoplasmic staining for laminin (1250X). D. Immunofluorescent localization of fibronectin in human fetal lung tissue from a 14-week gestational age human fetus. The fibronectin is especially prominent in the basement membrane beneath the ductal epithelium. The basement membrane is not continuous around the duct. Many cells in the connective tissue stain positively for fibronectin (1250X).

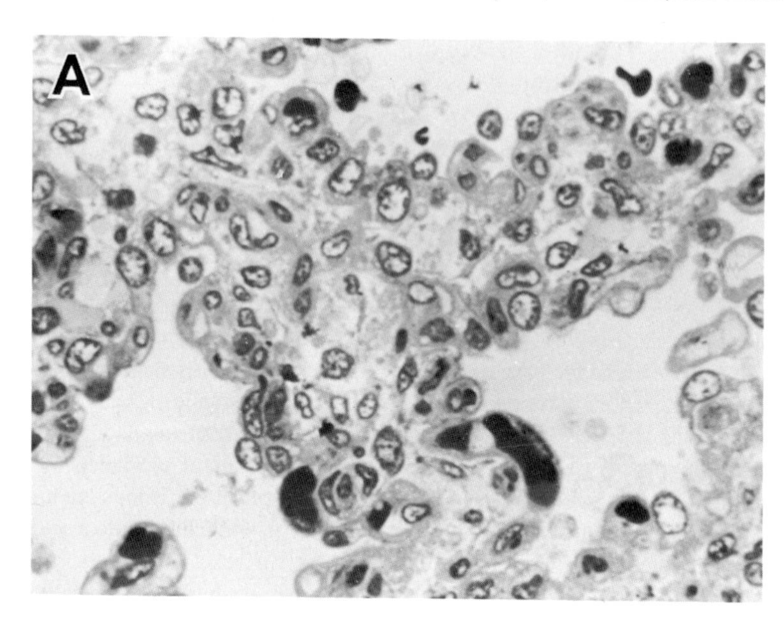

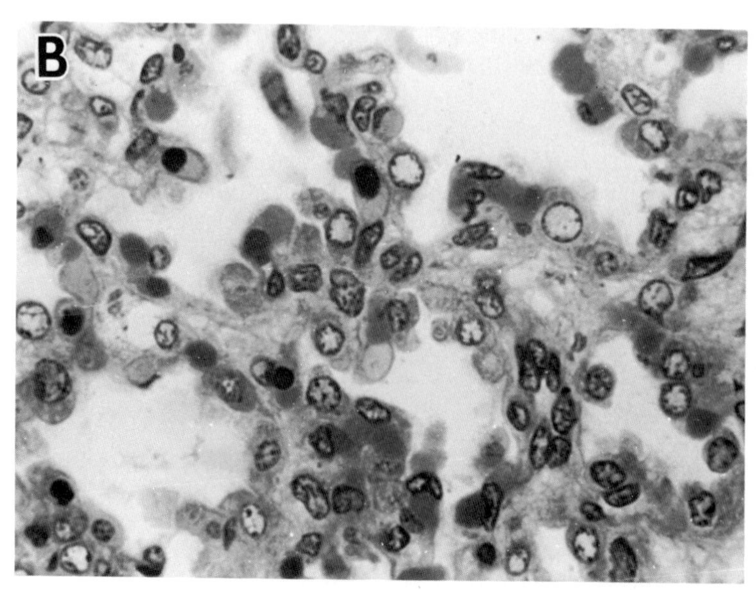

Figure 8 Light micrographs of human fetal lung tissues. A. Lung tissue from a 30-week gestational age fetus. The connective tissue septa between adjacent alveoli are very thick. The majority of capillaries lie directly beneath the epithelium lining the presumptive alveoli. The cells overlying these capillaries have

significantly until about the thirty-second week of gestation [38], it is presumed that secretion of lamellar bodies does not occur actively until that time.

The origin of the lamellar body is poorly understood. In view of the fact that numerous lysosomal enzymes have been detected in lamellar bodies, using both histochemical and biochemical techniques [40,41], it seems likely that the lamellar body is a modified lysosome. Using human fetal lung explants we have shown that during human fetal lung differentiation in vitro the tissue contains increased amounts of lysosomal enzymes and that this increase in enzymatic activity is shifted from a subcellular compartment resembling lysosomes to a lamellar body-enriched fraction (Fig. 9) [42]. The role of lamellar body lysosomal enzymes upon release of the lamellar body into the amniotic fluid-filled fetal lung or onto the alveolar surface in mature lung is not known. One unexplained finding is that some enzymes such as phosphatidate phosphohydrolase (PAPase), and phospholipase A_2, which are involved in the metabolism of phospholipids, are present in lamellar bodies [41]. However, no evidence of the function of these enzymes within the lamellar body or in the alveolus has ever been presented. Likewise, several glycosidases have been detected in lamellar bodies [41]. The major apoprotein in lamellar bodies is a glycoprotein [43]. It appears to have a similar molecular weight and isoelectric point in the lamellar body and in surfactant material obtained by lavage (V. Ng, C. Mendelson, and J. Snyder, unpublished observations).

The majority of proteins in lamellar bodies and surfactant are glycoproteins [43]. The transport of lysosomal proteins from the rough endoplasmic reticulum to lysosomes requires glycosylation of these proteins with a specific carbohydrate sequence that directs the proteins from the Golgi apparatus to the lysosomal compartment [44]. It seems likely that intracellular transport of lamellar body apoproteins involves a similar process. The transport of lipid to the lamellar body has not been investigated. In view of the current belief that membrane may be moved within the cell as small vesicles [45], it is possible that the vesicles that are observed within the lamellar body precursor, i.e., the multivesicular body [46], represent vesicles which have transported the enzymes and lipid characteristic of the mature lamellar body. The immature and mature lamellar body frequently contain dense core areas [47]. The

---

the thin flattened cytoplasm characteristic of type I pneumonocytes (575X). B. Lung tissue from a 40-week gestational age fetus. The alveolar septa are much thinner than in A. There appear to be more capillaries associated with the epithelium than in A. True alveoli are not present in lung tissue at this stage of development but are gradually formed during the first 8 years of life (575X).

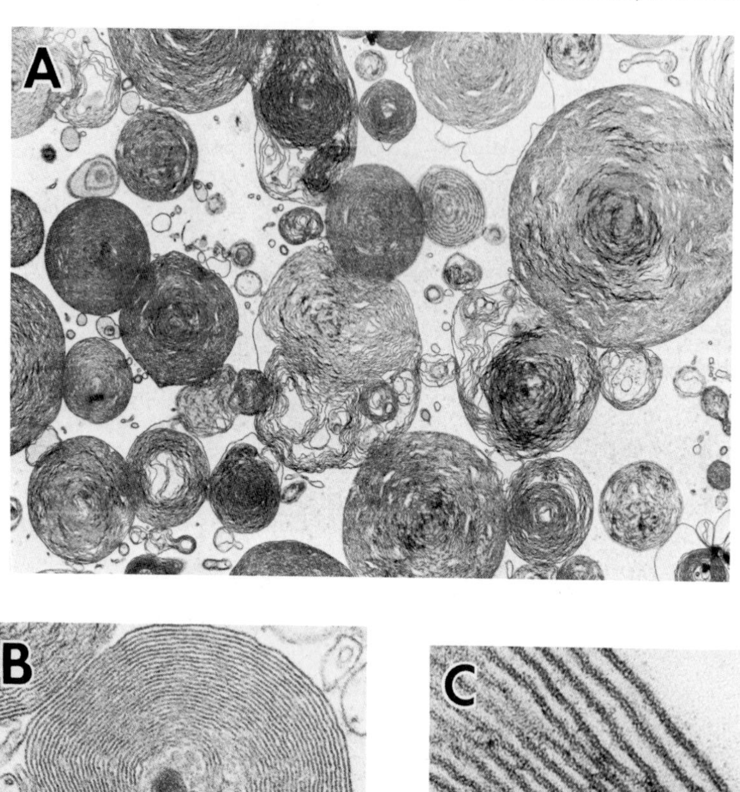

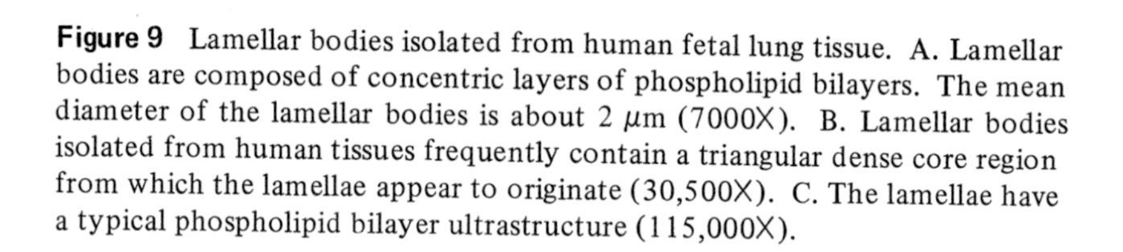

Figure 9 Lamellar bodies isolated from human fetal lung tissue. A. Lamellar bodies are composed of concentric layers of phospholipid bilayers. The mean diameter of the lamellar bodies is about 2 μm (7000X). B. Lamellar bodies isolated from human tissues frequently contain a triangular dense core region from which the lamellae appear to originate (30,500X). C. The lamellae have a typical phospholipid bilayer ultrastructure (115,000X).

lamellae of the lamellar body are frequently observed to originate from such dense core areas (Fig. 9A). Whether the dense cores represent areas of concentrated protein components or lamellar body lipid precursors is not known.

VI. Postnatal Lung Development

The connective tissue in lung undergoes many morphological changes after birth. Indentations of the septal wall into the air space results in the formation of true alveoli. This process begins before birth and continues up to the eighth year [8]. The number of alveoli increases from about 20 million at birth to 180 million in the adult. The increase in the number of alveoli increases the surface area of the lung devoted to gas exchange considerably. The thinning of the walls of the lung parenchyma at this stage of development has important physiological consequences. It probably permits the increase in lung distensibility necessary for aeration of the lungs during breathing.

Brody and Vaccaro have described "alveolarization" in the neonatal rat [48]. Alveolarization involves the differentiation of connective tissue cells to form the myofibroblasts, which secrete elastin and glycosaminoglycans. Some of the connective tissue cells at the base of the alveolar wall are filled with lipid droplets. The function of these lipid-containing cells is unknown [49]. The connective tissue at alveolar junctional areas is characterized by collagen fibrils interspersed with fibroblastlike cells. Macrophages are rarely observed in fetal lung. The macrophages do not appear in great abundance until after birth [50]. The reasons for this are not clear, but it is possible they are not necessary during life in utero.

VII. The Role of Hormones in Fetal Lung Development

The fetal lung is a hormonally responsive tissue [51]. In addition to biochemical criteria (see Chap. 3), many investigators have noted differentiation-characteristic morphological changes in hormonally treated lung tissues. The number of type II pneumonocytes in the lung and the number of lamellar bodies per type II pneumonocyte have been reported to be increased by agents such as glucocorticoids, thyroid hormone, estrogens, and epidermal growth factor [52-55]. The release of surfactant from the type II pneumonocytes also seems to be stimulated by hormonal treatment [56,57]. In addition, several investigators have reported a hormonally influenced decrease in the glycogen content of the presumptive alveolar pneumonocytes concomitant with the appearance of surfactant [20]. Type I pneumonocyte differentiation in vivo is also accelerated by hormone administration [52]. It has been reported that thinning of the alveolar septa is responsive to glucocorticoids [58]. Beck et al. [59] have reported that in the fetus of the *Rhesus* monkey glucocorticoids stimulate lung maturation by influencing connective tissue characteristics rather than type II pneumonocyte function. They report that alveolar diameter is increased in glucocorticoid-treated fetuses and that the lungs of such fetuses have an increased collagen to elastin ratio.

Most of these morphological criteria have been reported to be delayed in infants who develop RDS. The number of type II pneumonocytes and lamellar bodies per type II pneumonocyte are reduced [60]. The secretion of surfactant is also reduced in this disease [2]. This reduction in surfactant secretion probably results in the characteristic atelectasis observed in the lungs of infants dying from RDS. Edema of the interstitial tissues has also been reported in RDS [25], although the morphology of interstitial and capillary endothelial cells does not appear to be affected. Lauweryns [25] has reported that, in addition to hyaline membranes, there is an enlargement of pulmonary lymphatics and, as shown by perfusion studies, a filling defect in the arterial blood vessels of infants who die of RDS. Lauweryns [25] and Chu et al. [61] have suggested that a basic abnormality in infants who develop RDS may be a pathological vasoconstriction of pulmonary arterioles. Lauweryns [25] observed a narrowing of the diameter of small muscular pulmonary arteries and pulmonary arterioles in infants whose deaths were due to RDS. The fact that infants who develop RDS also frequently develop bronchopulmonary dysplasia (BPD) [62-64], a disease with a similar pathology, is suggestive that at least in some of the infants who develop RDS an underlying defect may be a developmental abnormality or immaturity in pulmonary blood vessels.

VIII. Neuroendocrine Cells in Fetal Lung

Neuroendocrine cells are numerous in human fetal lung, and they are associated primarily with airway epithelium as early as the eighth week of gestation [65, 66]. Neuroendocrine cells are analogous to the peptide hormone-producing cells found in the gut [67] and other tissues [68]. Serotonin and peptide hormones such as bombesin [69], calcitonin [70], and leu-enkephalin [71] have been identified in these cells. They are located in groups called neuroepithelial bodies or as single cells within the basement membrane of the airway epithelium, usually below the airway epithelial cells [65]. The cells rarely extend to the lumen. Neuroendocrine cells have been detected as far as the level of the alveolar ducts, but they are not found in the alveolar epithelium. They seem to occur at branching points in the pulmonary airways. The cells contain secretory granules at their basal pole, suggestive that they may secrete into the interstitial tissue (Fig. 10). Moody et al. [72] reported that cell lines from human oat-cell

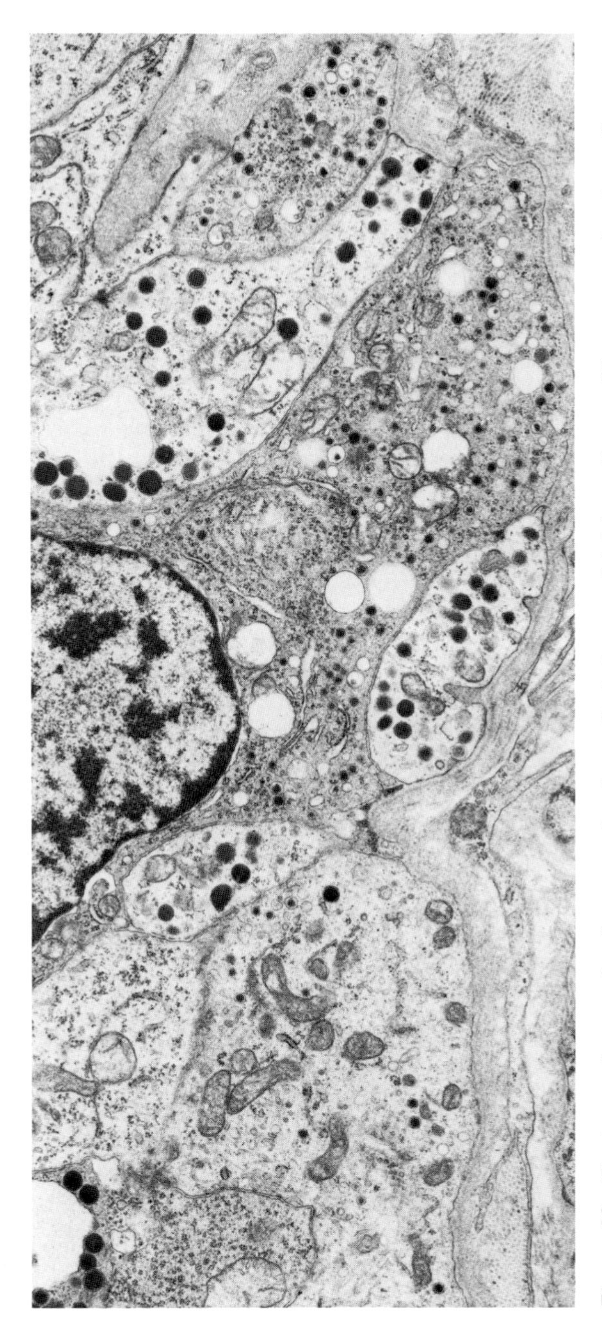

Figure 10 Electron micrograph of neuroendocrine cells in human fetal lung tissue. The neuroendocrine cells are usually detected within differentiated airways beneath the epithelial cells and adjacent to the basement membrane. At least three morphologically distinct cell types, characterized by hormone granules of varying densities and sizes, are distinguishable (15,000X). (Courtesy of E. Cutz.)

carcinomas produce bombesin, evidence that this type of lung cancer is derived from neuroendocrine cells of the pulmonary airway. In a recent study, Johnson et al. [73] have reported that the number and size of pulmonary neuroendocrine cells are increased in the lungs of infants who developed RDS or BPD.

The function of the neuroendocrine cells of the lung is unknown. Some investigators have suggested that these cells are transducers of O_2 tension in the pulmonary airway and alter pulmonary blood flow and the diameter of the airway by inducing contraction or relaxation of smooth muscle [74]. The observation of large numbers of these cells during fetal development (when the function proposed above is not necessary) is suggestive that these cells may also influence fetal lung development in some as yet unknown manner. Infants who develop RDS and BPD frequently also develop pulmonary hypertension [62]. These infants have narrowed pulmonary arterioles, presumably due to hypertrophy of the smooth muscle which surrounds these vessels [63]. They also frequently have a generalized fibrosis of the saccular septae [63]. A relationship between the neuroendocrine cells and the hypertrophy of connective tissue cells in the lung should be investigated.

IX. Conclusions

The morphological description of human fetal lung differentiation is well established, especially with respect to the morphology of the epithelium lining the airways and presumptive alveoli. However, the mechanisms by which the fetal lung differentiates are not well understood. By use of morphological and histochemical techniques a greater understanding of many functional aspects of fetal lung maturation could be achieved. Specific areas which could be addressed include:

1. The role of the mesenchyme in the differentiation of the alveolar epithelium has not been addressed. A detailed morphological description of the interaction between the connective tissue and epithelium during fetal lung differentiation is needed.

2. The basement membrane has been shown to be an important structure with respect to both differentiation and maintenance of differentiated function in many tissues. Studies concerning the localization of basement membrane components during fetal lung development may be informative.

3. The effects of hormones and other stimulatory factors on fetal lung connective tissue and basement membrane morphology should be examined.

4. The morphogenesis of the lamellar body is poorly understood. Correlative morphological and biochemical studies concerning the subcellular site of lamellar body lipoprotein synthesis, processing, and packaging should be undertaken.
5. Since surfactant recycling by the type II pneumonocyte may be physiologically important, especially in the newborn, an investigation of the differentiation of fetal lung cell structures which may be involved in surfactant recycling would be informative.

The contribution of morphological studies to our understanding of the development of human fetal lung has been great. However, many more aspects concerning human fetal lung maturation could be addressed using morphological techniques.

Acknowledgments

The authors wish to acknowledge the advice, support, and encouragement of Dr. P. C. MacDonald. The excellent editorial assistance of Dolly Tutton is also acknowledged.

References

1. Farrell, P. M., and M. E. Avery, Hyaline membrane disease, *Am. Rev. Respir. Dis.,* **111**:657 (1975).
2. Avery, M. E., and J. Mead, Surface properties in relation to atelectasis and hyaline membrane disease, *A.M.A.J. Dis. Child.,* **97**:517 (1959).
3. Clements, J. A., E. S. Brown, and R. P. Johnson, Pulmonary surface tension and the mucus lining of the lungs: Some theoretical considerations, *J. Appl. Physiol.,* **12**:262 (1958).
4. Charnock, E. L., and C. F. Doershuk, Developmental aspects of the human lung, *Pediat. Clin. North America,* **20**:275 (1973).
5. Burri, P. H., and E. R. Weibel, Ultrastructure and morphometry of the developing lung. In *Development of the Lung.* Edited by W. A. Hodson. New York, Marcel Dekker, 1977, p. 215.
6. Stahlman, M. T., and M. E. Gray, Anatomical development and maturation of the lungs, *Clin. Perinatol.,* **5**:181 (1978).
7. Inselman, L. S., and R. B. Mellins, Growth and development of the lung, *J. Pediatr.,* **98**:1 (1981).
8. Boyden, E. A., Development and growth of the airways. In *Development of the Lung.* Edited by W. A. Hodson. New York, Marcel Dekker, 1977, p. 3.

9. Breeze, R. G. and E. B. Wheeldon, Cells of the pulmonary airways, *Am. Rev. Respir. Dis.*, **116**:705 (1977).
10. Weibel, E. R., Morphological basis of alveolar-capillary gas exchange, *Physiol. Rev.*, **53**:419 (1973).
11. Loosli, C. G. and E. L. Potter, Pre- and postnatal development of the respiratory portion of the human lung, *Am. Rev. Respir. Dis.*, **80**:5 (1959).
12. Richardson, J. B., Nerve supply to the lungs, *Am. Rev. Respir. Dis.*, **119**: 785 (1979).
13. Jeffrey, P. K. and L. M. Reid, Ultrastructure of airway epithelium and submucosal gland during development. In *Development of the Lung*. Edited by W. A. Hodson. New York, Marcel Dekker, 1977, p. 87.
14. Masters, J. R. W., Epithelial-mesenchymal interaction during lung development: The effect of mesenchymal mass, *Devel. Biol.*, **51**:98 (1976).
15. Spooner, B. S. and N. K. Wessels, Mammalian lung development: Interactions in primordium formation and bronchial morphogenesis, *J. Exp. Zool.*, **175**:445 (1970).
16. Bluemink, J. G., P. Maurik, and K. A. Lawson, Intimate cell contacts at the epithelial/mesenchymal interface in embryonic mouse lung, *J. Ultra. Res.*, **55**:257 (1976).
17. Spooner, B. S. and J. M. Faubion, Collagen involvement in branching morphogenesis of embryonic lung and salivary gland, *Devel. Biol.*, **77**: 84 (1980).
18. Taderera, J. V., Control of lung differentiation *in vitro*, *Devel. Biol.*, **16**: 489 (1967).
19. Wessels, N. K., Mammalian lung development: Interactions in formation and morphogenesis of tracheal buds, *J. Exp. Zool.*, **175**:455 (1970).
20. Bourbon, J. and A. Jost, Control of glycogen metabolism in the developing fetal lung, *Pediatr. Res.*, **16**:50 (1982).
21. Hallman, M., B. L. Epstein, and L. Gluck, Analysis of labeling and clearance of lung surfactant phospholipids in rabbit. Evidence of bidirectional surfactant flux between lamellar bodies and alveolar lavage, *J. Clin. Invest.*, **68**:742 (1981).
22. Evans, M. J., L. J. Cabral, R. J. Stephens, and G. Freeman, Renewal of alveolar epithelium in the rat following exposure to NO_2, *Am. J. Pathol.*, **70**:175 (1973).
23. Adamson, I. Y. R. and D. H. Bowden, The type 2 cell as progenitor of alveolar epithelial regeneration. A cytodynamic study in mice after exposure to oxygen, *Lab. Invest.*, **30**:35 (1974).
24. Adamson, I. Y. R. and D. H. Bowden, Derivation of type 1 epithelium from type 2 cells in developing rat lung, *Lab. Invest.*, **32**:736 (1975).

25. Lauweryns, J. M., Hyaline membrane disease in newborn infants: Macroscopic, radiographic, and light and electron microscopic studies, *Hum. Pathol.*, **1**:175 (1970).
26. Snyder, J. M., J. M. Johnston, and C. R. Mendelson, Differentiation of type II cells of human fetal lung *in vitro*, *Cell Tissue Res.*, **220**:17 (1981).
27. Smith, B. T., Lung maturation in the fetal rat: Acceleration by injection of fibroblast pneumonocyte factor, *Science*, **204**:1094 (1979).
28. Diglio, C. A. and Y. Kikkawa, The type II epithelial cells of the lung. IV. Adaptation and behavior of isolated type II cells in culture, *Lab. Invest.*, **37**:622 (1977).
29. Hay, E. D., Extracellular matrix, *J. Cell Biol.*, **91**:205s (1981).
30. Vaccaro, C. A. and J. S. Brody, Structural features of alveolar wall basement membrane in the adult rat lung, *J. Cell Biol.*, **91**:427 (1981).
31. Heifetz, A. and J. M. Snyder, The effects of hydrocortisone on the biosynthesis of sulfated glycoconjugates by human fetal lung, *J. Biol. Chem.*, **256**:4957 (1981).
32. Yamada, K. M. and K. Olden, Fibronectin-adhesive glycoproteins of cell surface and blood, *Nature*, **275**:179 (1978).
33. Foidart, J. M., E. W. Bere, Jr., M. Yaar, S. I. Rennard, M. Gullino, G. R. Martin, and S. I. Katz, Distribution and immunoelectron microscopic localization of laminin, a noncollagenous basement membrane glycoprotein, *Lab. Invest.*, **42**:336 (1980).
34. Bender, B. L., R. Jaffe, B. Carlin, and A. E. Chung, Immunolocalization of enactin, a sulfated basement membrane component in rodent tissues, and comparison with GP-2 (laminin), *Am. J. Pathol.*, **103**:419 (1981).
35. Bernfield, M. R. and S. D. Banerjee, The basal lamina in epithelial-mesenchymal morphogenetic interactions. In *Biology and Chemistry of Basement Membranes*. Edited by N. A. Kefalides. New York, Academic Press, 1978, p. 137.
36. Ekbolm, P., K. Alitalo, A. Vaheri, R. Timpl, and L. Saxen, Induction of a basement membrane glycoprotein in embryonic kidney: Possible role of laminin in morphogenesis, *Proc. Natl. Acad. Sci. USA*, **77**:485 (1980).
37. Findlay-Jones, J. M., J. M. Papadimitrious, and R. A. Barter, Pulmonary hyaline membrane: Light and electron microscopic study of the early stage, *J. Pathol.*, **112**:117 (1974).
38. Hallman, M., M. Kulovich, E. Kirkpatrick, R. G. Sugarman, and L. Gluck, Phosphatidylinositol and phosphatidylglycerol in amniotic fluid: Indices of lung maturity, *Am. J. Obstet. Gynecol.*, **125**:613 (1976).
39. Snyder, J. M., K. J. Longmuir, J. M. Johnston, and C. R. Mendelson, Hormonal regulation of lamellar body phosphatidylglycerol and phosphatidylinositol in fetal lung tissue, *Endocrinology*, **112**:1012 (1983).

40. Heath, M. F., G. Gandy, and W. Jacobson, Lysosomes in the lung. In *Lysosomes in Biology and Pathology*. Vol. 5. Edited by J. T. Dingle and R. T. Dean. Amsterdam, Elsevier-North Holland, 1976, p. 33.
41. Hook, G. E. R. and L. B. Gilmore, Hydrolases of pulmonary lysosomes and lamellar bodies, *J. Biol. Chem.*, **257**:9211 (1982).
42. Okazaki, T., J. M. Johnston, and J. M. Snyder, Morphogenesis of the lamellar body in fetal lung tissue *in vitro*, *Biochim. Biophys. Acta*, **712**: 283 (1982).
43. Bhattacharyya, S. N., M. A. Passero, R. P. DiAugustine, and W. S. Lynn, Isolation and characterization of two hydroxyproline-containing glycoproteins from normal animal lung lavage and lamellar bodies, *J. Clin. Invest.*, **55**:914 (1975).
44. Rosenfeld, M. G., G. Kreibich, D. Popov, K. Kato, and D. D. Sabatini, Biosynthesis of lysosomal hydrolases: Their synthesis in bound polysomes and the role of co- and posttranslational processing in determining their subcellular distribution, *J. Cell Biol.*, **93**:135 (1982).
45. Bell, R. M., L. M. Ballas, and R. A. Coleman, Lipid topogenesis, *J. Lipid Res.*, **22**:391 (1981).
46. Sorokin, S. P., A morphologic and cytochemical study of the great alveolar cell, *J. Histochem. Cytochem.*, **14**:884 (1967).
47. Stratton, C. J., The ultrastructure of multilamellar bodies and surfactant in the human lung, *Cell Tissue Res.*, **193**:219 (1978).
48. Brody, J. S. and C. Vaccaro, Postnatal formation of alveoli: Interstitial events and physiologic consequences, *Fed. Proc.*, **38**:215 (1979).
49. Vaccaro, C. and J. S. Brody, Ultrastructure of developing alveoli: The role of the interstitial fibroblast, *Anat. Rec.*, **192**:467 (1978).
50. Kikkawa, Y., Morphology and morphologic development of the lung. In *Pulmonary Physiology of the Fetus, Newborn and Child*. Edited by E. Scarpelli. Philadelphia, Lea & Febiger, 1975, p. 37.
51. Ballard, P. L., Hormonal influences during fetal lung development. In *Metabolic Activities of the Lung*. London, Exerpta Medica, 1980, p. 251.
52. Kikkawa, Y., M. Kaibara, E. K. Motoyama, M. M. Orzalesi, and C. D. Cook, Morphologic development of fetal rabbit lung and its acceleration with cortisol, *Am. J. Pathol.*, **64**:423 (1971).
53. Wu, B., Y. Kikkawa, M. M. Orzalesi, E. K. Motoyama, M. Kaibara, C. J. Zigas, and C. D. Cook, The effect of thyroxine on the maturation of fetal rabbit lungs, *Biol. Neonate*, **22**:161 (1973).
54. Khosla, S. S., G. J. Walker-Smith, P. A. Parks, and S. A. Rooney, Effects of estrogen on fetal rabbit lung maturation: Morphological and biochemical studies, *Pediatr. Res.*, **15**:1274 (1981).

55. Sundell, H. W., M. E. Gray, F. S. Serenius, M. B. Escobedo, and M. T. Stahlman, Effects of epidermal growth factor on lung maturation in fetal lambs, *Am. J. Pathol.*, **100**:707 (1980).
56. Taeusch, H. W., Jr., M. Heitner, and M. E. Avery, Accelerated lung maturation and increased survival in premature rabbits treated with hydrocortisone, *Am. Rev. Respir. Dis.*, **105**:971 (1972).
57. Kotas, R. V. and M. E. Avery, Accelerated appearance of pulmonary surfactant in the fetal rabbit, *J. Appl. Physiol.*, **30**:358 (1971).
58. Motoyama, E. K., M. M. Orzalesi, Y. Kikkawa, M. Kaibara, B. Wu, C. J. Zigas, and C. D. Cook, Effect of cortisol on the maturation of fetal rabbit lungs, *Pediatrics*, **48**:547 (1971).
59. Beck, J. C., W. Mitzner, J. W. C. Johnson, G. M. Hutchins, J. M. Foidart, W. T. London, A. E. Palmer, and R. Scott, Betamethasone and the Rhesus fetus: Effect on lung morphometry and connective tissue, *Pediatr. Res.*, **15**:235 (1981).
60. Gandy, G., W. Jacobson, and D. Gairdner, Hyaline membrane disease. I. Cellular changes, *Arch. Dis. Child.*, **45**:289 (1970).
61. Chu, J., J. A. Clements, E. Cotton, M. H. Klaus, and A. Y. Sweet, The pulmonary hypoperfusion syndrome, *Pediatrics*, **35**:733 (1965).
62. Northway, W. H., Jr., R. C. Rosan, and D. Y. Porter, Pulmonary disease following respirator therapy of hyaline membrane disease: Bronchopulmonary dysplasia, *New Engl. J. Med.*, **276**:357 (1967).
63. Anderson, W. R., M. B. Strickland, S. H. Tsai, and J. J. Haglin, Light microscopic and ultrastructural study of the adverse effects of oxygen therapy on the neonate lung, *Am. J. Pathol.*, **73**:327 (1973).
64. Ehrenkranz, R. A., R. C. Ablow, and J. B. Warshaw, Oxygen toxicity. The complication of oxygen use in the newborn infant, *Clin. Perinatol.*, **5**:437 (1978).
65. Cutz, E. and P. E. Conen, Endocrine-like cells in human fetal lungs: An electron microscopic study, *Anat. Rec.*, **173**:115 (1972).
66. Hage, E., Endocrine cells in the bronchial mucosa of human foetuses, *Acta Pathol. Microbiol. Scand.*, Section A **80**:225 (1972).
67. Capella, C., E. Hage, E. Solcia, and L. Usellini, Ultrastructural similarity of endocrine-like cells of the human lung and some related cells of the gut, *Cell Tissue Res.*, **186**:25 (1978).
68. Pearse, A. G. E., The cytochemistry and ultrastructure of polypeptide hormone-producing cells of the APUD series and the embryologic, physiologic, and pathologic implications of the concept, *J. Histochem. Cytochem.*, **77**:303 (1969).

69. Wharton, J., J. M. Polak, S. R. Bloom, M. A. Ghatei, E. Solcia, M. R. Brown, and A. G. E. Pearse, Bombesin-like immunoreactivity in the lung, *Nature,* **273**:269 (1978).
70. Becker, K. L., K. G. Monaghan, and O. L. Silva, Immunocytochemical localization of calcitonin in Kultchitsky cells of human lung, *Arch. Pathol. Lab. Med.,* **104**:196 (1980).
71. Cutz, E., W. Chan, and N. S. Track, Bombesin, calcitonin and leu-enkephalin immunoreactivity in endocrine cells of human lung, *Experientia,* **37**: 765 (1981).
72. Moody, T. W., C. B. Pert, A. F. Gazdar, D. N. Carney, and J. D. Minna, High levels of intracellular bombesin characterize human small-cell lung carcinoma, *Science,* **214**:1246 (1981).
73. D. E. Johnson, J. E. Lock, R. P. Elde, and T. R. Thompson, Pulmonary neuroendocrine cells in hyaline membrane disease and bronchopulmonary dysplasia, *Pediatr. Res.,* **16**:446 (1982).
74. Lauweryns, J. M. and M. Cokelaere, Hypoxia-sensitive neuroepithelial bodies: Intrapulmonary secretory neuroreceptors modulated by the CNS, *Z. Zellforsch.,* **143**:521 (1973).

3

Developmental Biochemistry of Lung Surfactant

JOHN E. BLEASDALE and JOHN M. JOHNSTON

University of Texas Health Science Center at Dallas
Dallas, Texas

I. Introduction

The symptoms of respiratory distress syndrome (RDS) of the newborn were first described by Hochheim [1] at the turn of the century. It was not until 1959, however, that Avery and Mead [2] observed poor surface activity in extracts of the lungs of newborn infants who succumbed to respiratory distress syndrome, and they suggested that the disease results from an inadequate production of lung surfactant. It is not surprising, therefore, that most of the biochemical investigations of fetal lung development that have been undertaken in the last 2 decades have centered around the biochemistry of lung surfactant. Although the biochemistry of lung surfactant is the subject of this chapter, it should be emphasized that several other areas of the biochemistry of the lung are now being investigated actively and have been reviewed elsewhere. These areas include the biochemistry of other secretions of the lung, alveolar macrophage function, and the biochemistry of the extracellular matrix [3-5].

Investigations by the authors supported in part by USPHS grants HD 13912 and HD 14373.

II. The Composition of Lung Surfactant

In several species, the ability of fetal lungs to produce lung surfactant does not develop until gestation is more than 80% complete. It is generally agreed that the only sites of surfactant biosynthesis are the type II pneumonocytes of the alveoli. Lung surfactant is a lipoprotein and more than 90% of its dry weight is comprised of lipid. By far the largest fraction of surfactant lipids is composed of the glycerophospholipids. The glycerophospholipid composition of a typical mammalian lung surfactant is summarized in Figure 1, and is unusual in at least two respects. First, the most abundant glycerophospholipid and principal surface-active component of surfactant is 1,2-dipalmitoyl-*sn*-glycero-3-phosphocholine [6]. Such a disaturated phosphatidylcholine is uncommon in most mammalian tissues. Second, phosphatidylglycerol constitutes 7–16% of the glycerophospholipids of surfactant [7]. This lipid is found in only trace amounts in other mammalian tissues. The phosphatidylglycerol of surfactant (like the phosphatidylcholine) is enriched with saturated fatty acids [8]. During fetal lung development in several species, the earliest surfactant produced by immature lungs contains the full complement of disaturated phosphatidylcholine, but it is deficient in phosphatidylglycerol [9]. In place of phosphatidylglycerol, the surfactant from immature lungs is enriched with phosphatidylinositol. As the lung develops there is a change from the production of a surfactant rich in phosphatidylinositol to one rich in phosphatidylglycerol [9–11]. The biophysical properties of phosphatidylglycerol in surfactant and its physiological role in surfactant function are not well understood [12]. A number of investigators, however, have observed that preterm infants delivered before

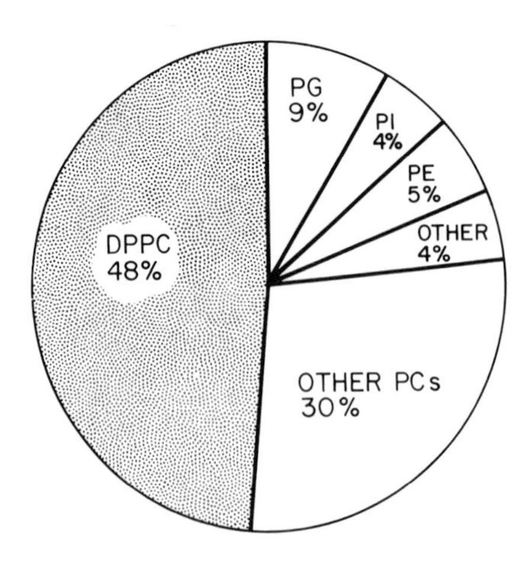

Figure 1 The glycerophospholipid composition of a typical mammalian lung surfactant. Abbreviations: PC, phosphatidylcholine; DPPC, dipalmitoylphosphatidylcholine (1,2-dipalmitoyl-*sn*-glycero-3-phosphocholine); PG, phosphatidylglyerol; PI, phosphatidylinositol; PE, phosphatidylethanolamine.

they can produce a surfactant that is rich in phosphatidylglycerol are at an increased risk of succumbing to respiratory distress syndrome (see Chap. 6).

Protein contributes approximately 10% to the dry weight of surfactant. In surfactant purified from material lavaged from lungs, as much as 50% or more of the recovered proteins are serum proteins. In addition, there is one (or more) integral apoprotein(s) of surfactant. The major integral apoprotein of the surfactant from several species is a glycoprotein with a molecular weight of 35,000-40,000 [13-15]. While the exact functions of surfactant apoproteins are unknown, there is evidence that they may be involved in adsorption and spreading of surfactant [16] (although this has been contested [17]).

III. The Biosynthesis of Lung Surfactant

The biosynthesis of lung surfactant occurs in only one cell type (i.e., the type II pneumonocytes), but within these cells several subcellular organelles are involved in the synthesis and/or assembly of surfactant [18]. Both rough endoplasmic reticulum (for apoprotein synthesis) and smooth endoplasmic reticulum (for synthesis of most of the glycerophospholipids) [19] are involved in surfactant biosynthesis. The Golgi apparatus is required for further glycosylation and processing of surfactant apoproteins. Several lysosomal acid hydrolases are associated with both the stored and secreted forms of surfactant [20]. Finally, it has been suggested that the phosphatidylglycerol component of surfactant may be synthesized in the mitochondria [18,21]. The integration of biosynthesis of the various components of surfactant is poorly understood. On the basis of data obtained largely from morphological investigations, it has been proposed that the intracellular sites for initial assembly of the lipid and protein components of surfactant are the multivesicular bodies [22]. Transport of glycerophospholipids from their sites of synthesis within type II pneumonocytes to the sites of surfactant assembly may involve phospholipid exchange proteins [23] or may occur by vesicle movement [24].

A. Biosynthesis of the Glycerophospholipids of Surfactant

The pathways for the biosynthesis of phosphatidylcholine, phosphatidylinositol, and phosphatidylglycerol are illustrated in Figure 2. The glycerol backbone of these glycerophospholipids is provided by either glycerol 3-phosphate or dihydroxyacetone phosphate. Glycerol 3-phosphate can originate from glucose via dihydroxyacetone phosphate or from glycerol in tissues in which glycerol kinase is active. Although glycerol can be incorporated into glycerophospholipids by type II pneumonocytes isolated from

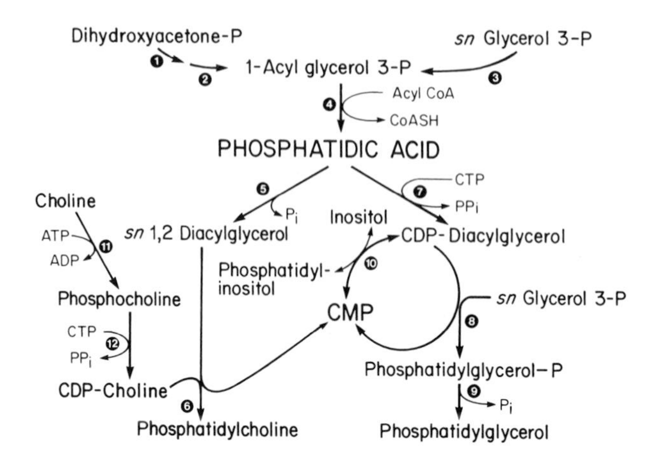

Figure 2 Integration of the biosynthesis of phosphatidylcholine, phosphatidylinositol, and phosphatidylglycerol for lung surfactant. The enzymes that catalyze the individual reactions are: (1) dihydroxyacetone phosphate acyltransferase; (2) 1-acyl dihydroxyacetone phosphate reductase; (3) glycerol 3-phosphate acyltransferase; (4) 1-acyl glycerol 3-phosphate acyltransferase; (5) phosphatidate phosphohydrolase (PAPase); (6) choline phosphotransferase; (7) CTP:phosphatidate cytidylyltransferase; (8) CDP-diacylglycerol:glycerol 3-phosphate phosphatidyltransferase; (9) phosphatidylglycerol phosphatase; (10) CDP-diacylglycerol:inositol phosphatidyltransferase; (11) choline kinase; and (12) CTP:phosphocholine cytidylyltransferase.

adult rat lung [25], it is doubtful that in vivo fetal rat lungs utilize much glycerol for surfactant biosynthesis. This is because lung tissue does not appear to have substantial glycerol kinase activity and because large amounts of glycerol do not appear in the circulation until after birth [26,27]. The glycerol 3-phosphate produced in type II pneumonocytes is acylated sequentially in reactions catalyzed by specific acyltransferases to yield phosphatidic acid. Alternatively, dihydroxyacetone phosphate can be acylated with a fatty acyl coenzyme A (CoA) to yield 1-acyl-dihydroxyacetone phosphate, which is then reduced to 1-acyl glycerol 3-phosphate. The 1-acyl glycerol 3-phosphate can be acylated readily in a reaction requiring fatty acyl CoA and catalyzed by a specific acyltransferase to produce phosphatidic acid. There is evidence that much of the phosphatidic acid that is used by type II pneumonocytes for surfactant lipid synthesis is itself synthesized via the dihydroxyacetone-phosphate pathway [28]. In most tissues, phosphatidic acid is synthesized with an unsaturated fatty acid at the *sn*-2 position. Although dipalmitoyl phosphatidylcholine is the major lipid product produced in the type II pneumonocyte, there is no evidence for a specific acyltransferase to catalyze the selective incorporation of palmitate into the *sn*-2 position of phosphatidic acid in lung tissue during the net synthesis of dipalmitoyl phosphatidylcholine [29]. It has been demonstrated, however, that pulmonary adenoma cells (derived from type II pneumonocytes) have a high capacity for fatty acid biosynthesis and that the major fatty acid synthesized is palmitic acid [30]. Therefore, a significant portion of the phosphatidic acid synthesized in lung tissue may be enriched with palmitic acid in the *sn*-1 and *sn*-2 positions. It is important to note that phosphatidic acid is a precursor not only of phosphatidylcholine, but also of phosphatidylglycerol and phosphatidylinositol. Therefore, the increased biosynthesis of glycerophospholipids for surfactant that occurs late in gestation depends upon an increased biosynthesis of phosphatidic acid. Despite the critical importance of phosphatidic acid, little is known about developmental changes in phosphatidic acid production by the lungs. In one study, it was reported that the rate of incorporation of [^{14}C]glycerol 3-phosphate into phosphatidic acid by fetal rabbit lung microsomes was nine-fold greater on day 28 of gestation than on day 21 [31].

For the biosynthesis of dipalmitoyl phosphatidylcholine, phosphatidic acid is hydrolyzed in a reaction catalyzed by phosphatidate phosphohydrolase (PAPase) to yield diacylglycerol. Diacylglycerol so formed serves as the cosubstrate with cytidine diphosphocholine (CDP-choline) in the formation of phosphatidylcholine and cytidine monophosphate (CMP) in a reaction catalyzed by choline phosphotransferase. The CDP-choline used in the reaction is formed through the sequential action of choline kinase (which gives rise to phosphocholine) and CTP:phosphocholine cytidylyltransferase (which catalyzes the formation of CDP-choline from phosphocholine and CTP). A significant amount of diacylglycerol containing palmitic acid in the *sn*-1 and *sn*-2 positions may be formed because of the high rate of synthesis of palmitic acid in the lung. Although it was once thought that dipalmitoylglycerol was a poor substrate for choline phosphotransferase in lung [32], there is evidence that dipalmitoylglycerol can be utilized effectively to produce dipalmitoyl phosphatidylcholine [33]. In addition, there are also two mechanisms in the lung for the remodeling of other phosphatidylcholines to form dipalmitoyl phosphatidylcholine [34]. The first reaction in each remodeling mechanism is catalyzed by a phospholipase A_2 and results in the removal of the fatty acid at the *sn*-2 position. The 1-palmitoyl glycerophosphocholine that is produced can be either reacylated with a molecule of palmitoyl-CoA or transacylated with another molecule of 1-palmitoyl glycerophosphocholine and in each case one product is dipalmitoyl phosphatidylcholine.

Much of the research aimed at understanding the mechanism by which lung surfactant production is initiated and stimulated during fetal lung development was based on the premise that the mechanism involved changes in the activities of biosynthetic enzymes that could be meaningfully monitored under optimal in vitro conditions. While it is now evident that optimal enzymatic activity in vitro can be quite different from physiological activity, much useful information was collected from such studies. For instance, it was observed that the specific activity of PAPase in the fetal rabbit lung tissue increased during gestation beginning at approximately the twenty-fifth day of gestation [35]. In fetal rat lung, PAPase activity does not increase until the time of birth [36]. Evidence that such an increase in PAPase activity occurs also in human fetal lung relied on the fortuitous observation that some PAPase activity is tightly associated with lamellar bodies and moves with the lamellar bodies that are secreted from type II penumonocytes into the amniotic fluid. It was found that PAPase activity in the amniotic fluid after the thirty-second week of gestation was much greater than that observed earlier in gestation [37]. PAPase activity in the nasopharyngeal fluid was significantly higher than that in amniotic fluid, a finding consistent with the proposition that much of the PAPase found in amniotic fluid originates in the fetal lung [38].

Possmayer and colleagues [39] characterized the PAPase activity in rat lung tissue. They reported that there were four experimentally distinguishable forms of the enzyme. The precise function of the various PAPase enzymes that are found in lung tissue is not readily apparent. We suggested previously that the PAPase activity present in lung tissue functions not only in the synthesis of phosphatidylcholine but also in the synthesis of phosphatidylglycerol [40]. Employing [^{32}P] phosphatidic acid and [^{14}C] phosphatidylglycerol phosphate as substrates, it was demonstrated that PAPase in lamellar bodies prepared from porcine lung catalyzed the hydrolysis of both substrates [40]. We observed also that a phosphonate analog of phosphatidic acid inhibits the hydrolysis of both phosphatidic acid and phosphatidylglycerol phosphate (Table 1) [41]. In contrast to these observations, Casola et al. [42] concluded that the hydrolysis of phosphatidic acid and phosphatidylglycerol phosphate was catalyzed by two distinct enzymes present in rat lung lamellar bodies. Although the substrate specificity of the PAPase activity associated with lamellar bodies is still controversial, Casola et al. [42] confirmed the observation that PAPase activity was closely associated with the lamellar body fraction.

The importance of CTP:phosphocholine cytidylyltransferase in the regulation of phosphatidylcholine biosynthesis in a number of tissues has been emphasized [43,44]. In several species there is a developmental increase in CTP:phosphocholine cytidylyltransferase specific activity in the lungs. The time course of the increase in activity of this enzyme, however, does not correlate well with the late gestational surge in phosphatidylcholine

Table 1 The Effect of Distearoylbutyl-Phosphonic Acid on the Hydrolysis of [^{32}P] Dioleoyl-Phosphatidate and Dipalmitoylphosphatidyl-[^{14}C] Glycerol 3-Phosphate by Pig Lung Lamellar Bodies

Additions	Total nmol hydrolyzed	Specific activity nmol × min^{-1} × mg^{-1} protein
1. [^{32}P] Phosphatidate	1.9	79.1
2. Phosphatidyl-[^{14}C] glycerol 3-phosphate	1.2	48.3
3. [^{32}P] Phosphatidate	0.8	33.7(57)
Plus		
Phosphatidyl-[^{14}C] glycerol 3-phosphate	0.8	31.3(35)
4. [^{32}P] Phosphatidate	0.9	38.2(52)
Plus Phosphonate analog		
5. Phosphatidyl-[^{14}C] glycerol 3-phosphate	0.5	22.1(54)
Plus Phosphonate analog		

Incubations were performed at 37°C for 20 min in a shaking water bath. Incubation vessels contained maleate buffer pH 6.0 (20 μmol), Triton X-100 (0.24 mg), lamellar body protein (2.5 μg), and a combination of racemic distearoylbutyl-phosphonate (40 nmol), [^{32}P] phosphatidate (20 nmol), and phosphatidyl-[^{14}C] glycerol 3-phosphate in a total volume of 0.2 ml. Numbers in parentheses are percentages of total inhibition achieved.

synthesis [45]. In fetal rabbit lung, the activity of CTP:phosphocholine cytidylyltransferase decreased between the twenty-first and thirty-first day of gestation [45]. In other species, developmental increases in CTP:phosphocholine cytidylyltransferase have been observed, but in general these do not occur until around the time of birth [45]. These findings do not preclude, however, the possibility that although enzymatic activity measured in vitro does not change appreciably during gestation, enzymatic activity in vivo may be regulated. Indeed, the activity appears to be regulated in part by the translocation of latent enzyme from the cytosol to the endoplasmic reticulum where it is active [44]. The positive effectors of this activation have been reported to be phosphatidylglycerol, other anionic glycerophospholipids, and unesterified fatty acids [44].

Weinhold and coworkers were the first to propose and to present supporting evidence that CTP:phosphocholine cytidylyltransferase may serve a regulatory function in lung surfactant phosphatidylcholine biosynthesis [46]. Recently, Post et al. [47] suggested that CTP:phosphocholine cytidylyltransferase activity is the rate-limiting reaction in the biosynthesis of surfactant phosphatidylcholine by type II pneumonocytes isolated from adult rat lung. While it is likely that CTP:phosphocholine cytidylyltransferase does catalyze a reaction that is a regulatory step in surfactant phosphatidylcholine biosynthesis in adult type II pneumonocytes, caution should be taken when extrapolating these findings to the development of phosphatidylcholine synthesis in fetal lungs.

Although several investigators have suggested that choline phosphotransferase in lung tissue may be a regulatory enzyme in the synthesis of surfactant phosphatidylcholine, the activity of this enzyme (at least under optimal in vitro conditions) does not change in parallel with changes in the rate of phosphatidylcholine biosynthesis during fetal lung development [48]. It has been suggested, however, that choline phosphotransferase activity is affected by certain hormones [48].

There is little evidence that choline kinase activity ever limits the synthesis of phosphatidylcholine for surfactant [49]. Although various enzymes have been proposed to catalyze *the* rate-limiting step in phosphatidylcholine biosynthesis, it is clear that during fetal lung development supplies of both CDP-choline (produced by the action of CTP:phosphocholine cytidylyltransferase) and diacylglycerol (produced by the action of PAPase) must be provided in amounts adequate to support increased synthesis of phosphatidylcholine. If either of these two substrates were present in limited amounts, then synthesis of phosphatidylcholine would be restricted. Therefore, it is possible that both CTP:phosphocholine cytidylyltransferase and PAPase perform regulatory roles in phosphatidylcholine biosynthesis during fetal lung development.

In addition to being hydrolyzed to diacylglycerol for phosphatidylcholine biosynthesis, phosphatidic acid may react with CTP to form CDP-diacylglycerol in a reaction catalyzed by CTP:phosphatidate cytidylyltransferase (Fig. 2). It was found that the specific activity of this enzyme in fetal rabbit lung remains relatively constant between the twenty-third and twenty-eighth day of gestation [50]. The specific activity of CTP:phosphatidate cytidylyltransferase then increased approximately 2.4-fold between the twenty-eighth day of gestation and 1 day after birth. CDP-diacylglycerol synthesized in this manner may react with free *myo*-inositol to form phosphatidylinositol and CMP in a reversible reaction catalyzed by CDP-diacylglycerol:inositol phosphatidyltransferase. Alternatively, CDP-diacylglycerol may react with glycerol 3-phosphate in a reaction catalyzed by CDP-diacylglycerol:glycerol 3-phosphate phosphatidyltransferase to produce phosphatidylglycerol phosphate and CMP. The phosphatidylglycerol phosphate is then hydrolyzed by a phosphohydrolase to yield phosphatidylglycerol. We have discussed previously the role of PAPase in the hydrolysis of both phosphatidic acid and phosphatidylglycerol phosphate.

It is clear that the developmental change from the biosynthesis of phosphatidylinositol-rich surfactant to the production of a surfactant rich in phosphatidylglycerol that occurs near birth in several species is not a consequence of developmental changes in the maximal activities of the enzymes involved in the biosynthesis of these two lipids [51,52]. Therefore, an alternative explanation must be sought for the developmental increase in the amount of phosphatidylglycerol in surfactant at the expense of its phosphatidylinositol content.

B. Integration of the Biosynthesis of Phosphatidylinositol, Phosphatidylglycerol, and Phosphatidylcholine for Surfactant—The Cytidine Monophosphate Cycle

The reciprocal developmental changes in the amounts of phosphatidylinositol and phosphatidylglycerol in surfactant are suggestive of regulation at the level of a common precursor, CDP-diacylglycerol. A mechanism that can account for this regulation is illustrated in Figure 2. In this mechanism cytidine monophosphate (CMP) plays an important role.

In the biosynthesis of the glycerophospholipids of surfactant, we envision the following sequence of events to occur: (1) A stimulation of phosphatidylcholine biosynthesis occurs possibly due to increases in the activities of CTP-phosphocholine cytidylyltransferase and PAPase. (2) Augmented phosphatidylcholine biosynthesis is accompanied by an increased formation of CMP in the developing type II pneumonocyte. (3) CMP in elevated concentrations within the type II pneumonocytes facilitates the reverse reaction catalyzed by CDP-diacylglycerol:inositol phosphatidyltransferase resulting in a decreased net flux of CDP-diacylglycerol to phosphatidylinositol and an increased availability of CDP-diacylglycerol for phosphatidylglycerol biosynthesis. During the course of the synthesis of phosphatidylglycerol phosphate CMP is regenerated. Thus, the elevated levels of CMP that were initially a result of increased phosphatidylcholine biosynthesis are maintained by this *CMP cycle*. In this regulatory mechanism, it is envisioned that PAPase serves a second important function by catalyzing the irreversible hydrolysis of phosphatidylglycerol phosphate to phosphatidylglycerol.

According to the proposed mechanism, enhanced phosphatidylcholine biosynthesis is accompanied by increased intracellular amounts of CMP in lung tissue during fetal lung development. We have measured the amounts of CMP, CDP, CTP, CDP-choline, and CDP-ethanolamine in rabbit lung tissue obtained at various times during development [53]. On the twenty-first day of gestation it was found that the CTP levels were relatively high and only small amounts of CMP and CDP-choline were present in fetal lung. By the twenty-sixth day of gestation, the CTP levels fell dramatically with a concomitant increase in CDP-choline. No change was observed in the levels of CMP during this developmental period. Subsequently, CDP-choline levels decreased and CMP levels increased at a time concomitant with the observed surge in phosphatidylcholine biosynthesis in fetal rabbit lung tissue. Augmented phosphatidylcholine biosynthesis is due most likely to the increased availability of diacylglycerol as a result of increased PAPase activity [35]. Thus, it appears that during *this* critical time of fetal rabbit lung development it is not the availability of CDP-choline but rather the availability of diacylglycerols that restricts phosphatidylcholine biosynthesis. No changes in the amounts of AMP in fetal lung tissue or CMP in fetal liver tissue were observed during this developmental period. It should be emphasized that although PAPase activity may be critical at this time of development, it can not be assumed that in adult type II pneumonocytes this enzyme catalyzes a regulatory reaction. Further support for the proposed importance of CMP in the regulation of the biosynthesis of surfactant glycerophospholipids was provided by the observation that CMP stimulated the incorporation of [^{14}C]-glycerol 3-phosphate into phosphatidylglycerol by adult rabbit lung microsomes [54]. CMP-dependent incorporation of [^{14}C]glycerol 3-phosphate into phosphatidylglycerol appeared to require CDP-diacylglycerol:inositol phosphatidyltransferase activity as predicted from the mechanism described above.

The competition for CDP-diacylglycerol to support the biosynthesis of both phosphatidylinositol and phosphatidylglycerol is influenced not only by CMP but also by *myo*-inositol. It was found that as gestation advances, fetal rabbit lungs have a decreased ability not only to synthesize *myo*-inositol but also to take up *myo*-inositol from the blood [55]. This may result in a decreased availability of *myo*-inositol for phosphatidylinositol biosynthesis by the fetal lungs. Such a situation favors the production of surfactant enriched with phosphatidylglycerol and this effect of *myo*-inositol complements the influence of CMP described in the above mechanism. The proposition that *myo*-inositol availability influences surfactant composition received support from the results of experiments in which the incorporation of [^{14}C] glycerol into glycerophospholipids by adult rat type II pneumonocytes was measured (Fig. 3). It was found that as the concentration of *myo*-inositol in the medium was increased, the incorporation of radioisotope into phosphatidylglycerol relative to the incorporation into phosphatidylinositol was reduced. The concentration of *myo*-inositol at which the effect on the ratio [^{14}C] phosphatidylglycerol: [^{14}C] phosphatidylinositol was half maximal was similar to the concentration at which half maximal uptake of *myo*-inositol into type II pneumonocytes was observed (Fig. 3).

The concentration of *myo*-inositol in human fetal serum also decreases as gestation advances [56]. The influence of *myo*-inositol on surfactant lipid biosynthesis may explain the delayed appearance of phosphatidylglycerol-rich

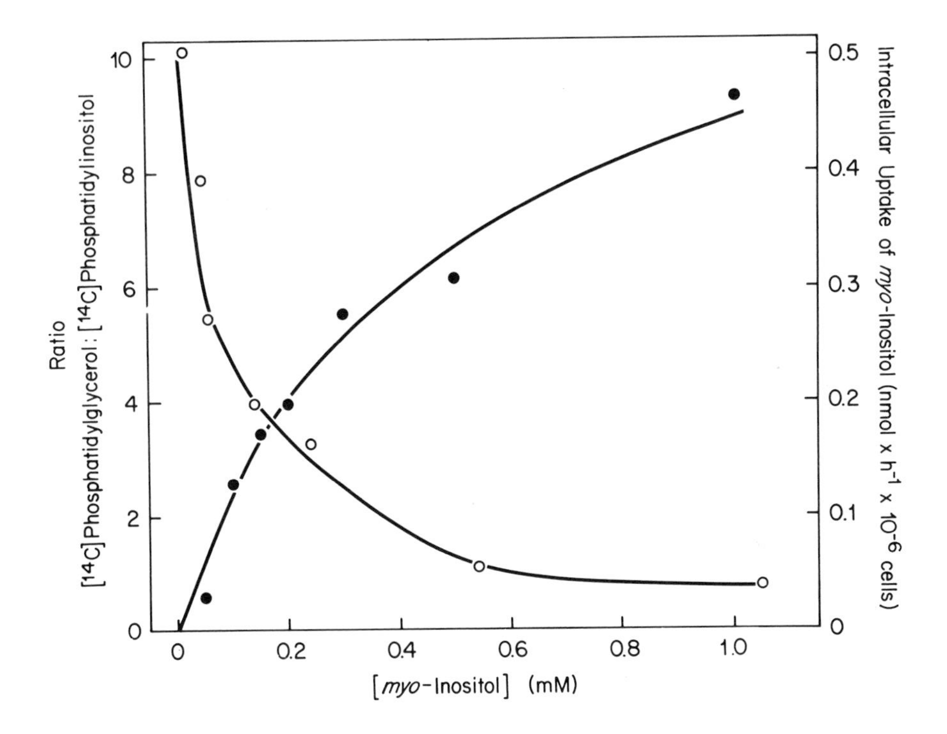

Figure 3 The relative rates of biosynthesis of phosphatidylglycerol and phosphatidylinositol when the rate of *myo*-inositol uptake by type II pneumonocytes is altered by changing the concentration of *myo*-inositol in the medium. Type II pneumonocytes isolated from adult rat lung were incubated for 24 hr in medium containing [^{14}C] glycerol (0.1 mM) and *myo*-inositol at various concentrations. Lipids were extracted, then separated using two-dimensional thin-layer chromatography and the ratio of ^{14}C incorporated into phosphatidylglycerol to ^{14}C incorporated into phosphatidylinositol was measured. In other experiments the type II pneumonocytes were incubated for 20 min in medium supplemented with *myo*-[^{3}H] inositol and nonradiolabeled *myo*-inositol at various concentrations. The intracellular uptake of *myo*-inositol by type II pneumonocytes was then measured using methods described [55]. The data are mean values obtained from three experiments. Ratio [^{14}C] Phosphatidylglycerol: [^{14}C] Phosphatidylinositol, (–○–); Intracellular uptake of *myo*-inositol, (–●–). (Data derived from Bleasdale, J. E., N. E. Tyler, F. N. Busch, and J. G. Quirk, The influence of *myo*-inositol on phosphatidylglycerol synthesis by rat type II pneumonocytes, *Biochem. J.*, **212**:811, 1983.)

surfactant in the fetus of the mother with mild diabetes mellitus. It is known that the patient with diabetes mellitus, in addition to being glucose intolerant, is also *myo*-inositol intolerant, i.e., urinary excretion and circulating concentrations of *myo*-inositol are abnormally increased and there is an apparent defect in the uptake of *myo*-inositol into various tissues [57]. We have proposed that an imbalance in *myo*-inositol homeostasis in the pregnant woman with diabetes mellitus affects adversely *myo*-inositol homeostasis in her fetus. As a consequence, the normal developmental decline in *myo*-inositol availability to the fetal lung is retarded and production of surfactant rich in phosphatidylinositol persists.

C. Biosynthesis of the Apoproteins of Surfactant

Compared to the biosynthesis of surfactant lipids, relatively little is known about the synthesis of surfactant apoproteins. King and coworkers have examined the kinetics of incorporation of radioactive precursors into the apoproteins of dog and rat lung surfactant [58,59]. [^{3}H] Leucine was incorporated in vivo into two surfactant apoproteins, one of molecular weight 35,000 (apoprotein A) and the other of molecular weight 10,000 (apoprotein B). Incorporation of [^{14}C] palmitate into saturated phosphatidylcholine followed a similar time course to that for the incorporation of [^{3}H] leucine into apoprotein A. On the other hand, the incorporation of [^{3}H] leucine into apoprotein B exhibited a different time course. Evidence was obtained that apoprotein A may be a precursor of apoprotein B. When surfactant apoprotein synthesis by isolated type II pneumonocytes was suppressed employing cycloheximide, the synthesis and secretion of dipalmitoyl phosphatidylcholine remained unaltered as did the secretion of previously synthesized apoprotein [60].

With the advent of improved techniques for isolating surfactant apoproteins and the availability of specific antibodies to these proteins, immunocytochemical investigations of surfactant apoprotein biosynthesis are now feasible. Using such techniques, Williams and Benson [61] observed that antibodies to the apoprotein bound to the rough endoplasmic reticulum, Golgi apparatus, and multivesicular bodies of type II pneumonocytes of adult rat lung. Phagosomes of alveolar macrophages and type I pneumonocytes also contained the specific antigen [61]. These investigators concluded that only type II pneumonocytes synthesize surfactant and that the initial intracellular sites of association of apoprotein with lipid may be the multivesicular bodies [61]. They also concluded that alveolar macrophages are important sites of surfactant apoprotein catabolism [61]. It is now clear, however, that a substantial portion of secreted surfactant is not catabolized but may be recycled. The possible role of apoproteins in the cellular recognition of surfactant for re-uptake and their role in recycling remain exciting topics for further investigation.

IV. Secretion of Surfactant by Type II Pneumonocytes

Little is known of the mechanism of surfactant secretion by adult or developing type II pneumonocytes. Delahunty and Johnston [62] reported evidence that the secretion of surfactant by the adult hamster lung may require an intact microtubule system. Prior treatment of adult hamsters with colchicine or vinblastine markedly decreased the release of surfactant from slices of adult hamster lung incubated in vitro. Similar results have been reported recently by Longmore and Brown [63]. The secretion of surfactant is influenced by adrenergic effectors [64], cholinergic agonists [65], and prostaglandins [66]. Type II pneumonocytes possess β-adrenergic receptors [67,68], and β-adrenergic agonists have been reported to stimulate surfactant secretion [69], presumably by a cyclic AMP-dependent mechanism.

V. Hormonal Regulation of Surfactant Lipid Biosynthesis

Liggins [70] and Kotas and Avery [71] were the first to obtain direct evidence that fetal lung maturation could be accelerated hormonally by the administration of glucocorticosteroids. Many investigators have adopted the view that fetal hormones may provide the stimulus for the observed surge in surfactant biosynthesis that occurs late in gestation. In addition, hormones may increase surfactant secretion. Hormones that have been proposed to influence surfactant production include glucocorticoids, adrenocorticotropic hormone, thyroid hormones, thyrotropin releasing hormone, estrogens, prolactin, catecholamines, insulin, epidermal growth factor, fibroblast pneumonocyte factor, and prostaglandins (see Ref. 72 for review).

A. Glucocorticoids

The effect of glucocorticoids on the morphological development of fetal lung tissue has been discussed in Chapter 2. A major effect of glucocorticoids is to increase the rate of glycerophospholipid synthesis at a critical time in lung development. During the course of normal lung development in several species, the rate of choline incorporation into phosphatidylcholine increases severalfold near the end of gestation at a time when liver and lung glycogen is being depleted. It appears that the mechanism of action of glucocorticoids involves acceleration of both glycogen depletion and glycerophospholipid biosynthesis. Although it has been reported that glucocorticoid treatment in vivo or in vitro increases the activities of CTP:phosphocholine cytidylyltransferase [73], choline phosphotransferase [74], and PAPase [75], other investigators have been unable to detect such effects of glucocorticoids on the fetal lungs of a number of species [76]. The precise biochemical mechanism by which glucocorticoids affect fetal lung maturation has not been established. Glucocorticoid receptors, however, have been identified in the lung tissue of several species, including the human as well as in isolated type II pneumonocytes [77-79]. Since approximately 24 hr of treatment is required in order to demonstrate increased phosphatidylcholine biosynthesis in response to glucocorticoids, it is likely that the mechanism of action involves protein synthesis. In agreement with this conclusion was the observation that cycloheximide blocks the effect of glucocorticoid treatment in vivo and in vitro [72].

Although the administration of glucocorticoids in large amounts has proved under certain circumstances to be beneficial in increasing surfactant production in fetal lung tissue, it is not clear that glucocorticoids function physiologically to initiate surfactant production in fetal lungs. It is known, however, that the concentration of free cortisol in the fetal blood of several species does not increase until surfactant biosynthesis has already been initiated (e.g., 80). On the other hand, the apparent ability of cortisol to stimulate surfactant production after surfactant synthesis has been initiated may be an explanation for the observed effect of fetal stress in promoting lung surfactant production [81]. The concentration of cortisol in cord serum and in amniotic fluid are abnormally low in infants who suffer respiratory distress syndrome [82,83]. Further evidence that glucocorticoids may modulate but not initiate surfactant production comes from investigations of the in vitro "differentiation" of fetal lung tissue. It was found that explants of human fetal lung obtained during the twentieth to twenty-second week of gestation (i.e., before the initiation of surfactant production) underwent a marked morphological and biochemical differentiation after only 4 days in culture in vitro [84]. This in vitro differentiation was accompanied by increased phosphatidylcholine biosynthesis for surfactant and occurred in the absence of added serum or hormones. Cortisol plus prolactin, when added to the fetal lung explants on the first day of culture, caused an accelerated appearance of enhanced phosphatidylcholine biosynthesis (Fig. 4) [84].

The failure to observe a universal glucocorticoid-induced increase in the activities of enzymes involved in phosphatidylcholine synthesis may be due to species differences in the response to glucocorticoids. In addition, it has been suggested [72,84] that glucocorticoids act not alone but synergistically with other hormones. Specifically, we have observed that cortisol in concert with prolactin (but not by itself) increased greatly the incorporation of [^{3}H]choline into phosphatidylcholine by explants of human fetal lung [84]. Finally, it must be considered that glucocorticoids may indirectly influence surfactant biosynthesis in the fetal lung by modulating the release of factors from other lung cell types such as lung fibroblasts (see below) [85].

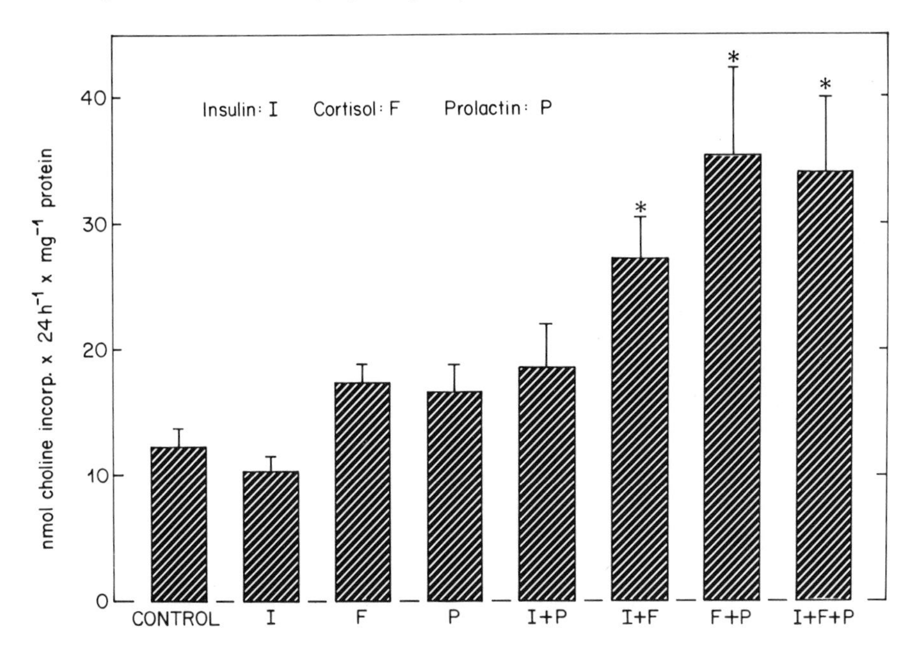

Figure 4 The effect of cortisol, prolactin, and insulin on the rate of incorporation of [^{3}H] choline into disaturated phosphatidylcholine by explants of human fetal lung. Lung explants obtained from 22-week gestational age abortuses were incubated for 4 days in medium lacking serum but supplemented with one or more of the hormones indicated in the figure. [^{3}H] Choline was added to the explants for the last 24 hr of incubation. Lipids were extracted and then separated by thin-layer chromatography and the incorporation of radioisotope into disaturated phosphatidylcholine was measured. Treatment with hormones did not alter the ratio of disaturated phosphatidylcholine to total phosphatidylcholine (not shown). The data are mean values ± SEM obtained from three experiments and are derived from data reported elsewhere [84]. Asterisks denote the values that are significantly different ($p < 0.05$) from the control value.

B. Thyroid Hormones

It has been reported that the in vitro treatment of lung tissue with thyroid hormones results in the stimulation of the rate of choline incorporation into phosphatidylcholine [76]. In addition, the direct administration of thyroxine (to the fetal rat) has been reported to accelerate both morphological development and increased surfactant synthesis [86]. A proposed effect of thyroid hormones on fetal lung maturation in vivo has received support from investigations employing 3,5-dimethyl-3′-isopropyl-*L*-thyronine (DIMIT) (a synthetic analog of T_3 which readily crosses the rabbit placenta). The injection of DIMIT into pregnant rabbits caused a dose-dependent increase in the in vitro incorporation of choline into phosphatidylcholine by the fetal lungs obtained from treated animals [87]. In the same study, DIMIT administration resulted in a small increase in phosphatidate phosphohydrolase activity in fetal lung and a decrease in the amount of glycogen in this tissue [75]. In several species, the fetal serum concentrations of thyroid hormones increase late in gestation [88]. Like cortisol concentrations, however, the increase in concentrations of thyroid hormones in fetal serum occurs largely *after* the initiation of surfactant production. Although receptors for thyroid hormones are present in fetal lung [89], it is not yet established whether thyroid hormones act directly on the lung or modulate the action of other hormones.

C. Estrogens

The intramuscular administration of estradiol for 48 hr to pregnant rabbits, beginning on the twenty-fifth day of gestation, increased the amount of total glycerophospholipid (and specifically the amount of phosphatidylcholine) in fetal lung tissue and lung lavage [90]. In addition, it was also demonstrated that there is an increased rate of choline incorporation into slices of fetal rat lung from animals that had been pretreated with estradiol prior to the assay [91]. In the latter investigation, however, the optimal in vitro activities of several enzymes involved in phosphatidylcholine biosynthesis were not increased in the lungs of treated fetuses. Rooney and Brehier [45] have suggested that the estrogen-induced increase in incorporation of choline into phosphatidylcholine is mediated by in vivo changes in CTP:phosphocholine cytidylyltransferase activity, possibly by an increase in the relative amount of the high molecular weight (more active) form of this enzyme. The presence of estrogen-binding proteins in fetal lung tissue has been established in several species, including the human [92]. However, whether or not these represent specific estrogen-binding receptors capable of permitting a physiological response of fetal and adult lung tissue to estrogens remains undetermined.

D. Prolactin

Late in gestation there is an increase in the concentration of prolactin in fetal serum of several species (e.g., 93). This increase occurs before the concentration of glucocorticoids in fetal serum increases and before the appearance of surfactant in tracheal fluid. In addition, a correlation between low concentrations of prolactin in serum from human umbilical cord and the incidence of respiratory distress syndrome of the newborn has been described [93]. On the basis of such a correlation, however, it can not be concluded that prolactin alone influences surfactant production. Although in vivo treatment of fetal rabbits with prolactin for 2 days resulted in an increase in total phospholipid and saturated phosphatidylcholine in their lungs [94], only in combination with cortisol or insulin could prolactin affect the synthesis of surfactant lipids by explants of human fetal lung tissue maintained in vitro [84].

The likelihood that the influence of prolactin on surfactant production involves synergism with other hormones is strengthened by several reports of a lack of an effect of prolactin alone either in vivo or in vitro (e.g., [95,96]). Prolactin-binding proteins (possibly functioning as lactogenic hormone receptors) have been described in fetal lung tissue from the monkey [97] and human [98]. In addition to influencing the fetal lungs directly, prolactin has the potential for affecting the lungs indirectly by promoting steroidogenesis in the fetal adrenal [99].

E. Insulin

There are a number of reasons for suspecting that insulin may antagonize the normal development of surfactant production. First, as mentioned above, the initiation of surfactant production is accompanied by depletion of glycogen in the fetal lungs and liver. Insulin, however, promotes glycogen *deposition* in the liver. Second, many of the actions of glucocorticoids on liver are antagonized by insulin. Glucocorticoids appear to play a role in facilitating surfactant production. Third, there is an apparent delay in fetal lung surfactant production in pregnancies complicated by mild diabetes mellitus (see Chap. 9). In such pregnancies the fetus is often hyperinsulinemic.

The experimental evidence of such an antagonistic role of insulin has, however, been inconclusive. Smith et al. [100] found that cortisol stimulated the incorporation of [^{3}H]choline into phosphatidylcholine by monolayers of fetal rabbit lung cells and that this effect of cortisol was reduced by insulin. This inhibition by insulin of cortisol-stimulated [^{3}H]choline incorporation was apparently specific, since a cortisol-induced reduction in cellular growth was not antagonized by insulin. Although insulin suppressed cortisol-stimulated incorporation of [^{3}H] choline into phosphatidylcholine, its effect in the absence of cortisol was to stimulate incorporation. Furthermore, no inhibitory effect of insulin on surfactant synthesis by explants of human fetal lung maintained in vitro could be observed [84]. Indeed, the incorporation of [^{3}H]choline into disaturated phosphatidylcholine by explants exposed to insulin plus cortisol was more than three times greater than that observed for explants exposed to cortisol alone [84]. Gross et al. [101] investigated the effect of insulin on [^{3}H]-choline incorporation into phosphatidylcholine by fetal rat lung in organ culture. They observed that insulin had no influence on the rate of [^{3}H]choline incorporation and did not antagonize a dexamethasone-induced stimulation of [^{3}H]choline incorporation into phosphatidylcholine. In the same study, the effects of insulin on the activities of several enzymes involved in phosphatidylcholine biosynthesis were investigated. The only significant insulin-dependent changes in enzymatic activity were small increases (< 30%) in the activities of choline kinase and 1-acyl glycerophosphocholine acyltransferase. While there appear to be few (if any) effects of insulin on the enzymes involved in surfactant phosphatidylcholine biosynthesis, it was found that insulin antagonized the corticosterone-induced increase in PAPase activity in isolated rat hepatocytes [102]. Insulin receptors have been identified in fetal rat lung and the density of insulin receptors was found to increase fivefold during the last trimester of gestation [103]. The importance of insulin in normal lung maturation is unclear and the issue of whether the effects of insulin are direct or indirect (e.g., via antagonism of another hormone) remains controversial.

F. Catecholamines

In the third trimester of human gestation, increases in the concentrations of several catecholamines in the fetal circulation are reflected as increased concentrations in amniotic fluid [104]. One of the most abundant catecholamines in human amniotic fluid late in gestation is dopamine (and its metabolite 3,4-dihydroxyphenylacetic acid). The influence of dopamine on fetal lung maturation (possibly by modulating fetal prolactin release) remains unknown. There is evidence, however, that β-adrenergic catecholamines may stimulate surfactant synthesis in addition to their effects on surfactant secretion noted earlier. The administration of the β-sympathomimetic isoxsuprine to pregnant rabbits resulted in increased synthesis of saturated phosphatidylcholine in fetal lungs [105]. On the otherhand, chronic administration of another β-sympathomimetic, ritodrine, to pregnant rabbits was found to have no effect on either synthesis or secretion of surfactant [106]. Any effect of β-agonists on surfactant synthesis is presumably mediated by cyclic AMP. Indeed, there are several reports that cyclic AMP and phosphodiesterase inhibitors stimulate surfactant synthesis both in vivo and in vitro (e.g., 107,108). The mechanism by which cyclic AMP might stimulate surfactant synthesis is unknown but may involve the effect of cyclic AMP in stimulating glycogen degradation that has been well described in the liver.

G. Other Factors

A variety of other effectors have been reported to influence surfactant synthesis. Smith has described a heat-stable, dialyzable polypeptide whose synthesis in human fetal lung fibroblasts is induced by steroids [85]. The partially purified material when injected intraperitoneally into pregnant rats on day 17 of gestation caused an increase in the proportion of phosphatidylcholine, disaturated phosphatidylcholine, and phosphatidylglycerol in total lipids of the fetal lungs [85]. The same polypeptide material enhanced the stimulation of [^{3}H]choline into saturated phosphatidylcholine by human fetal type II pneumonocytes that was induced by oxygen stress [109]. It was speculated that fetal type II pneumonocytes require a fibroblast-derived polypeptide in order to respond to steroids and increase surfactant production. Other peptides that have been proposed to influence surfactant production directly or indirectly include thyrotropin releasing hormone [110], adrenocorticotropic hormone [111], and epidermal growth factor [112].

VI. Conclusions

While the developmental biochemistry of lung surfactant production is still not understood completely, the advances made by many investigators have revealed new complexities of this biological process.

1. The established concept of a single rate-limiting or regulatory enzyme in surfactant lipid biosynthesis appears to be an oversimplification. Thus, for unrestricted synthesis of phosphatidylcholine to occur, an adequate supply of both diacylglycerol and CDP-choline must be maintained enzymatically. Since phosphatidic acid is the precursor of all the glycerophospholipids of surfactant, regulation of phosphatidic acid production is a critical but neglected aspect of the regulation of surfactant lipid synthesis.
2. The individual components of surfactant have too often been investigated separately, but it is increasingly evident that the synthesis of surfactant is a complex, integrated process. Information about the mechanism by which type II pneumonocytes achieve *metabolic* integration and the effectors involved may lead to a better understanding of how the synthesis of individual components is controlled. More detailed investigation of the *spatial* integration of the various subcellular sites contributing to surfactant synthesis and assembly also may have important implications with regard to regulation of surfactant production.
3. Characteristics of the regulation of surfactant synthesis that have been deduced from investigations employing adult lung tissue or adult type II pneumonocytes are not necessarily relevant to regulation of surfactant synthesis by the developing fetal lung.
4. The results of many investigations of the hormonal control of surfactant biosynthesis support the conclusion that it is not a single hormone or factor but rather a total hormonal milieu that is conducive to the normal development of fetal lung surfactant production.

Acknowledgment

The authors are grateful to Ms. D. Tutton for help in the preparation of this manuscript.

References

1. Hochheim, K., Ueber eimige Befunde in den Lungen von Neugeborenen und die Beziehung derselben zur Aspiration von Fruchtwasser, *Zentralbl. Pathol.*, **14**:537 (1903).
2. Avery, M. E. and J. Mead, Surface properties in relation to atelectasis and hyaline membrane disease, *Am. J. Dis. Child.*, **97**:517 (1959).
3. Gallagher, J. T. and P. S. Richardson, Respiratory mucus: Structure, metabolism and control of secretion, *Adv. Exp. Med. Biol.*, **144**:335 (1982).
4. Van Ould Alblas, A. B. and R. Van Furth, Origin, kinetics, and characteristics of pulmonary macrophages in the normal steady state, *J. Exp. Med.*, **149**:1504 (1979).
5. Vaccaro, C. A. and J. S. Brody, Ultrastructural localization and characterization of proteoglycans in the pulmonary alveolus, *Am. Rev. Respir. Dis.*, **120**:901 (1979).
6. Klaus, M. H., J. A. Clements, and R. J. Havel, Composition of surface-active material isolated from beef lung, *Proc. Natl. Acad. Sci. USA*, **47**:1858 (1961).
7. Pfleger, R. C., R. F. Henderson, and J. Waide, Phosphatidylglycerol–A major component of pulmonary surfactant, *Chem. Phys. Lipids*, 9:51 (1972).
8. Sanders, R. L. and W. J. Longmore, Phosphatidylglycerol in rat lung. II. Comparison of occurrence, composition and metabolism in surfactant and residual lung fractions, *Biochemistry*, **14**:835 (1975).
9. Hallman, M. and L. Gluck, Formation of acidic phospholipids in rabbit lung during perinatal development, *Pediatr. Res.*, **14**:1250 (1980).
10. Hallman, M., M. Kulovich, E. Kirkpatrick, R. G. Sugarman, and L. Gluck, Phosphatidylinositol and phosphatidylglycerol in amniotic fluid: Indices of lung maturity, *Am. J. Obstet. Gynecol.*, **125**:613 (1976).
11. Hallman, M., B. H. Feldman, E. Kirkpatrick, and L. Gluck, Absence of phosphatidylglycerol (PG) in respiratory distress syndrome in the newborn. Study of the minor surfactant phospholipids in newborns, *Pediatr. Res.*, **11**:714 (1977).
12. King, R. J. and M. C. MacBeth, Interaction of the lipid and protein components of pulmonary surfactant. Role of phosphatidylglycerol and calcium, *Biochim. Biophys. Acta*, **647**:159 (1981).

13. King, R. J., The surfactant system of the lung, *Fed. Proc.*, **33**:2238 (1974).
14. King, R. J., J. Ruch, E. G. Gikas, A. C. G. Platzker, and R. K. Creasy, Appearance of apoproteins of pulmonary surfactant in human amniotic fluid, *J. Appl. Physiol.*, **39**:735 (1975).
15. Katyal, S. L. and G. Singh, An immunologic study of the apoproteins of rat lung surfactant, *Lab. Invest.*, **40**:562 (1979).
16. King, R. J. and J. A. Clements, Surface active materials from dog lung. II. Composition and physiological correlations, *Am. J. Physiol.*, **223**:715 (1972).
17. Metcalfe, I. L., G. Enhorning, and F. Possmayer, Pulmonary surfactant-associated proteins: Their role in the expression of surface activity, *J. Appl. Physiol.*, 49:34 (1980).
18. Jobe, A., M. Ikegami, I. Sarton-Miller, S. Jones, and G. Yu, Characterization of phospholipids and localization of some phospholipid synthetic and subcellular marker enzymes in subcellular fractions from rabbit lung, *Biochim. Biophys. Acta*, **666**:47 (1981).
19. Higgins, J. A., Studies on the biogenesis of smooth endoplasmic reticulum membranes in hepatocytes of phenobarbital-treated rats, *J. Cell Biol.*, **62**: 635 (1974).
20. Hook, G. E. R. and L. B. Gilmore, Hydrolases of pulmonary lysosomes and lamellar bodies, *J. Biol. Chem.*, **257**:9211 (1982).
21. Mavis, R. D. and M. J. Vang, Optimal assay and subcellular location of phosphatidylglycerol synthesis in lung, *Biochim. Biophys. Acta*, **664**:409 (1981).
22. Chevalier, G. and A. J. Collet, *In vivo* Incorporation of choline-^{3}H, leucine-^{3}H and galactose-^{3}H in alveolar type II pneumonocytes in relation to surfactant synthesis. A quantitative radioautographic study in mouse by electron microscopy, *Anat. Rec.*, 174:289 (1972).
23. Engle, M. J., Cellular and subcellular sites of lung lipid metabolism. In *Lung Development: Biological and Clinical Perspectives.* Vol. I. Edited by P.M. Farrell. New York, Academic Press, 1982, p. 239.
24. Bell, R. M., L. M. Ballas, and R. A. Coleman. Lipid topogenesis, *J. Lipid Res.*, 22:391 (1981).
25. Mason, R. J. and L. G. Dobbs, Synthesis of phosphatidylcholine and phosphatidylglycerol by alveolar type II cells in primary culture, *J. Biol. Chem.*, **255**:5101 (1980).
26. Scholz, R. W., B. M. Woodward, and R. A. Rhoades, Utilization *in vitro* and *in vivo* of glucose and glycerol by rat lung, *Am. J. Physiol.*, **223**:991 (1972).
27. Persson, B. and J. Gentz, The pattern of blood lipids, glycerol and ketone bodies during the neonatal period, infancy and childhood, *Acta Paediatr. Scand.*, **55**:353 (1966).

28. Mason, R. J., Importance of the acyl dihydroxyacetone phosphate pathway in the synthesis of phosphatidylglycerol and phosphatidylcholine in alveolar type II cells, *J. Biol. Chem.*, **253**:3367 (1978).
29. Hendry, A. T. and F. Possmayer, Pulmonary phospholipid biosynthesis: Properties of a stable microsomal glycerophosphate acyltransferase preparation from rabbit lung, *Biochim. Biophys. Acta,* **369**:156 (1974).
30. Voelker, D. R., T.-C. Lee, and F. Snyder, Fatty acid biosynthesis and dietary regulation in pulmonary adenomas, *Arch. Biochem. Biophys.* , **176**: 753 (1976).
31. Acebal, C., R. Arche, C. Casals, J. Castro, and S. Rodriguez, Biosynthesis of phosphatidic acid by liver and lung of maternal and fetal rabbits, *Int. J. Biochem.,* **10**:463 (1979).
32. Sarzala, M. G., and L. M. G. Van Golde, Selective utilization of endogenous unsaturated phosphatidylcholine and diacylglycerols by cholinephosphotransferase of mouse lung microsomes, *Biochim. Biophys. Acta,* **441**:423 (1976).
33. Miller, J. C., and P. A. Weinhold, Cholinephosphotransferase in rat lung. The *in vitro* synthesis of dipalmitoylphosphatidylcholine from dipalmitoylglycerol, *J. Biol. Chem.,* **256**:12662 (1981).
34. Van Heusden, G. P. H., G. M. Vianen, and H. Van den Bosch, Differentiation between acyl coenzyme A:lysophosphatidylcholine acyltransacylase and lysophosphatidylcholine:lysophosphatidylcholine transacylase in the synthesis of dipalmitoylphosphatidylcholine in rat lung, *J. Biol. Chem.,* **255**:9312 (1980).
35. Schultz, F. M., J. M. Jimenez, P. C. MacDonald, and J. M. Johnston, Fetal lung maturation. I. Phosphatidic acid phosphohydrolase in rabbit lung, *Gynecol. Invest.,* **5**:222 (1974).
36. Ravinuthala, M. R., J. C. Miller, and P. A. Weinhold, Phosphatidate phosphatase: Activity and properties in fetal and adult rat lung, *Biochim. Biophys. Acta,* **530**:347 (1978).
37. Jimenez, J. M., F. M. Schultz, P. C. MacDonald, and J. M. Johnston, Fetal lung maturation. II. Phosphatidic acid phosphohydrolase in human amniotic fluid, *Gynecol. Invest.,* **5**:245 (1974).
38. Jimenez, J. M., and J. M. Johnston, Fetal lung maturation. IV: The release of phosphatidic acid phosphohydrolase and phospholipids into the human amniotic fluid, *Pediatr. Res.,* **10**:767 (1976).
39. Yeung, A., P. G. Casola, C. Wong, J. F. Fellows, and F. Possmayer, Pulmonary phosphatidic acid phosphatase: A comparative study of the aqueously dispersed phosphatidate-dependent and membrane-bound phosphatidate-dependent phosphatidic acid phosphatase activities of rat lung, *Biochim. Biophys. Acta,* **574**:226 (1979).
40. Johnston, J. M., G. Reynolds, M. B. Wylie, and P. C. MacDonald, The phosphohydrolase activity in lamellar bodies and its relationship to phospha-

tidylglycerol and lung surfactant formation, *Biochim. Biophys. Acta,* **531**: 65 (1978).
41. Johnston, J. M., M. B. Wylie, and G. Reynolds, The substrate specificity of glycerophospholipid phosphomonoesterase(s) activity in porcine lung tissue, unpublished observations.
42. Casola, P. G., P. M. MacDonald, W. C. McMurray, and F. Possmayer, Concerning the coidentity of phosphatidic acid phosphohydrolase and phosphatidylglycerophosphate phosphohydrolase in rat lung lamellar bodies, *Exp. Lung. Res.,* **3**:1 (1982).
43. Pelech, S. L. and D. E. Vance, Regulation of phosphatidylcholine biosynthesis, *Biochim. Biophys. Acta,* **779**:217 (1984).
44. Weinhold, P. A., M. E. Rounsifer, S. E. Williams, P. G. Brubaker, and D. A. Feldman, CTP:phosphorylcholine cytidylyltransferase in rat lung, *J. Biol. Chem.* **259**:10315 (1984).
45. Rooney, S. A., and A. Brehier, The CDP-choline pathway:choline phosphate cytidylyltransferase. In *Lung Development: Biological and Clinical perspectives.* Vol. I. Edited by P. M. Farrell. New York, Academic Press, 1982, p. 317.
46. Weinhold, P. A., R. S. Skinner, and R. D. Sanders, Activity and some properties of choline kinase, cholinephosphate cytidylyltransferase and choline phosphotransferase during liver development in the rat, *Biochim. Biophys. Acta,* **326**:43 (1973).
47. Post, M., J. J. Batenburg, E. A. J. M. Schuurmans, and L. M. G. Van Golde, The rate-limiting step in the biosynthesis of phosphatidylcholine by alveolar type II cells from adult rat lung, *Biochim. Biophys. Acta,* **712**:390 (1982).
48. Van Golde, L. M. G., The CDP-choline pathway: Cholinephosphotransferase. In *Lung Development: Biological and Clinical Perspectives.* Vol. I. Edited by P. M. Farrell. New York, Academic Press, 1982, p. 337.
49. Ulane, R. E., The CDP-choline pathway: Choline kinase. In *Lung Development: Biological and Clinical Perspectives,* Vol. I. Edited by P. M. Farrell. New York, Academic Press, 1982, p. 295.
50. Longmuir, K. J., and J. M. Johnston, Changes in CTP:phosphatidate cytidylyltransferase activity during rabbit lung development, *Biochim. Biophys. Acta,* **620**:500 (1980).
51. Bleasdale, J. E., P. Wallis, P. C. MacDonald, and J. M. Johnston. Changes in CDP-diglyceride:inositol transferase activity during rabbit lung development, *Pediatr. Res.,* **13**:1182 (1979).
52. Hallman, M., and L. Gluck, Formation of acidic phospholipids in rabbit lung during perinatal development, *Pediatr. Res.,* **14**:1250 (1980).
53. Quirk, J. G., J. E. Bleasdale, P. C. MacDonald, and J. M. Johnston, A role for cytidine monophosphate in the regulation of the glycerophospholipid

composition of surfactant in developing lung, *Biochem. Biophys. Res. Commun.*, **95**:985 (1980).
54. Bleasdale, J. E., and J. M. Johnston, CMP-dependent incorporation of [^{14}C] glycerol 3-phosphate into phosphatidylglycerol and phosphatidylglycerol phosphate by rabbit lung microsomes, *Biochim. Biophys. Acta*, **710**:377 (1982).
55. Bleasdale, J. E., M. C. Maberry, and J. G. Quirk, *myo*-Inositol homeostasis in foetal rabbit lung, *Biochem. J.*, **206**:43 (1982).
56. Quirk, J. G., and J. E. Bleasdale, *myo*-Inositol homeostasis in the human fetus, *Obstet. Gynecol.*, **62**:41 (1983).
57. Clements, R. S., and R. Reynertson, Myoinositol metabolism in diabetes mellitus, *Diabetes*, **26**:215 (1977).
58. King, R. J., H. Martin, D. Mitts, and F. M. Holmstrom, Metabolism of the apoproteins in pulmonary surfactant, *J. Appl. Physiol.*, **42**:483 (1977).
59. King, R. J., and H. Martin, Intracellular metabolism of the apoproteins of pulmonary surfactant in rat lung, *J. Appl. Physiol.*, **48**:812 (1980).
60. King, R. J., and H. Martin, Effects of inhibiting protein synthesis on the secretion of surfactant by type II cells in primary culture, *Biochim. Biophys. Acta*, **663**:289 (1981).
61. Williams, M. C., and B. J. Benson, Immunocytochemical localization and identification of the major surfactant protein in adult rat lung, *J. Histochem. Cytochem.*, **29**:291 (1981).
62. Delahunty, T. J., and J. M. Johnston, The effect of colchicine and vinblastine on the release of pulmonary surface active material, *J. Lipid Res.*, **17**: 112 (1976).
63. Brown, L. S., and W. J. Longmore, Effects of β-adrenergic agents on tubulin pools in the isolated perfused rat lung, *Fed. Proc.*, **41**:1423 (1982).
64. Olson, D. B., Neurohumoral-hormonal secretory stimulation of pulmonary surfactant in the rat, *Physiologist*, **15**:230 (1972).
65. Oyarzun, M. J., and J. A. Clements, Ventilatory and cholinergic control of pulmonary surfactant in the rabbit, *J. Appl. Physiol.*, **43**:39 (1977).
66. Oyarzun, M. J., and J. A. Clements, Control of lung surfactant by ventilation, adrenergic mediators and prostaglandins in the rabbit, *Amer. Rev. Respir. Dis.*, **117**:879 (1978).
67. Sommers Smith, S. K., and G. Giannopoulos, Beta-adrenergic receptor binding in isolated fetal, neonatal and adult alveolar type II cells, *Fed. Proc.*, **40**:407 (1981).
68. Barnes, P. J., C. B. Basbaum, J. A. Nadel, and J. M. Roberts, Localization of β-adrenoreceptors in mammalian lung by light microscopic autoradiography, *Nature*, **299**:444 (1982).
69. Brown, L. S., and W. J. Longmore, Adrenergic and cholinergic regulation of lung surfactant secretion in the isolated perfused rat lung and in the alveolar type II cell in culture, *J. Biol. Chem.*, **256**:66 (1981).

70. Liggins, G. C., Premature delivery of foetal lambs infused with glucocorticoids, *J. Endocrinol.*, **45**:515 (1969).
71. Kotas, R. V., and M. E. Avery, Accelerated appearance of pulmonary surfactant in the fetal rabbit, *J. Appl. Physiol.*, **30**:358 (1971).
72. Ballard, P. L., Hormonal aspects of fetal lung development. In *Lung Development: Biological and Clinical Perspectives.* Vol. II. Edited by P. M. Farrell. New York, Academic Press, 1982, p. 205.
73. Rooney, S. A., L. I. Gobran, P. A. Marino, W. M. Maniscalco, and I. Gross, Effects of betamethasone on phospholipid content, composition and biosynthesis in the fetal rabbit lung, *Biochim. Biophys. Acta,* **572**:64 (1979).
74. Brehier, A. and S. A. Rooney, Phosphatidylcholine synthesis and glycogen depletion in fetal mouse lung. Developmental changes and the effects of dexamethasone, *Exp. Lung Res.*, **2**:273 (1981).
75. Brehier, A., B. J. Benson, M. C. Williams, R. J. Mason, and P. L. Ballard, Corticosteroid induction of phosphatidic acid phosphatase in fetal rabbit lung, *Biochem. Biophys. Res. Commun.*, **77**:883 (1977).
76. Gross, I., C. M. Wilson, L. D. Ingleson, A. Brehier, and S. A. Rooney, Fetal lung in organ culture. III. Comparison of dexamethasone, thyroxine and methylxanthines, *J. Appl. Physiol.*, **48**:872 (1980).
77. Ballard, P. L., Glucocorticoid receptors in the lung, *Fed. Proc.*, **36**:2660 (1977).
78. Ballard, P. L., R. J. Mason, and W. H. J. Douglas, Glucocorticoid binding by isolated lung cells, *Endocrinology,* **102**:1570 (1978).
79. Giannopoulos, G., Variations in the levels of cytoplasmic glucocorticoid receptors in lungs of various species at different developmental stages, *Endocrinology,* **94**:450 (1974).
80. Murphy, B. E. P., M. Sebenick, and M. E. Patchell, Cortisol production and metabolism in the human fetus and its reflection in the maternal urine, *J. Steroid Biochem.*, **12**:37 (1980).
81. Gluck, L. and M. V. Kulovich, The evaluation of functional maturity in the human fetus. In *Modern Perinatal Medicine*. Edited by L. Gluck. Chicago, Year Book, 1974, p. 195.
82. Murphy, B. E. P., Cortisol and cortisone levels in the cord blood at delivery of infants with and without the respiratory distress syndrome, *Am. J. Obstet. Gynecol.*, **119**:1112 (1974).
83. Fencl, M. D. and D. Tulchinsky, Total cortisol in amniotic fluid and fetal lung maturation, *N. Engl. J. Med.*, **292**:133 (1975).
84. Mendelson, C. R., J. M. Johnston, P. C. MacDonald, and J. M. Snyder, Multihormonal regulation of surfactant synthesis by human fetal lung *in vitro, J. Clin. Endocrinol. Metab.*, **53**:307 (1981).
85. Smith, B. T., Lung maturation in the fetal rat: Acceleration by injection of fibroblast-pneumonocyte factor, *Science,* **204**:1094 (1979).

86. Hitchcock, K. R., Hormones and the lung. I. Thyroid hormones and glucocorticoids in lung development, *Anat. Rec.*, **194**:15 (1979).
87. Ballard, P. L., B. J. Benson, A. Brehier, J. P. Carter, B. M. Kriz, and E. C. Jorgensen, Transplacental stimulation of lung development in the fetal rabbit by 3,5-dimethyl-3′-isopropyl-L-thyronine, *J. Clin. Invest.*, **65**: 1407 (1980).
88. Fisher, D. A., J. H. Dussault, J. Sack, and I. J. Chopra, Ontogenesis of hypothalamic-pituitary-thyroid function and metabolism in man, sheep and rat, *Recent Prog. Horm. Res.*, **33**:59 (1977).
89. Lindberg, J. A., A. Brehier, and P. L. Ballard, Triiodothyronine nuclear binding in fetal and adult rabbit lung and cultured lung cells, *Endocrinology*, **103**:1725 (1978).
90. Khosla, S. S. and S. A. Rooney, Stimulation of fetal lung surfactant production by administration of 17β-estradiol to the maternal rabbit, *Am. J. Obstet. Gynecol.*, **133**:213 (1979).
91. Gross, I., C. M. Wilson, L. D. Ingleson, A. Brehier, and S. A. Rooney, The influence of hormones on the biochemical development of fetal rat lung in organ culture. I. Estrogen, *Biochim. Biophys. Acta*, **575**:375 (1979).
92. Mendelson, C. R., P. C. MacDonald, and J. M. Johnston, Estrogen binding in human fetal lung tissue cytosol, *Endocrinology*, **106**:368 (1980).
93. Hauth, J. C., C. R. Parker, P. C. MacDonald, J. C. Porter, and J. M. Johnston, A role of fetal prolactin in lung maturation, *Obstet. Gynecol.*, **51**:81 (1978).
94. Hamosh, M. and P. Hamosh, The effect of prolactin on the lecithin content of fetal rabbit lung, *J. Clin. Invest.*, **59**:1002 (1977).
95. Ballard, P. L., P. G. Gluckman, A. Brehier, J. A. Kitterman, S. L. Kaplan, A. M. Rudolph, and M. M. Grumbach, Failure to detect an effect of prolactin on pulmonary surfactant and adrenal steroids in fetal sheep and rabbits, *J. Clin. Invest.*, **62**:879 (1978).
96. Cox, M. A. and J. S. Torday, Pituitary oligopeptide regulation of phosphatidylcholine synthesis by fetal rabbit lung cells: Lack of effect with prolactin, *Am. Rev. Respir. Dis.*, **123**:181 (1981).
97. Josimovich, J. B., K. Merisko, L. Boccella, and H. Tobon, Binding of prolactin by fetal rhesus cell membrane fractions, *Endocrinology*, **100**:557 (1977).
98. Mendelson, C. R., C. W. Bryan, and J. M. Snyder, Lactogenic receptors in human fetal lung tissue, *Proc. Soc. Gynecol. Invest.*, p. 185 (1982) (abstract).
99. Winters, A. J., C. Colston, P. C. MacDonald, and J. C. Porter, Fetal plasma prolactin levels, *J. Clin. Endocrinol. Metab.*, **41**:626 (1975).
100. Smith, B. T., C. J. P. Giroud, M. Robert, and M. E. Avery, Insulin antagonism of cortisol action on lecithin synthesis by cultured fetal lung cells, *J. Pediatr.*, **87**:953 (1975).

101. Gross, I., G. J. Walker-Smith, C. M. Wilson, W. M. Maniscalco, L. D. Ingleson, A. Brehier, and S. A. Rooney, The influence of hormones on the biochemical development of fetal rat lung in organ culture. II. Insulin, *Pediatr. Res.*, **14**:834 (1980).
102. Lawson, N., R. J. Jennings, R. Fears, and D. N. Brindley, Antagonistic effects of insulin on the corticosterone-induced increase of phosphatidate phosphohydrolase activity in isolated rat hepatocytes, *F.E.B.S. Lett.*, **143**:9 (1982).
103. Ulane, R. E., J. E. Graeber, J. W. Hansen, L. Liccini, and M. Cornblath, Insulin receptors in the developing fetal lung, *Life Sci.*, **31**:3017 (1982).
104. Divers, W. A., M. M. Wilkes, A. Babaknia, and S. S. C. Yen, An increase in catecholamines and metabolites in the amniotic fluid compartment from middle to late gestation, *Am. J. Obstet. Gynecol.*, **139**:483 (1981).
105. Kanjanapone, V., I. Hartig-Beecken, and M. F. Epstein, Effect of isoxsuprine on fetal lung surfactant in rabbits, *Pediatr. Res.*, **14**:278 (1980).
106. Bichler, A., H. Wiesinger, and P. Mayr, Investigations of the effect and mechanism of action of the β-sympathomimetic ritodrine on the synthesis and release of dipalmitoyl-lecithin in the fetal rabbit lung, *Arch. Gynecol.*, **227**:29 (1979).
107. Barrett, C. T., A. Sevanian, N. Lavin, and S. A. Kaplan, Role of adenosine 3′,5′ monophosphate in maturation of fetal lungs, *Pediatr. Res.*, **10**:621 (1976).
108. Korotkin, E. H., M. Kido, W. J. Cashore, R. A. Redding, W. J. Douglas, L. Stern, and W. Oh, Acceleration of fetal lung maturation by aminophyllin in pregnant rabbits, *Pediatr. Res.*, **10**:722 (1976).
109. Tanswell, A. K. and B. T. Smith, Human fetal lung type II pneumonocytes in monolayer cell culture: The influence of oxidant, stress, cortisol environment, and soluble fibroblast factors, *Pediatr. Res.*, **13**:1097 (1979).
110. Rooney, S. A., P. A. Marino, L. I. Gobran, I. Gross, and J. B. Warshaw, Thyrotropin-releasing hormone increases the amount of surfactant in lung lavage from fetal rabbits, *Pediatr. Res.*, **13**:623 (1979).
111. Ekelund, L., G. Arvidson, S. Kullander, and B. Astedt, Effect of cortisone and ACTH on the phospholipids of human amniotic fluid and lung tissue in early gestation, *Scand. J. Clin. Lab. Invest.*, **36**:257 (1976).
112. Sundell, H., M. E. Gray, F. S. Serenius, M. B. Escobedo, and M. T. Stahlman, Effects of epidermal growth factor on lung maturation in fetal lambs, *Am. J. Pathol.*, **100**:707 (1980).

4

Fetal Breathing Activity

GEOFFREY S. DAWES

The Nuffield Institute for Medical Research
University of Oxford
Oxford, England

JOHN E. PATRICK

St. Joseph's Hospital Research Institute
University of Western Ontario
London, Ontario, Canada

I. Introduction

Pregnant women and obstetricians have long recognized the significance of fetal movements as a sign of life and health. During the last 10 years two developments have permitted physiological investigation of fetal activity and in particular fetal breathing. Chronic preparations were developed to permit systematic investigations of fetal breathing and other muscular activity during the last half of pregnancy in fetal lambs [1]. Secondly, the introduction of real-time ultrasonic scanners has provided the means for direct measurement of fetal breathing movements and body movements in man. The purpose of this chapter will be to review the physiology of fetal breathing activity and its influence on pulmonary function in the newborn. Observational data gathered from studies of human fetal breathing activity will be reviewed in detail, and where possible we will attempt to supplement these data with hypotheses developed from carefully controlled studies of animals.

II. Patterns of Fetal Breathing Movements During Human Pregnancy

It is convenient to observe human fetal breathing movements using linear array real-time ultrasonic scanners which display echoes on a small oscilloscope screen representing a two-dimensional cross section (Fig. 1). Fetal breathing and body movements are recognized on a video display and coded on chart recorders using event markers.

Longitudinal scanning of human fetuses permits visualization of fetal chest and abdominal wall echoes. During each fetal breathing movement the anterior chest wall echoes move inward 0.5–5.0 mm and the anterior fetal abdominal wall echoes move outward 0.5–8.0 mm. When posterior chest wall echoes are not over or near the fetal spine both chest walls can be observed to move inward toward each other by 0.5–5.0 mm during breathing movements. Following each inspiratory movement the fetal chest wall echoes move outward and the anterior fetal abdominal wall echoes move inward to their resting positions. These paradoxical movements of chest and abdominal wall echoes permit identification of each breath. The amplitude of chest and abdominal wall movements during episodes of breathing is variable. During fetal breathing, echoes which represent the fetal diaphragm and

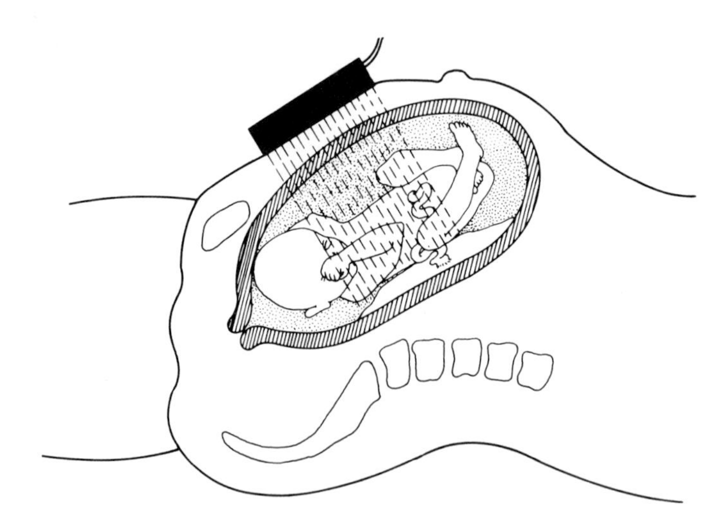

Figure 1 Illustration of longitudinal scanning of a human fetus in utero. (From J. Patrick, W. Fetherston, H. Vick, and R. Voegelin, Human fetal breathing movements and gross fetal body movements at weeks 34 to 35 of gestation, *Am. J. Obstet. Gynecol., 130*:693, 1978.)

liver descend downward into the fetal abdomen; they return after each breathing movement. Recently, it has become possible to make chart recordings of fetal chest and abdominal wall echo movement using a phase-locked tracking system developed by Cousin et al. [2]. Figure 2 is a chart recording which demonstrates fetal chest and abdominal wall movement during an episode of fetal breathing activity. It also is possible to identify and time fetal breaths by using Doppler ultrasound measurements to detect respiratory changes in blood flow velocity in the inferior vena cava, hepatic veins, or umbilical veins [3].

A second type of chest and abdominal wall movement is characterized by rapid inward and outward movement of the fetal chest and abdominal wall echoes. Movements of this kind appear to be episodes of fetal hiccoughs, which occur every 2–6 sec and are sensed by mothers as gentle regular fetal movements. During the last 10 weeks of pregnancy fetuses exhibit two to four episodes of hiccoughs each 24 hr. Such episodes are not related to time of day and last on average 6–11 min. It is interesting that fetal hiccoughs are usually preceded by marked enlargement of the fetal stomach.

Fetal body movements also can be measured using real-time ultrasonic scanners. During the last 30 weeks of pregnancy fetuses move passively and actively within the amniotic cavity. With each maternal respiration they

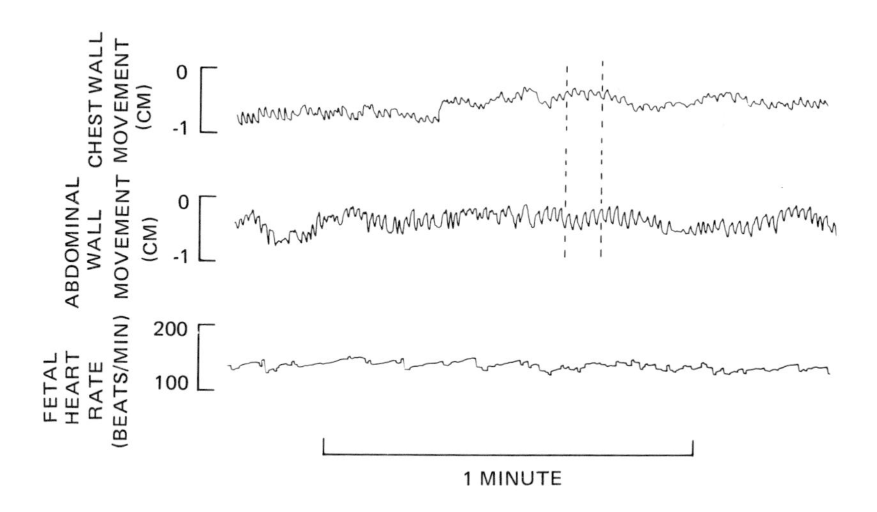

Figure 2 Chart recording of simultaneous measurements of chest and abdominal wall diameters during an episode of fetal breathing in a healthy fetus near term. Note that as chest wall moves inward (downward deflection) the abdominal wall moves outward in the opposite direction.

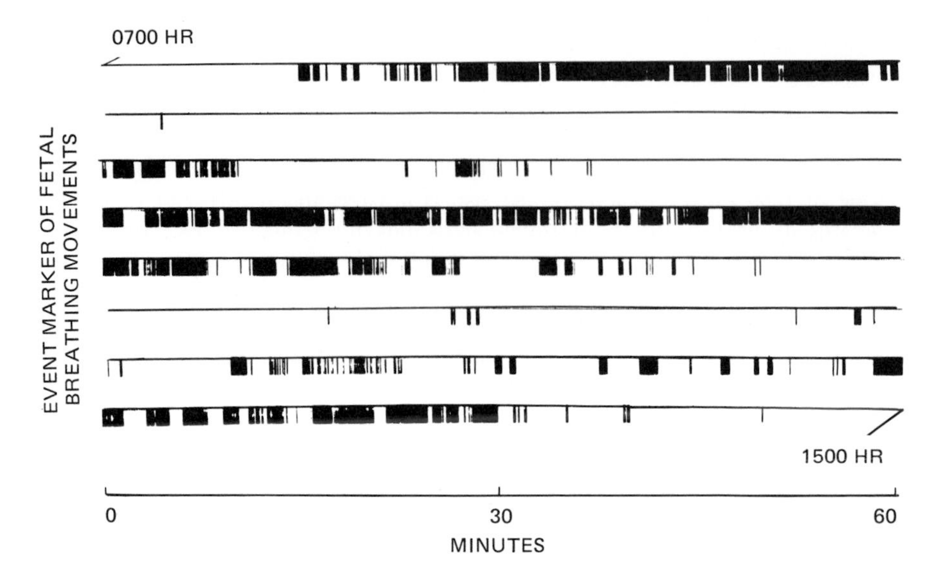

Figure 3 Chart recording of event marker indicating fetal breathing movements from 0700 to 1500 hr in a healthy fetus at 35 weeks' gestation. Fetal breathing movements were episodic and separated by periods of apnea.

move passively in a longitudinal axis superiorly and inferiorly with respect to the mother. Maternal arterial pulsations move some fetuses anteriorly and posteriorly within the uterus. Maternal coughing, laughing, or gross movement also cause passive movement within the amniotic cavity. At least three types of active fetal movements can be observed. Stretching movements are detected from observation of extension of the echoes from the region of the thoracic and cervical vertebrae. Fetal rolling movements are observed about a longitudinal axis and active movements of the fetal extremities can be seen. Fetal breathing movements can be observed during times of passive fetal activity and during isolated fetal limb movements. However, fetal breathing movements are not observed during rolling or stretching movements. In fact, using the phase-locked tracking system developed by Cousin et al. [2] it was unusual to detect fetal breathing movements during gross fetal body movements.

The most remarkable difference between fetal breathing during the last 10 weeks of pregnancy and breathing after birth is that the human fetus only makes breathing movements episodically. Episodes of fetal breathing activity are separated by periods of fetal apnea (Fig. 3).

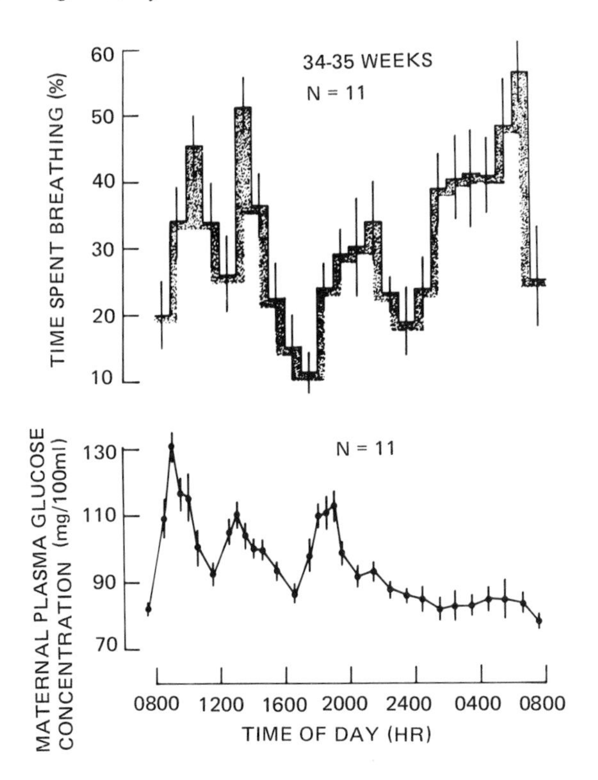

Figure 4 The percentage of time spent breathing each hour of the day in 11 healthy fetuses at 34–35 weeks' gestation and maternal plasma glucose concentrations were plotted. Fetuses made breathing movements a greater percentage of the time during the second and third hour following breakfast, lunch, and supper. There was a prolonged significant increase in the percentage of time spent breathing between 0100 and 0700 hr. (From Ref. 5. J. Patrick, R. Natale, and B. Richardson, Patterns of human fetal breathing activity at 34 to 35 weeks' gestational age, *Am. J. Obstet. Gynecol.*, **132**: 507, 1978.)

There is evidence of maturation in the control of patterns of fetal breathing movements during pregnancy. Using real-time ultrasonic scanners isolated fetal breaths can be seen by 11 weeks' gestation. Because of the mobility of the human fetus between 11 and 20 weeks' gestation no comprehensive investigation of the pattern of breathing has been performed. Recent reports of studies of human fetuses under 20 weeks' gestation have suggested that breathing movements occur either as isolated breaths or groups of breaths which last for a few seconds. There are similar reports in sheep very early in gestation.

Trudinger and Knight studied eight patients serially from 20 weeks' gestational age and reported that at 20 and 24 weeks fetal breathing movements occurred as rapid, isolated bursts of four to 10 breaths [4]. By 28–30 weeks' gestational age fetal breathing movements began to occur in episodes.

During the last 10 weeks of human pregnancy fetal breathing movements occur episodically about 30% of the time [5]. The incidence does not normally change during this period, but the frequency distribution of breath intervals (during episodes of breathing) alters and hence provides evidence of maturation. We analyzed 165,786 breath intervals in four fetuses at 30–31 weeks' gestation and four fetuses at 38–39 weeks' gestation [6]. The mean rate during episodes of breathing at 30–31 weeks (59 ± 4 breaths/min) was significantly greater than at 38–39 weeks (47 ± 2 breaths/min). Histograms of breath-to-breath intervals demonstrated a peak at 1.0–1.5 sec in the 38–39-week group and at 0.5–1.0 sec in the 30–31-week group. The distribution of breath intervals was much broader in the 30–31 week group than at 38-39 weeks. Hence breathing when present was more regular in older fetuses. Trudinger and Knight reported similar observations in a group of eight fetuses studied serially from 33 to 40 weeks' gestational age [4]. Furthermore, episodes of fetal apnea of up to 2 hr were normal events in healthy human fetuses near term.

During the last 10 weeks of human pregnancy the time of day and relationship to maternal meals are further factors which influence fetal breathing activity. Groups of healthy human fetuses were studied at 30–31, 34–35, and 38–39 weeks' gestational age [5,7]. Studies were conducted continuously over 24-hr observation intervals using a real-time ultrasonic scanner. Mothers rested in bed in a quiet room exposed to normal daylight and darkness and were given 800-K cal meals at 0800, 1200, and 1700 hr. Fetuses in the three groups made breathing movements approximately 30% of the time on average. At 30–31 and 34–35 weeks the percentage of time spent breathing was significantly increased during the second and third hour following breakfast, lunch, and supper (Fig. 4). At all three gestational ages there was a prolonged significant increase in fetal breathing movements observed between 0100 and 0700 hr while mothers were asleep. The increase overnight occurred while maternal blood glucose concentrations were stable. It was hypothesized that the increase in fetal breathing movements overnight was due to a circadian rhythm as had been shown in fetal sheep. The changes after meals were attributed to changes in blood glucose concentrations and will be discussed subsequently.

III. Influence of Carbon Dioxide on Fetal Breathing Movements

A. Hypercapnia

Few studies on the influence of increased concentrations of carbon dioxide on fetal breathing activity have been conducted during human pregnancy. Ritchie and Lakhani administered 5% carbon dioxide in the air to pregnant women for 15 min and measured a three-fold increase in the incidence of fetal breathing movements in uncomplicated pregnancies [8]. They conducted some studies with maternal radial arterial catheters in place for simultaneous blood gas sampling. Under the conditions of their experiment, maternal arterial P_{CO_2} increased from 29.9 to 33.8 mmHg. At the same time, maternal arterial P_{O_2} increased from 92 to 105 mmHg and maternal arterial pH did not change from a resting value of 7.45.

Similar observations were made by a group who used a 10% mixture of carbon dioxide for 5-min intervals and noted that the incidence of fetal breathing movements usually increased. They reported that some fetuses, which were small for gestational age, made no breathing movements in response to this stimulus, but it is noteworthy that the study time was short.

Richardson et al. studied the effect of administering a 4% carbon dioxide mixture in air to healthy pregnant women over 15-min observation intervals at 30, 34, and 38 weeks' gestational age [9]. They reported a significant increase in the incidence of fetal breathing movements at all three gestational ages after administration of carbon dioxide, but the increase was significantly greater in fetuses at 34 and 38 weeks compared to the same fetuses at 30 weeks' gestational age. They did not observe any change in the rate of fetal breathing movements during breathing episodes. They concluded that a maturational change in the sensitivity of the fetal respiratory center to carbon dioxide may occur during the last 10 weeks of human pregnancy.

In chronic experiments on pregnant sheep the principal effects of hypercapnia were to cause more regular and deeper fetal breathing movements with recruitment of intercostal muscular activity, as recorded by direct measurements of tracheal pressure and diaphragmatic electromyography (EMG) over a wide range of arterial P_{CO_2} [10]. There was a small increase in the incidence of breathing, but no significant change in frequency because of the large range of variation in eucapnia. Recent experiments in sheep have also shown that the effects of hypercapnia are due to a direct action of carbon dioxide on the central chemoreceptors in fetal medulla, as in adults. The effects persist after section of the brain stem above the medulla and can be reproduced by perfusion from the cerebral ventricles to the cisterna magna with a fluid low in bicarbonate [11].

It is notable that human studies have concentrated on the incidence of fetal breathing rather than on changes in the depth of breathing which would be expected to be more relevant. This may well be due to the difficulty in measuring the depth of breathing using present ultrasound equipment. It is an area which would justify further investigation.

B. Hypocapnia

It is known that maternal hyperventilation during human pregnancy sufficient to reduce maternal arterial P_{CO_2} results in a reduction in the incidence of fetal breathing movements. Similarly, fetal hypocapnia is associated with a reduction or arrest of breathing in sheep.

IV. Influence of Maternal Oxygen on Fetal Breathing Movements

A. Hypoxemia

There are no data available on the influence of hypoxemia during human pregnancy on fetal breathing movements. Studies have been reported on the influence of 8-12% oxygen mixtures given to pregnant women before and during labor on fetal heart rate. Wood et al. investigated effects on the fetal heart rate of administration of 10% oxygen and nitrogen for periods of 3-20 min on 14 patients during labor [12]. They abandoned the study when large decelerations were observed in two patients, and severe fetal acidosis was measured in a third without significant change in the fetal heart rate. These data suggest that further experiments with such low O_2 mixtures to determine the effects of hypoxemia on the human fetus would be unethical.

In sheep an abrupt reduction of fetal arterial P_{O_2} by 4-5 mmHg decreases, and by 7-9 mmHg abolishes both fetal breathing movements and other skeletal muscular movements. The abolition of fetal breathing is not due to a direct effect upon the central chemoreceptors in the medulla since, after cutting the brain stem in the upper pons, hypoxemia causes an increase in the amplitude and frequency of fetal breathing. The center involved, which is required to be intact and connected to the medulla for the normal inhibition of fetal breathing by hypoxia, lies between the inferior colliculus and the caudal hypothalamus [11]. Whether this is also true of man will be difficult to establish.

B. Hyperoxia

Ritchie and Lakhani [8] found no change in the incidence of fetal breathing movements in healthy fetuses whose mothers were given 50% oxygen by mask.

V. Influence of Asphyxia and Acidemia on Fetal Breathing Movements

In fetal sheep and in other animal species gasping movements immediately precede death from acute asphyxia. Anecdotal reports have appeared from time to time suggesting that the human fetus may make gasping movements prior to death in utero. Clinically, one characteristic of the asphyxiated human fetus is the presence of meconium which has been inhaled deeply into the airway before death. Manning reported that when real-time ultrasound observations were made on dying fetal Rhesus monkeys gasping activity could not be differentiated from normal breathing movements by real-time ultrasound scanning despite repeated detailed videotape analysis [13]. Direct recordings with newer ultrasound tracking devices may provide an opportunity for examining the structure of fetal gasping movements in dying human fetuses. However, it is clear that no comprehensive investigation of these phenomena can be expected from clinical investigators.

VI. Effects of Maternal Glucose Concentrations on Fetal Breathing Movements

Analysis of 24-hr studies of human fetal breathing movements suggested that there was an increase in fetal breathing activity during the second and third hour after maternal meals (Fig. 4). In the same studies maternal glucose concentrations were determined 31 times from maternal venous plasma; the increase in fetal breathing activity during the second and third hour following maternal meals seemed to follow postprandial increase in maternal plasma glucose concentrations (5,7).

Fox and Hohler, using real-time ultrasound, reported a significant increase in fetal breathing movements in eight of nine patients given an oral glucose load [14]. Lewis et al. observed fetal breathing movements in 24 singleton pregnancies between 34 and 38 weeks' gestation and reported that the percentage of time spent breathing increased following an oral glucose load [15].

Natale et al., in a well controlled study, examined the effects of glucose concentrations in maternal plasma on human fetal breathing movements [16]. They used an ADR real-time scanner to observe human fetal breathing movements and gross fetal body movements in 22 patients at 32–34 weeks' gestational age. After a 2-hr control period of observation, patients were given either a 50-g oral glucose drink or an equal volume of tap water. Observers were not aware of the solution given. The percentage of time fetuses made breathing movements was 23% in the control period in both groups. The incidence of breathing movements decreased significantly in the water-treated group, but in the glucose-treated group fetal breathing movements increased to 40.0 ± 4.5% during the 3-hr study period. It was interesting that maternal plasma glucose concentrations reached a peak at 45 min after the glucose load, but fetal breathing movements did not reach a peak until 105 min afterward, 60 min later than the peak in maternal glucose concentrations (Fig. 5). This confirmed that the increase in fetal breathing movements after breakfast, lunch, and supper in normal fetuses at 34-35 weeks could be reproduced at 32–34 weeks by giving fasted women glucose; no similar increases occurred in women who were not fed or given glucose during the day. Hence, maternal carbohydrate intake must be known to permit proper interpretation of human fetal breathing studies.

Recently, Harding et al. [17] examined fetal breathing activity following maternal ingestion of a meal containing only fat and protein with a total caloric intake of 600 K cal. Maternal plasma glucose concentrations did not change after this meal and no significant increase in fetal breathing activity was measured [17]. This is further evidence that maternal carbohydrate intake is the primary factor responsible for increased fetal breathing activity following meals.

Similar increases in fetal breathing activity also occurred after injections of glucose in women near full term. Bocking et al. demonstrated that the incidence of fetal breathing movements increased from 16.5% during a 3-hr control period before injection, to a peak of 54.9% between 30 and 75 min following injections of 25 g of glucose intravenously [18]. No such increases were observed after injections of normal saline in the same patients.

Adamson et al. [19] in a parallel study continuously measured fetal chest and abdominal wall echo diameters using an ultrasonic tracking device developed by Cousin and Rapoport [2]. They measured a 100% increase in amplitude of fetal chest and abdominal wall excursions during the first 80 min following maternal glucose injection [19]. There was no significant change in the frequency or variability of fetal breathing movements after glucose injection. There was a negative correlation between fetal breath amplitude and breath interval for data averaged over hourly intervals.

These data were compatible with the hypothesis that maternal glucose injections during human pregnancy may influence fetal respiratory drive. The mechanism involved is unknown and there appears to be no analogy

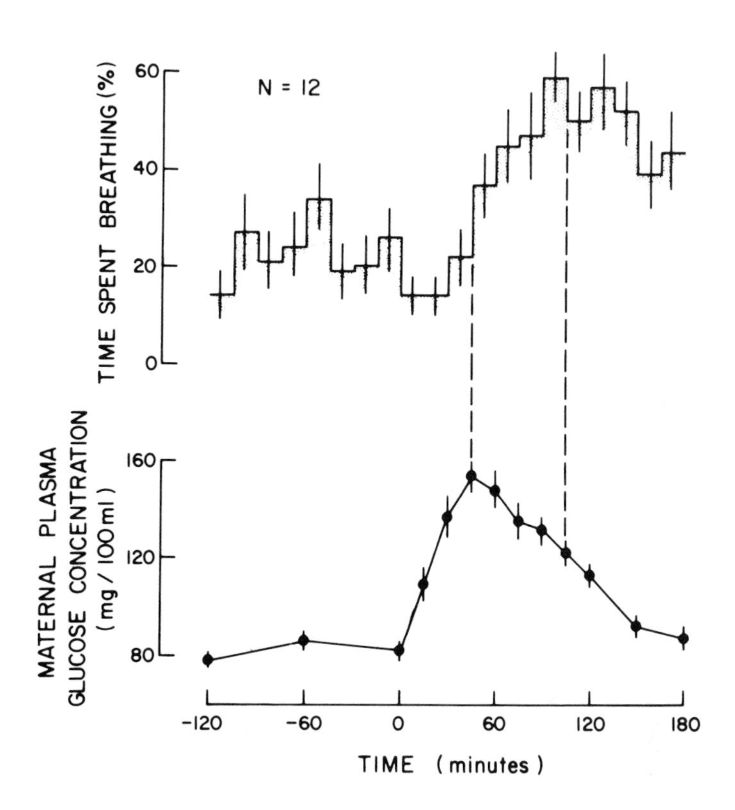

Figure 5 The relationship between maternal plasma glucose concentration and fetal breathing activity. Peak maternal plasma glucose concentrations occurred at t + 45 min. Fetal breathing activity began to increase at t + 60 min but did not reach a maximum until t + 105 min, which was 60 min after the peak maternal plasma glucose concentration. (From Ref. 16. Natale, R., J. Patrick, and B. Richardson, Effects of human maternal venous plasma glucose concentrations on fetal breathing movements, *Am. J. Obstet. Gynecol.*, **132**:36, 1978.)

postnatally in man or animals. There is no evidence of a similar effect in fetal sheep over the normal physiological range of blood glucose concentrations, though it was established 10 years ago that hypoglycemia causes an arrest of fetal breathing in this species. The fact that there is a delay of 20 min or more between the rise in maternal plasma glucose and in fetal breathing suggests the effect may be indirect on the fetal respiratory center.

VII. Influence of Time of Day on Fetal Breathing Movements

We measured a prolonged significant increase in the incidence of fetal breathing movements observed between 0100 and 0700 hrs while mothers were asleep during continuous observations conducted over 24-hr observation intervals [5,7]. The overnight increase in the incidence of fetal breathing movements during the last 10 weeks of pregnancy occurred during a time when maternal blood glucose concentrations were stable or falling (Fig. 4). It is possible that the increase in fetal breathing movements overnight is part of a circadian rhythm in fetal breathing activity during human pregnancy.

At 34-35 weeks' gestation we demonstrated that a significant circadian rhythm existed in the concentrations of cortisol and estriol in maternal venous plasma and that there was an inverse relationship between these steroids [20]. These data were consistent with the hypothesis that maternal glucocorticoids may influence fetal hypothalamic pituitary adrenal function. It was interesting that the overnight increase in fetal breathing movements at 30-31, 34-35 and 38-39 weeks occurred at about the same time as the overnight increase in maternal glucocorticoid concentrations [5,7,20].

In order to test the hypothesis that maternal glucocorticoids may influence fetal breathing activity, we examined changes in fetal breathing movements in a group of six women at 34-35 weeks' gestational age who were treated with synthetic glucocorticoid throughout pregnancy and in whom the endogenous circadian rhythm of cortisol was absent or had been suppressed [21]. Each patient was studied continuously for two 24-hr observation periods. In the steroid-treated women there was a significant increase in fetal breathing movements during the second and third hours after each meal. However, there was no overnight increase in the incidence of fetal breathing movements. It was interesting that a peak in fetal breathing activity was measured at 2400-0200 hr and this was most pronounced in women who received glucocorticoid at 2200 hr. These data suggested that fetal breathing movements may be increased by increases in maternal glucocorticoid, whether synthetic or natural. It is possible that glucocorticoids may cross the placenta and act to increase fetal breathing movements directly or indirectly, perhaps by increasing fetal glucose concentrations.

VIII. Influence of Parturition on Fetal Breathing Activity

There is evidence from human pregnancies at full term to suggest that patterns of fetal breathing activity are changed in two ways by parturition. Firstly, there is some evidence to suggest that the incidence of fetal breathing movements diminishes during the last 3 days before spontaneous parturition. Secondly, there is strong evidence to suggest that human fetal breathing activity is virtually abolished during active labor at full term, as in sheep.

Richardson et al. measured human fetal breathing movements before and during elective induction of labor in uncomplicated term pregnancies [22]. They measured fetal breathing movements during a control period prior to induction of labor by rupture of membranes or oxytocin infusion. They continued to measure fetal breathing movements throughout the first stage of labor. Episodes of fetal breathing activity were observed during the control period and continued until the onset of accelerated labor as defined by the Friedman curve. After accelerated labor began, no episodes of normal rapid irregular fetal breathing movements were observed throughout the first stage of labor (Fig. 6). Richardson et al. [22] examined the effects of epidural anesthesia, ruptured membranes, oxytocin infusions, maternal blood sugar, and maternal venous blood gases but could not explain the arrest for many hours of fetal breathing movements during active labor. The fetuses in their study had good outcomes by all clinical criteria, and the authors concluded that rapid irregular fetal breathing movements do not normally occur after the onset of active labor during human pregnancy [22].

Carmichael et al. demonstrated that there is a decrease in the incidence of fetal breathing movements at full term in fetuses within 3 days of spontaneous parturition compared to similar groups of term fetuses who delivered more than 7 days following study [23]. Furthermore, they reported that just before spontaneous labor without spontaneous rupture of membranes at term there is a marked decrease in fetal breathing movements compared to fetuses about to enter labor following spontaneous rupture of membranes. These investigators [23] found no similar differences in the incidence of gross fetal body movements prior to spontaneous labor. Their report is further evidence that a significant decrease normally occurs in the incidence of fetal breathing movements during human pregnancy just prior to spontaneous parturition at term.

It has been demonstrated in sheep that the infusion of prostaglandin synthetase inhibitors into fetal lambs or pregnant ewes results in a dramatic increase in fetal breathing activity during the first 12 hr following infusion (24, 25). Conversely, Kitterman et al. [26] reported a significant decrease in fetal breathing activity following infusion of prostaglandin E_2 intravenously into

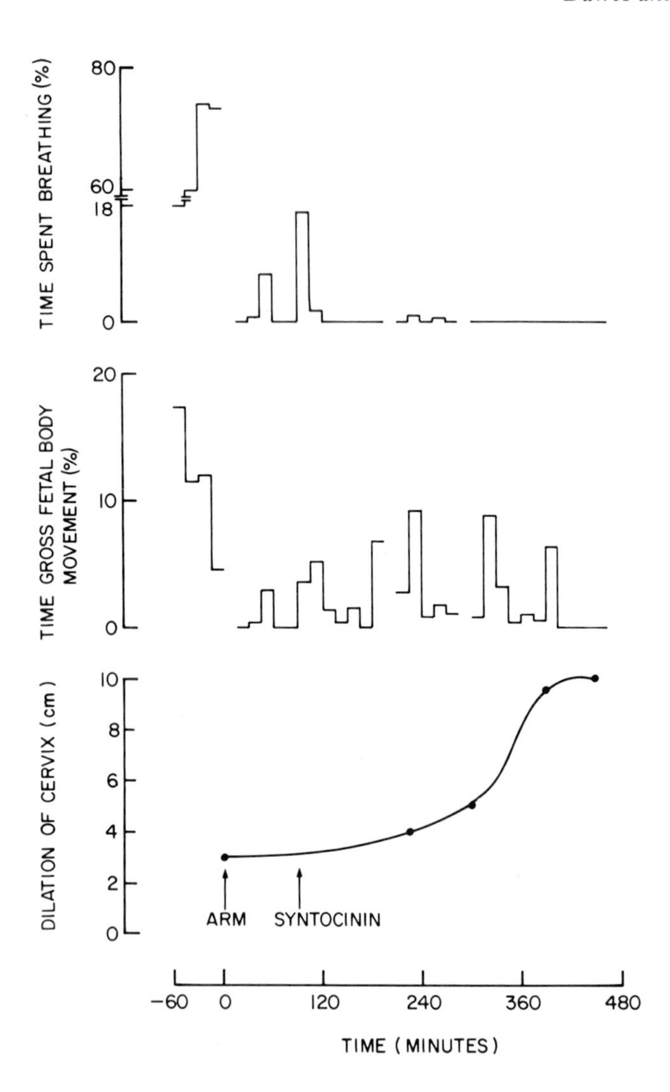

Figure 6 The incidence of fetal breathing and gross body movements in one fetus were plotted in 15-min intervals. During the control period before induction of labor and during prelatent-phase labor, episodes of breathing activity occurred during episodes of increased gross fetal body movements. During latent and active-phase labor, episodes of gross fetal body movements continued every 60–90 min but fetal breathing movements were absent. (From Ref. 22. Richardson, B., R. Natale, and J. Patrick, Human fetal breathing activity during electively induced labor at term, *Am. J. Obstet. Gynecol.*, **133**:247, 1979.)

healthy fetal lambs. They reported that intravenous infusions of prostaglandin $F_{2\alpha}$ caused slightly diminished fetal breathing activity and measured no decrease in fetal breathing activity following fetal intravenous infusions of endoperoxides [26]. It has been suggested that the decrease in fetal breathing activity normally observed just before and during active labor in sheep, Rhesus monkeys, and humans may be due to an increase in fetal prostaglandin concentrations. However, Patrick et al. have reported that increased fetal breathing movements, measured within 4 hr of the onset of indomethacin infusions into ewes, seemed to return to normal incidence after 12 hr despite normal fetal blood gas measurements and continuing indomethacin infusions [25]. These investigators reported an increase in maternal and fetal plasma glucose concentrations during the first 16 hr following indomethacin infusions.

It is possible that fetal prostaglandin concentrations may increase before human parturition and it has been demonstrated that prostaglandin concentrations increase in amniotic fluid during active labor in humans. It is tempting to speculate that prostaglandins may play a role in the control of fetal breathing movements in the human based on physiological observations in chronic fetal lamb preparations. In the latter, the effects are central; they persist after denervation of the systemic arterial chemoreceptors (the aortic and carotid bodies) and after section of the vagi or of the brainstem in the upper pons.

IX. Influence of Drugs on Fetal Breathing Movements

A. Nicotine—Cigarette Smoking

Thaler et al. measured fetal breathing movements using continuous Doppler ultrasound in 10 healthy pregnant women before and after their smoking two cigarettes and in the same women on a second day when under the same conditions no cigarettes were taken [27]. They observed no change in the incidence of fetal breathing movements before or after cigarette smoking, but they measured a change in the distribution of breath intervals following cigarette smoking. The mean rate of fetal breathing movements before cigarettes and on the control day was 46 breaths/min and this increased to a maximum of 57 breaths/min between 20 and 25 minutes following cigarette smoking. Fox et al. recently confirmed these observations in 19 women using real-time ultrasound [28]. They reported an increase in the frequency of fetal breathing movements from 42 breaths/min before to 56 breaths/min following cigarette smoking. They observed no effect on the incidence of fetal breathing movements by cigarette smoking.

B. Maternal Ethanol Ingestion

Fox et al. reported that fetal breathing activity diminished following ingestion of alcohol by pregnant women [29]. They demonstrated that a single ounce of vodka (80 proof) resulted in diminished fetal breathing movements for approximately 1 hr, following which time breathing activity resumed. These observations have been extended by McLeod et al. in a carefully controlled study of healthy pregnant women between 37 and 40 weeks' gestational age [30]. They administered ethanol, 0.25 g/kg, in soda as a 15% solution or an equal volume of soda water on consecutive days. The maternal venous blood alcohol concentration was 0.33 ng/ml 30 min after alcohol ingestion; thereafter it declined until ethanol was only detectable in two patients after 3 hr. The incidence of fetal breathing decreased from 38% of the time during the control period to 1.6% during the 3 hr following alcohol administration. Fetal breathing was virtually abolished at the time of maximum maternal venous ethanol concentration. Three hours after giving ethanol and soda, or soda alone, there was no significant difference in the incidence of fetal breathing activity. There was no change in fetal gross body movements or in fetal heart rate after alcohol ingestion. McLeod et al. [31] also injected 25 g glucose intravenously into pregnant women 30 min after alcohol ingestion; there was no increase in the incidence of fetal breathing movements. Hence, the suppression of fetal breathing by maternal alcohol could not be reversed by maternal glucose infusion; yet in the same fetuses, giving glucose after maternal ingestion of soda water produced large increases in the incidence of fetal breathing movements within 20 min. Careful examination of gross body movements recorded during the studies of McLeod et al. [31] did not suggest any change in periods of fetal rest and activity.

Kitterman et al. injected PGE_2 intravenously into fetal lambs and reported a marked decrease in the incidence of fetal breathing movements [26]. It has been reported that in humans ethanol enhances conversion of dihomogamma-linoleic acid to PGE_1 in platelets. If this effect occurs in human fetal tissues or blood in response to ethanol it might explain the decrease in human fetal breathing movements measured following alcohol ingestion by pregnant women. Other studies on prostaglandins and prostaglandin synthetase inhibitors have already been described.

C. Catecholamines

No systematic studies concerning effects of catecholamines on human fetal breathing movements are available. It has been reported that infusions of epinephrine, norepinephrine, and isoproterenol into the fetal jugular vein result in an increase in the incidence of fetal breathing movements in sheep [32]. Murata et al. reported an increase in fetal breathing activity in chronic fetal Rhesus monkey preparations following injections of isoproterenol [33]. It is not yet clear whether catecholamines have a direct effect on fetal breathing movements or whether they increase fetal breathing movements by effects on fetal plasma glucose or electrocorticol activity.

D. Analgesic Drugs

No comprehensive studies on the influence of analgesic drugs on human fetal breathing activity are available. In sheep, Boddy et al. reported that injections of meperidine (Pethidine), 100–200 mg, into ewes caused no consistent change in fetal breathing activity but reduced the response to hypercapnia [34].

Recently, Richardson et al. measured human fetal breathing movements with real-time ultrasound in eight patients on a methadone treatment program at the University of Oregon [35]. They administered a 5% mixture of carbon dioxide in air to women before and after their daily methadone treatment. Before methadone administration fetal breathing movements increased from 4.7 to 30.7% following CO_2 stimulation. Two hours after methadone treatment fetal breathing movements were virtually abolished; they were restored to 20.7% of the time following carbon dioxide administration. It was concluded that both the incidence of fetal breathing movements and ventilatory response to carbon dioxide are depressed in human fetuses by maternal methadone administration.

Wittmann et al. recently reported observations of fetal breathing and body movements 1 hour before and after administration of methadone (40 mg/24 hr) to pregnant women [36]. They observed a significant decrease in the incidence of both fetal body movements and fetal breathing movements.

In chronic fetal lamb preparations, Szeto administered methadone and morphine intravenously to ewes (5 μg/kg/min) or to fetuses (0.5 μg/maternal kg/min) for 2-5 hours [37]. She reported that both drugs produced suppression of high-voltage slow-wave electrocortical activity, sustained nuchal tone and sustained fetal breathing movements and eye movements, and an increase in the fetal heart rate. The observations by Szeto [37] are very different from those of Richardson and Wittmann made during human pregnancy. In addition to the possibility of significant species difference it seemed possible that morphine or methadone might have a biphasic effect with generalized stimulation of breathing activity, nuchal tone, and central nervous system at low doses such as those administered by Szeto [37] and suppression of fetal breathing activity at higher doses. Indeed, recent results obtained by George Olsen (personal communication) have shown a primary stimulation of fetal breathing in sheep, followed 2-3 hr later by a secondary depression during prolonged infusions of morphine.

Several groups of investigators have shown that administration of naloxone to normal fetal lambs has no effect on breathing movements. But the fact that morphine can affect fetal breathing implies that natural opiates may play a part in control in pathophysiological circumstances.

E. Hypnotic Drugs

It has been reported that in chronic fetal lamb preparations diaphragmatic electromyographic activity ceased within 2 min of induction of anesthesia in the ewe with thiopental sodium. It has been reported that small doses of pentobarbitone (4 mg/kg) given intravenously to pregnant ewes caused a decrease in fetal breathing activity in mature fetuses at 116-137 days' gestation, but that in immature fetuses at 87-97 days there was no effect on fetal breathing activity during the first hour following injection [34]. These investigators measured electrocortical activity in mature fetuses and reported dramatic decreases in the incidence of low-voltage electrocortical activity following pentobarbitone injections to ewes, which suggested the effect of pentobarbitone on fetal breathing movements was secondary to its effect on electrocortical activity.

X. The Epidsodic Nature and Significance of Fetal Breathing Movements

The mechanism and significance of the episodic mature of human fetal breathing are unexplained and indeed largely unexplored. In sheep, the pattern of intermittent fetal breathing very early in gestation is succeeded by almost continuous breathing movements 0.7 of the way through gestation, with brief episodes of apnea lasting 2 min or less [38]. Then, after 0.8 of full term, the periods of apnea increase in association with the development of episodes of high-voltage electrocortical activity characteristic of quiet sleep. Ultimately, these episodes of apnea may last an hour or more near term as in man.

Yet, there are some differences between these episodes in man and sheep. First, in man no period of gestation has yet been identified during which there are almost continuous fetal breathing movements. And second, such indirect evidence as there is does not support the view that human fetal apnea is normally related to quiet sleep. Human infants born prematurely show clearly defined episodes of quiet or rapid eye movement sleep or wakefulness by 36 weeks' gestation and possibly earlier. Such quiet sleep is associated with low heart rate variability. Episodes of low heart rate variability, interspersed with episodes of higher variability, are easily identified by 36 weeks' gestation, and are first discernible at 28 weeks. But human fetal breathing is not correlated with such episodes of lower or higher heart rate variability at 36-38 weeks' gestation. No direct test of the relation between fetal breathing and electrocortical activity in labor is possible when access to the fetal scalp to place electroencephalographic (EEG) electrodes is feasible, since fetal breathing is arrested in labor, as already mentioned. So the basic physiology and the significance of this episodic phenomenon in man is not yet established.

There are some other phenomena which have been observed in sheep and which are relevant to human perinatal medicine, but which have not yet been explored in man for technical or ethical reasons. For instance, it is not uncommon to observe sheep in which there is growth retardation, occurring either naturally or as a result of surgical interference with the development of the placenta. In such sheep there is commonly a considerable degree of hypoxemia; the arterial PO_2 may be as low as 10–12 mmHg, yet the incidence and pattern of fetal breathing is normal for gestational age. The explanation for this phenomenon is that the lambs have largely compensated for their hypoxemia by increasing their red cell concentration; it can be doubled. Secondly, it should be mentioned that abnormal patterns of breathing are not uncommonly seen before fetal death in sheep. At the time when these observations were first made in the early 1970s there was no obvious mechanism [39]. We would now speculate that they may be due to unusual effects on the central chemoreceptors, derived through prostaglandin activity, perhaps in part by an effect on local blood flow pattern. Thirdly, in man, postnatally as in other species, it is known that the carotid chemoreceptors play a most important role in regulating breathing movements in response to changes in the blood gases, especially of oxygen. Such indirect or direct evidence as has been available in the past suggested that the carotid bodies were inactive in the fetal lamb near term. However, recent observations have shown that they are indeed active, and we must suppose that their central activity is inhibited by some so far unknown mechanism in order to explain the lack of normal responsiveness to abrupt, brief episodes of hypoxemia in fetal breathing.

XI. Production of Fetal Pulmonary Fluid

Fetal tracheal fluid flow in lambs has been measured by electromagnetic flow meters implanted in the trachea. The inward and outward movement of tracheal fluid is small, rarely exceeding ±1 ml, commensurate with the relatively high density and viscosity of the tracheal fluid compared with air. The dead space of the trachea is 8–10 ml in fetal lambs near term, and as a result in healthy fetuses individual breaths are insufficient to actually inhale amniotic fluid into the lung.

In some animals, large amplitude breathing movements may be associated with a net inward tracheal flow of several ml over 2-3 min. However, outward fluid flow is most common. Total net outward tracheal flow increases with gestational age from 110 to 145 days' gestation to reach volumes of up to 100 ml/kg/day near term. Outward flow occurs in small amounts (1–2 ml), especially accompanying brief expiratory efforts indicated by a rise in fetal intrathoracic pressure. Larger flows of fluid (20–40 ml) occur in outward gushes 6–12 times per day over periods of 3-5 min and are often associated with rises in fetal carotid arterial pressure of 20 mmHg. Outward gushes of fluid are not necessarily associated with episodic rapid irregular breathing movements.

XII. Fetal Breathing Movements and Fetal Lung Growth

Recently evidence in fetal lambs has accumulated to show that fetal breathing movements [40], and the maintenance of a positive pressure in the tracheobronchial tree before birth [41], are essential to the development of the future airways. So the possibility arises that pulmonary hypoplasia may result from inadequate practice in the respiratory musculature prenatally. Though the mechanism is still conjectural, we can recall that such pulmonary hypoplasia arises naturally in man in association with space-occupying lesions of the thorax (e.g., diaphragmatic hernia), in Potter's syndrome when the low amniotic fluid volume limits fetal movements, and in congenital disorders of phrenic nerve or cervical cord development.

XIII. Conclusions

Major advances have taken place in identifying and understanding the normal physiology of human fetal breathing movements since the introduction of real-time ultrasound scanners in 1975. However, this should not blind us to the fact that the results so far described are limited. Almost too much emphasis has been placed on measurements of the incidence of fetal breathing, and much less attention has been given to accurate measurement of changes in breathing interval and amplitude. Yet, these latter are the variables which medical scientists would put weight on postnatally. Secondly, when human fetal breathing movements were rediscovered using pulse-echo and other methods in 1971 it looked at first as though they might immediately give useful clinical indications of health, but this reasonable expectation has not been fulfilled. The principal reason is the episodic nature of fetal breathing. Notwithstanding this, it is evident that if a full picture of fetal activity is to be established as a guide to health, then measurements of fetal breathing as well as of heart rate and body movements are desired, as judged by postnatal experience. The crucial question in all such obstetrical studies is how long the investigator is prepared to give to the examination of a fetus which may be sick, and may be very sick.

References

1. Dawes, G. S., H. E. Fox, B. M. Leduc, G. C. Liggins, and R. T. Richards, Respiratory movements and rapid eye movement sleep in the foetal lamb, *J. Physiol. (Lond.)*, **220**:119 (1972).
2. Cousin, A. J., Advanced methods for measurement of fetal breathing movements in the human fetus, *Semin. Perinatol.*, **4**(4): (1980).

3. Goodman, J. D. S. and C. D. Mantell, A second means of identifying fetal breathing movements using Doppler ultrasound, *Am. J. Obstet. Gynecol.*, **136**:73 (1980).
4. Trudinger, B. J. and P. C. Knight, Fetal age and patterns of human fetal breathing movements, *Am. J. Obstet. Gynecol.*, **137**:724 (1980).
5. Patrick, J., R. Natale, and B. Richardson, Patterns of human fetal breathing activity at 34 to 35 weeks' gestational age, *Am. J. Obstet. Gynecol.*, **132**: 207 (1978).
6. Patrick, J., K. Campbell, L. Carmichael, R. Natale, and B. Richardson, A definition of human fetal apnea and the distribution of fetal apneic intervals during the last 10 weeks of pregnancy, *Am. J. Obstet. Gynecol.*, **136**:471 (1981).
7. Patrick, J., K. Campbell, L. Carmichael, R. Natale, and B. Richardson, Patterns of human fetal breathing during the last 10 weeks of pregnancy, *Obstet. Gynecol.*, **56**:24 (1980).
8. Ritchie, J. W. K. and K. Lakhani, Fetal breathing movements in response to maternal inhalation of 5% carbon dioxide, *Am. J. Obstet. Gynecol.*, **136**:386 (1980).
9. Richardson, B. S., J. P. O'Grady, and K. Johnson, The fetal response to carbon dioxide studied serially during the last 10 weeks of pregnancy, *Soc. Gynecol. Invest.*, Dallas, Abstr. 11 (1982).
10. Dawes, G. S., W. N. Gardner, B. M. Johnston, and D. W. Walker, Effects of hypercapnia on tracheal pressure, diaphragm and intercostal electromyograms in unanesthetized fetal lambs, *J. Physiol. (Lond.)*, **326**:461 (1982).
11. Dawes, G. S., W. N. Gardner, B. M. Johnston, and D. W. Walker, Breathing in fetal lambs: The effect of brain stem section, *J. Physiol. (Lond.)*, **335**:535 (1983).
12. Wood, C., J. Hammond, J. Lumley, et al., Effect of maternal inhalation of 10% oxygen upon the human fetus, *Aust. NZ Obstet. Gynaecol.*, **11**: 85 (1971).
13. Manning, F. A., Y. Murata, C. B. Martin, K. Miyaki, and G. Danzler, Breathing movements before death in the primate fetus (Macaca mulatta), *Am. J. Obstet. Gynecol.*, **135**:71 (1979).
14. Fox, H. E. and C. W. Hohler, Fetal evaluation by real-time imaging, *Clin. Obstet. Gynecol.*, **20**:339 (1977).
15. Lewis, P. J., B. J. Trudinger, and J. Mangez, Effect of maternal glucose ingestion on fetal breathing and body movements in late pregnancy, *Br. J. Obstet. Gynaecol.*, **85**:86 (1978).
16. Natale, R., J. Patrick, and B. Richardson, Effects of maternal venous plasma glucose concentrations on fetal breathing movements, *Am. J. Obstet. Gynecol.*, **132**:36 (1978).

17. Harding, P. G., M. Harding, A. Charbonneau, and J. Patrick, Unpublished observations.
18. Bocking, A., L. Adamson, A. Cousin, K. Campbell, L. Carmichael, R. Natale, and J. Patrick, Effects of intravenous glucose injections on human fetal breathing movements and gross fetal body movements at 38–40 weeks' gestational age, *Am. J. Obstet. Gynecol.,* **142**:606 (1982).
19. Adamson, L., A. Bocking, A. Cousin, I. Rapoport, and J. Patrick, Ultrasonic measurement of rate and depth of human fetal breathing: Effect of glucose, *Am. J. Obstet. Gynecol.,* **147**:288 (1983).
20. Patrick, J., J. Challis, K. Campbell, L. Carmichael, R. Natale, and B. Richardson, Circadian rhythms in maternal plasma cortisol and estriol concentrations at 30 to 31, 34 to 35, and 38 to 39 weeks' gestational age, *Am. J. Obstet. Gynecol.,* **136**:325 (1980).
21. Patrick, J., J. Challis, K. Campbell, L. Carmichael, B. Richardson, and G. Tevarrwerk, Effects of synthetic glucocorticoid administration on human fetal breathing movements at 34 to 35 weeks' gestational age, *Am. J. Obstet. Gynecol.,* **139**:324 (1981).
22. Richardson, B., R. Natale, and J. Patrick, Human fetal breathing activity during induced labour at term, *Am. J. Obstet. Gynecol.,* **133**:247 (1979).
23. Carmichael, L., K. Campbell, R. Natale, J. Patrick, and B. Richardson, Decrease in human fetal breathing movements prior to spontaneous labour at term, *Am. J. Obstet. Gynecol.,* **148**:675 (1984).
24. Kitterman, J. A. and G. C. Liggins, Fetal breathing movements and inhibitors of prostaglandin synthesis, *Semin. Perinatol.* **4**(2):97 (1980).
25. Patrick, J., J. R. G. Challis, and J. Cross, *Effects of Indomethacin Infusion Given to Pregnant Ewes on Glucose Concentrations and Fetal Breathing Movements.* Presented at Canadian Investigators in Reproduction, Quebec (1981).
26. Kitterman, J. A., G. C. Liggins, J. E. Fewell, J. A. Clements, and W. H. Tooley, Inhibitions of breathing movements in fetal lambs by prostaglandins, *Seventh International Symposium on Fetal Breathing*, Oxford, England (1980).
27. Thaler, J. S., J. D. S. Goodman, and G. S. Dawes, The effect of maternal smoking on fetal breathing rate and activity patterns, *Am. J. Obstet. Gynecol.,* **138**:282 (1980).
28. Fox, H. E., T. Soulos, J. M. Hutson, A. Higgins, and L. S. James, Cigarette smoking and real-time linear array B-scan observations of fetal activity, *Ninth International Symposium on Fetal Breathing*, London, Ontario, Canada (1982).
29. Fox, H. E., M. Steinbrecher, D. Pessle, J. Inglis, L. Medvid, and E. Angel, Maternal ethanol ingestion and the occurrence of human fetal breathing movements, *Am. J. Obstet. Gynecol.,* **132**:354 (1978).

30. McLeod, W., J. Brien, L. Carmichael, C. Probert, and J. Patrick, Effect of maternal alcohol ingestion on fetal breathing movements, body movements, and heart rate at 37–40 weeks' gestational age, *Am. J. Obstet. Gynecol.,* **145**:251 (1983).
31. McLeod, W., J. Brien, L. Carmichael, C. Probert, N. Steenaart, and J. Patrick, Maternal glucose injections do not alter the suppression of fetal breathing following maternal alcohol ingestion, *Am. J. Obstet. Gynecol.* **148**:634 (1984).
32. Jones, C. T. and J. W. Ritchie, The cardiovascular effects of circulating catecholamines in fetal sheep, *J. Physiol. (Lond.).,* **285**:381 (1978).
33. Murata, Y., C. B. Martin, K. Miyake, M. Socol, and M. Druzin, Effect of catecholamine on fetal breathing activity in rhesus monkeys, *Am. J. Obstet. Gynecol.,* **139**:942 (1981).
34. Boddy, K., G. S. Dawes, R. L. Fisher, S. Pinter, and J. S. Robinson, The effects of pentabarbitone and pethidine on foetal breathing movements in sheep, *Br. J. Pharmacol.,* **57**:311 (1976).
35. Richardson, B. S., J. P. O'Grady, and G. D. Olsen, Fetal breathing movements and the response to CO_2 in patients on methadone maintenance, *Am. J. Obstet. Gynecol.* **150**:400 (1984).
36. Wittmann, B. K., S. Brown, S. Segal, and W. O. C. Young, Fetal activity in patients on methadone maintenance, *Ninth International Symposium on Fetal Breathing,* London, Ontario, Canada (1982).
37. Szeto, H. H., Effects of methadone and morphine on fetal electrocortical activity, heart rate and body movements, *Soc. Gynecol. Invest.,* Dallas, Abstr. 161 (1982).
38. Bowes, G., T. M. Adamson, B. C. Ritchie, M. Dowling, M. H. Wilkinson, and J. E. Maloney, Developmental patterns of respiratory activity in unanesthetized fetal sheep in utero, *J. Appl. Physiol.,* **50**:693 (1981).
39. Patrick, J. E., K. J. Dalton, and G. S. Dawes, Breathing patterns before death in fetal lambs, *Am. J. Obstet. Gynecol.,* **125**:73 (1976).
40. Liggins, G. C. and J. A. Kitterman, Development of the fetal lung. CIBA Foundation Symposium 86, London, Pitman, 1981, p. 308.
41. Fewell, J. E., A. A. Hislop, J. A. Kitterman, and P. Johnson, Effect of tracheostomy on lung development in fetal lambs, *J. Appl. Physiol.,* **55**:1103 (1983).

Part Two

METHODS OF EVALUATION

5

Gestational Age Estimation and Amniocentesis

DONALD L. LEVY and PRESTON LEA WILDS*

Eastern Virginia Medical School
Norfolk, Virginia

I. Gestational Age Estimation

A. Introduction

Nowhere in medical care is the age of the patient more important than in the case of the human fetus. This is because (1) the fetal period is characterized by the most rapid anatomical and physiological growth, and (2) virtually all important management decisions in obstetrics are made on the basis of an accurate estimate of fetal age. As survival rates for very low birth weight infants have improved so has the need increased to date pregnancies accurately. Current obstetrical estimates of gestational age have been shown to correlate well with subsequent pediatric assessments [1]. This chapter will review the clinical and ultrasonographic methods of estimating gestational age and will emphasize the most recently proven techniques and the potential for error associated with each method. Amniocentesis for the purpose of obtaining fluid for fetal pulmonary maturity studies will be covered in the second part of this chapter.

**Present affiliation*: Virginia Department of Health, Virginia Beach, Virginia

B. Clinical Methods

Menstrual History

Pregnancy is most often diagnosed after a woman has skipped one or more menstrual periods. If the patient normally bleeds in a 28-day cycle, conception has occurred about 14 days before the missed period. In obstetrics, when one estimates gestational age using the last menstrual period [LMP] as a marker, the number of weeks denoted is actually that from the first day of the LMP and not from conception. In effect, obstetricians calculate gestational age as if the patient were already 2 weeks pregnant on the date of conception. All further indications of gestational age in this section refer to the interval from the LMP, from which the mean length of gestation is assumed to be 280 days.

Various investigators have suggested the predictive accuracy of the LMP to range from 60 to 90%, involving at best an error of ±3 weeks [2-6]. There are numerous causes for error in using the LMP as a single source of information. Not all women bleed (or ovulate) at regular intervals. This is particularly true in women who have recently discontinued oral contraceptives. Furthermore, even in those patients whose cycles are regular reporting is often inaccurate. Zador and associates reviewed the records of 889 patients and found that they gave days 1, 5, and 15 of the month most frequently as the start of their LMP [7].

Quickening

Another historical marker used to predict fetal age is quickening. Pregnant women usually first experience fetal movement at approximately 16-17 weeks' gestation, but this is entirely too variable to be of any real value as a single marker in dating [8].

Fetal Heart Tones

Fetal heart tones should be audible with a fetoscope by 20 weeks' gestation [2] and with Doppler ultrasound by as early as 8-10 weeks.

Fundal Height

Measurement of the height of the uterine fundus, usually from the symphysis pubis, has received conflicting evaluations of its accuracy in dating pregnancy [9-12]. Sources of potential error include normal biological variation in abdominal length, which translates to an age difference of 8 weeks [9], variation in fundal height due to the fullness of the urinary bladder [10], and the differences due to amount of abdominal wall fatty tissue. Uterine size estimated by bimanual examination prior to 12 weeks is helpful only when it closely correlates with an accurate LMP. A single fundal height measurement between 12 and 20 weeks is probably most helpful in prompting initial suspicion of multiple pregnancy. With a singleton pregnancy at 12 weeks' gestation the fundus of the uterus should be palpable just above the symphysis pubis. At about 15 weeks the fundus lies approximately one-half the distance between the symphysis and the umbilicus, a point which is reached by 20 weeks' gestation and may be used as an important marker in dating the pregnancy. Up until early in the third trimester serial measurements of fundal height may first suggest abnormalities in fetal growth, but they are of little value in accurately dating the pregnancy.

Overall Usefulness

If one combines the date of the LMP with other clinical data, including first auscultation of fetal heart tones, the accuracy does not improve sufficiently over that reached by LMP alone [2,13]. However, where the LMP date is uncertain, a gestational age estimate as accurate as that predicted from a reliable LMP date can be made by averaging clinical data (time of quickening, time when fetal heart tones are first audible, and time at which the uterus reaches the umbilicus) [13].

C. Roentgenography

Prior to the advent of ultrasound various skeletal measurements via roentgenograms were used to date pregnancies [14]. These methods have been shown to be at best only as accurate as the use of the LMP [15,16], and because they add the potential risk of x-ray exposure to the developing fetus they have no current application in pregnancy dating.

D. Ultrasound

Introduction

With a combination of improved technology and the accumulated clinical experience, obstetrical ultrasound currently allows accurate estimates of gestational age with a small margin of error. The instruments used in diagnostic ultrasound emit sound waves having a frequency ranging from 1 to 10 MHz, with the imaging resulting from the reflected waves. The quality of the image is limited by the fact that when the frequency is increased the resolution improves but the penetration of the beam decreases.

Up until recently obstetrical ultrasound scanning was done using a static B-mode instrument with a linear array transducer (3.5 MHz). Today most imaging done for the purpose of pregnancy dating is accomplished with a real-time scanner, which has the distinct advantage of picturing movements while only slightly sacrificing resolution. Although there are theoretical risks associated with the use of ultrasound, no untoward biological effects have been confirmed that resulted from the use of ultrasound with the usual intensities and frequencies.

Gestational Sac

The earliest sonographic evidence of intrauterine pregnancy is the gestational sac (see Fig. 1), first seen at about 5 weeks' gestation. Originally thought to grow with a linear relationship to gestational age [17], the sac now is believed to grow in a curvilinear fashion between the fifth and eleventh week [18]. Variation in configuration of the sac secondary to uterine tonus, uterine position, and bladder fullness explains in part the potential error in estimating age by this method [18]. Bulic and Vrtar showed an accuracy of ±6 days in 95% of cases studied between 5 and 11 weeks using thread planimetry to measure sac area [18]. Using an average of 2 diameters will increase accuracy. It is also useful to study the gestational sac for the purpose of diagnosing pregnancy and predicting outcome in cases complicated by first-trimester bleeding.

Crown-Rump Length

A more accurate method of dating pregnancy in the first trimester was first reported by Robinson using crown-rump length (CRL) measurements (see Fig. 2)

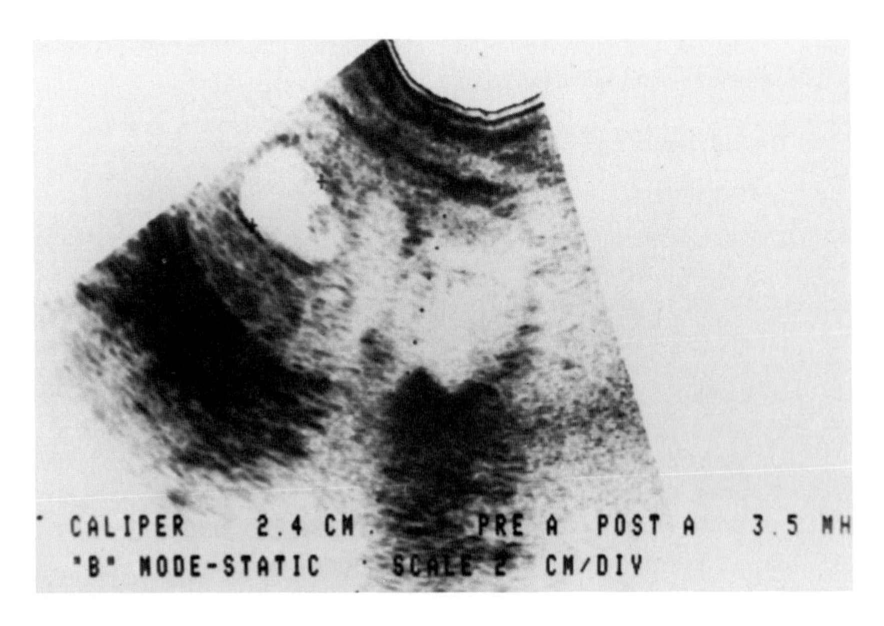

Figure 1 Gestational sac, 7–8 weeks.

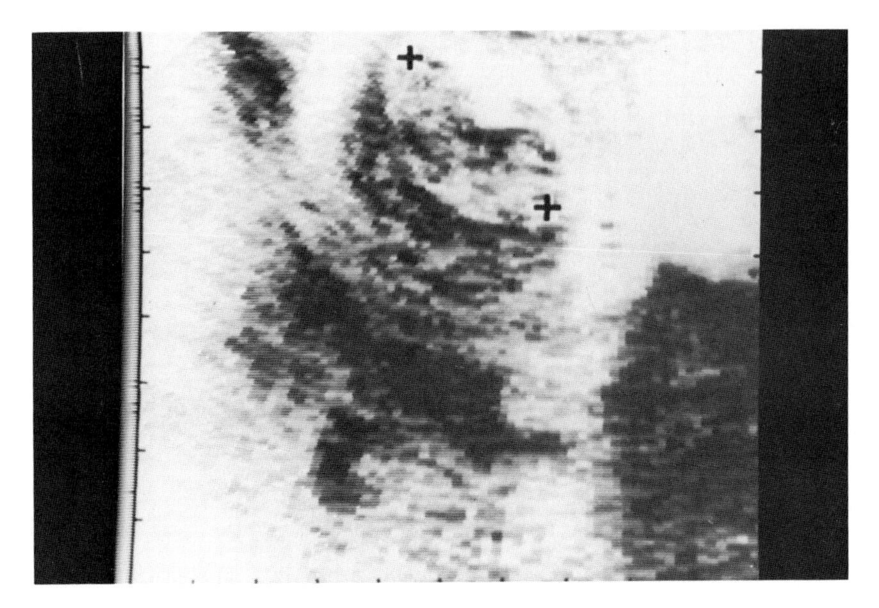

Figure 2 Crown-rump length, 12–13 weeks.

[19]. He later confirmed and refined his earlier studies using a static method which resulted in an error by only ±4–5 days when dating a pregnancy between 6 and 14 weeks (see Table 1) [16–20]. Subsequent studies measuring CRL with real-time scanners resulted in a comparable degree of accuracy [21,22].

Biparietal Diameter

After 14 weeks' gestation the CRL is no longer applicable to estimation of gestational age and is replaced by measurements of the fetal biparietal diameter (BPD) (see Fig. 3). Since the early reports of Campbell [23], Campbell and Newman [24], and Thompson and Makowski [25], a multitude of studies which include tables and graphs have flooded the literature [26–29]. As the technology has improved so has the accuracy, including that with real-time imaging [28–30]. The table presented here is abstracted from Sabbagha and Hughey's paper in which they produced a composite table from four separate studies using uniform methodology (see Table 2) [28]. It is important to note that if this table is used, the BPD should be measured from the outer to the inner aspect of the fetal skull. The accuracy of a single BPD measurement is greatest (±7–10 days) in the second trimester and falls off considerably after that (±14–21 days). Combining measurements of various other diameters (e.g., abdominal) or repeating the determination of the same diameter will lead to an improved accuracy even in the third trimester [25,31,32]. Growth of the BPD's in twin

Table 1 Fetal Crown-Rump Length vs. Menstrual Age

Menstrual age (weeks + days)	Corrected CRL[a] Mean values (mm)	Menstrual age (weeks + days)	Corrected CRL[a] mean values (mm)
6 + 2	5.5	10 + 2	33.2
6 + 3	6.1	10 + 3	34.6
6 + 4	6.8	10 + 4	36.0
6 + 5	7.5	10 + 5	37.4
6 + 6	8.1	10 + 6	38.9
7 + 0	8.9	11 + 0	40.4
7 + 1	9.6	11 + 1	41.9
7 + 2	10.4	11 + 2	43.9
7 + 3	11.2	11 + 3	45.1
7 + 4	12.0	11 + 4	46.7
7 + 5	12.9	11 + 5	48.3
7 + 6	13.8	11 + 6	50.0
8 + 0	14.7	12 + 0	51.7
8 + 1	15.7	12 + 1	53.4
8 + 2	16.6	12 + 2	55.2
8 + 3	17.6	12 + 3	57.0
8 + 4	18.7	12 + 4	58.8
8 + 5	19.7	12 + 5	60.6
8 + 6	20.8	12 + 6	62.5
9 + 0	21.9	13 + 0	64.3
9 + 1	23.1	13 + 1	66.3
9 + 2	24.2	13 + 2	68.2
9 + 3	25.4	13 + 3	70.2
9 + 4	26.7	13 + 4	72.2
9 + 5	27.9	13 + 5	74.2
9 + 6	29.2	13 + 6	76.3
10 + 0	30.5	14 + 0	78.3
10 + 1	31.8	14 + 0	78.3

[a]Derived from regression analysis after correction for the systematic errors (1.0 mm + 3.7%) of the technique.
Source: Ref. 20.

Table 2 Fetal Biparietal Diameter vs. Menstrual Age

Menstrual age (weeks)	Composite mean[a] BPD (cm)
14	2.8
15	3.2
16	3.6
17	3.9
18	4.2
19	4.5
20	4.8
21	5.1
22	5.4
23	5.8
24	6.1
25	6.4
26	6.7
27	7.0
28	7.2
29	7.5
30	7.8
31	8.0
32	8.2
33	8.5
34	8.7
35	8.8
36	9.0
37	9.2
38	9.3
39	9.4
40	9.5

[a]Sonographic BPDs representing four studies with uniform methodology.
Source: Ref. 28.

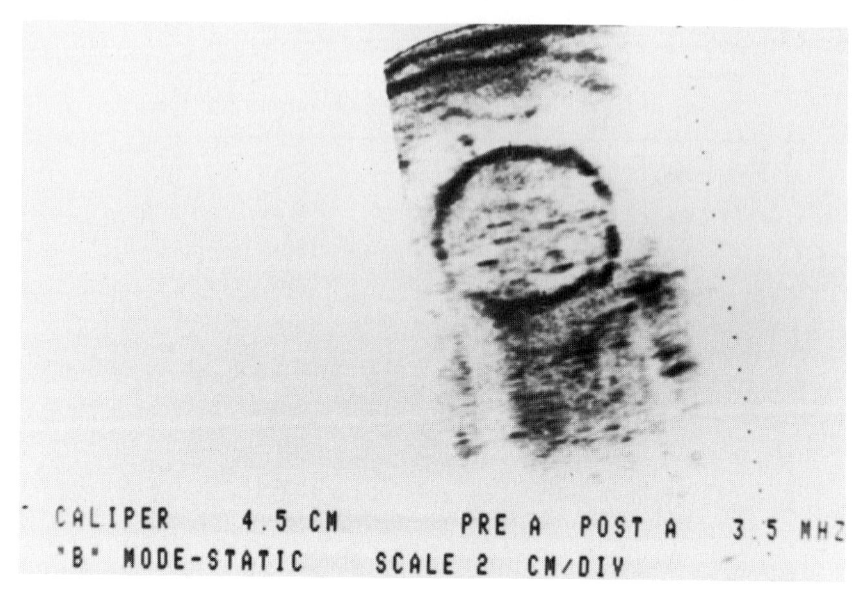

Figure 3 Biparietal diameter, 19–20 weeks.

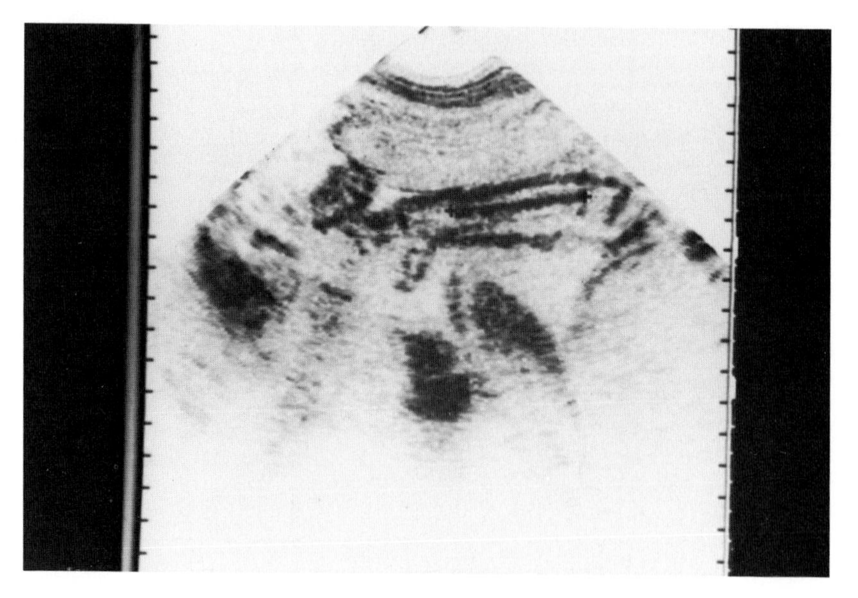

Figure 4 Femoral length, 22–23 weeks.

Table 3 Femur Length vs. Menstrual Age

	Femur length (mm)	
Menstrual age (weeks)	mean	± 2 SD
14	16.6	2.5
15	19.9	2.3
16	22.0	3.0
17	25.2	2.9
18	29.6	3.1
19	32.4	3.1
20	34.8	2.5
21	37.5	4.1
22	40.9	3.9
23	43.5	3.6
24	46.4	3.5
25	48.0	4.6
26	51.1	5.0
27	53.0	3.2
28	54.4	4.1
29	57.3	4.3
30	58.7	3.8
31	61.5	4.5
32	62.8	4.2
33	64.9	4.6
34	65.7	4.4
35	67.7	4.8
36	69.5	4.6
37	70.8	4.3
38	71.8	5.6
39	74.2	5.1
40	75.4	5.6

Source: Ref. 36.

gestations has been shown to be very similar to that of singletons prior to 30 weeks [33], and thus is associated with a similar accuracy in estimating fetal age(s).

Femoral Length

More recently, measurement of the fetal femoral length (see Fig. 4) has been used to date pregnancies between 12 and 40 weeks' gestation [34-37]. Hohler and Quetel [37] suggest that the accuracy of this method extends to term, while O'Brien and Queenan [36] suggest that an error of ±6-7 days applies only up to 24 weeks prior to the time when normal biological variation results in a widening of the growth curve limits (see Table 3). Hohler and Quetel [37] also showed a linear relationship between femoral length (FL) and BPD after 22 weeks–FL/BPD = 0.79 ± 0.08. Both groups stressed that multiple measurements should be made at the time of the sonographic examination in order to achieve the appropriate levels of accuracy [34-37].

E. Summary

Documenting quickening and time of the first audible fetal heart tones is not particularly helpful in pregnancy dating. Roentgenograms should not be used at all. Ultrasound visualization of the gestational sac is most helpful in diagnosing pregnancy rather than specifically for dating. The ideal approach to an accurate estimate of fetal age would include a reliable history of the LMP plus compatible determination of uterine size in the first 20 weeks. Adding to this a single sonogram measuring CRL between 7 and 14 weeks should accurately date the pregnancy to within a few days. Where the LMP date is uncertain and/or early exams are missed, at least two BPD and femoral length measurements prior to the third trimester would be indicated.

II. Amniocentesis

A. Introduction

Third-trimester amniocentesis for diagnostic purposes was first reported more than 50 years ago when Menees et al. described amniocentesis for amniography as a diagnostic procedure [38]. Amniocentesis to obtain amniotic fluid for laboratory analysis became established as a diagnostic procedure during the 1950s after Bevis demonstrated that analysis of amniotic fluid for blood pigments was useful in managing Rh-sensitized pregnancies [39]. During the past decade, third-trimester amniocentesis has been eclipsed in the public mind and in the medical literature by second-trimester amniocentesis performed for the antepartal detection of genetic disorders. Clearly, the indications, technique, risks, and laboratory procedures associated with third-trimester amniocentesis differ in many ways from genetic amniocentesis performed at 4 months of pregnancy. Most of the literature has emphasized the techniques and risks of second-trimester amniocentesis to the relative neglect of the older procedure. Many of the technical developments in recent years, although directed mainly toward improving the safety of second-trimester amniocentesis, have been adapted and modified for use in the third trimester to improve its safety [40,41].

B. Safety

Amniocentesis is an everyday occurrence on most large obstetrical services. Its performance is often delegated to physicians of limited experience who are unfamiliar with the risks they incur by failure to adhere to strict techniques. Certainly, each time the procedure is performed the benefits derived should outweigh the risks of the procedure. At times the best measure of expert skill and judgment in amniocentesis may be a decision to postpone the test or not to do it at all. The available information on the safety of third-trimester amniocentesis is very different from that available on the safety of amniocentesis performed for genetic indications in the second trimester. To establish the safety of the latter procedure, large-scale prospective and retrospective studies have been reported in which the outcome for patients undergoing amniocentesis was compared with the outcome in similar groups of patients who did not have an amniocentesis [42–44]. Studies involving thousands of patients were carried out in second-trimester amniocentesis because (1) extensive genetic screening programs often involved substantial outlays of public funds; (2) second-trimester amniocentesis was thought to be more difficult and hazardous than the third-trimester procedure, and if it were to receive public support, its risks had to be quantified; and (3) genetic amniocentesis was performed for a single indication using techniques which differed relatively little from one institution to the next. In contrast, third-trimester amniocentesis is performed for a variety of indications by operators using substantially different techniques, incurring risks that vary significantly from operator-to-operator and from patient-to-patient. In reviews summarizing case reports up to 1968, Burnett and Anderson [45] and Creasman and his colleagues [46] concluded that the incidence of serious fetal complications in over 8500 reports of amniocentesis found in the literature was <0.4%. A more recent review by Rome et al. [47] suggests a similar figure. This number of 0.4% is comparable to the 0.5% figure often used in discussing the safety of second-trimester amniocentesis, but it is in fact far less meaningful in counseling individual patients facing third-trimester amniocentesis. For example, the risk of injury from amniocentesis when the patient has a posterior placenta and mild polyhydramnios, as is often seen in diabetes mellitus, is quite different from the risks of amniocentesis in a patient with an anterior placenta and oligohydramnios with no readily accessible pocket of amniotic fluid; and yet in statistical studies cases with readily identifiable differences in risk are lumped together.

C. Complications

Most of the case reports of the hazards of third-trimester amniocentesis antedate the general availability of ultrasound in the performance of the procedures. This should not be construed to mean that with the use of ultrasound complications do not occur. Rather, it suggests that reports of complications are rarely published because the literature is already replete with such reports.

Ultrasound used appropriately can reduce the risk of injury. Serious consequences of amniocentesis are caused by injury to fetal vessels in the placenta or umbilical cord with resultant fetal bleeding, exsanguination, or maternal isoimmunization, direct injury to the fetus from puncture or laceration by the needle, introduction of microorganisms into the amniotic sac, premature rupture of the membranes, and induction of premature labor.

Fetal Hemorrhage

Fetal bleeding from transplacental amniocentesis may be unavoidable when the placenta is located on the anterior uterine wall and the only accessible pocket of amniotic fluid lies beneath it. Massive fetal bleeding may result from puncture or laceration of a vessel on the fetal surface of the placenta. When this occurs, the amniotic fluid is grossly bloody. On the other hand, injury to fetal vessels within the body of the placenta may cause fetal blood loss from fetal–maternal hemorrhage with no bleeding into the amniotic cavity [48]. Thus, obtaining clear amniotic fluid during transplacental amniocentesis is insufficient assurance against fetal hemorrhage. An Apt or Kleihauer–Betke test for fetal–maternal hemorrhage should also be done [49]. Fetal heart rate monitoring after potential injury to the placenta or umbilical cord may be helpful in identifying fetal distress, but it may be inadequate to detect blood loss at a slow rate, leading to gradual exsanguination and fetal death [48], and it has not been effective in preventing sudden death when the exsanguination is rapid [50].

Fetal Injury

Accidental injuries to third-trimester fetuses from diagnostic amniocentesis are presumably rare events, but such injuries have included intraperitoneal hemorrhage from laceration of the fetal spleen [51] and pneumothorax and tension pneumothorax as a consequence of lung injury after thoracic puncture [52–54]. Fetal death from cardiac tamponade after accidental pericardial puncture has also been reported [55]. Fetal intracranial hemorrhage in a term infant has occurred as a result of amniocentesis [56]. Fetal puncture and laceration may occur as a result of the operator's manipulation of the needle, or the fetus may impale itself on the needle, or fetal movement may convert a puncture into a laceration.

Chorioamnionitis

Amniotic fluid infection after diagnostic amniocentesis was reported by Liley as early as 1960 [57]. It is a rare complication, however, and the occurrence of infection can be virtually eliminated by strict adherence to aseptic technique whenever amniocentesis is attempted.

Premature Rupture of the Membranes

Adequately controlled studies to determine whether or not third-trimester amniocentesis is associated with an increased incidence of premature ruptured membranes have not been reported. Studies comparing the relationship of different sites or techniques of amniocentesis to the occurrence of premature ruptured membranes permit no conclusions to be drawn as the reported studies [58-60] do not clearly favor one site over another as being safest with regard to this complication.

Premature Labor

Amniocentesis per se has not been associated with an increased incidence of premature labor over that which might be expected to occur spontaneously in similar patients who did not receive amniocentesis, but randomized, prospective, controlled studies have not been reported and are probably unjustifiable from the ethical standpoint. In earlier years, when amniocentesis was used chiefly for amniography with injection of substantial quantities of hyperosmolar radiopaque solutions into the amniotic sac, there was a similar lack of evidence that the procedure was associated with an increased incidence of premature labor. Obviously, when amniocentesis is associated with hemorrhagic complications there is an associated risk of premature labor or premature termination of pregnancy, but these complications are rare. Most third-trimester amniocenteses are performed close to term in order to evaluate fetal lung maturity. Under these circumstances, the effect—if any—of amniocentesis in accelerating the onset of labor is probably too small to measure.

Other

Serious maternal complications have also been reported. They include maternal death, amniotic fluid embolism, abruption of the placenta, febrile morbidity, peritonitis, hemorrhagic complications, and isoimmunization from fetal-maternal hemorrhage [45,57,61-64]. For the most part, information on maternal complications of amniocentesis takes the form of isolated case reports. The exception is maternal isoimmunization, which is dealt with in more detail in a later section.

D. Technique

The nature of the risks associated with amniocentesis makes it clear that most of them can be greatly reduced or eliminated entirely by careful planning and strict attention to technique. Before beginning the procedure, the obstetrician should weigh carefully the value and timing of the information to be gained from amniotic fluid analysis in comparison with the risks of obtaining the fluid.

Consent

Although amniocentesis is a routine procedure for the obstetrician, it is rarely seen as such by the patient or by members of her family. There is no substitute for detailed and careful discussion with the patient, and with family members if present, of the reasons the procedure is being recommended, the nature of the information being sought and how soon it will be available, and the procedure to be used. A written consent form covering all these points and individualized to fit the patient's special circumstances would be a very long document and is obviously impractical in most clinical settings. Nevertheless, some form of written consent is highly desirable [49]. It should at least include a list of the topics covered in the discussion and should be signed by the patient and the person providing the information.

Amniocentesis Without Ultrasound

Tens of thousands of amniocenteses have been performed "blindly" without ultrasonic guidance and with a very low rate of complications. The risk-benefit ratio for amniocentesis for proper indications was established as favorable long before sonography came into widespread use. In the present decade, however, performance of amniocentesis without ultrasonic guidance at the time of the procedure should be condemned as unacceptable [65] except in unusual circumstances when ultrasound is absolutely unavailable and the performance of amniocentesis cannot be delayed. When these circumstances prevail, the technique of amniocentesis and the selection of the site for puncture differ substantially from what should be done under ultrasonic guidance. Past studies have shown that the suprapubic approach is associated with fewer failures and fewer complications than the periumbilical "small parts" approach. There appears to be no difference in the two approaches in the incidence of premature rupture of the membranes [58,59]. On the other hand, in one study, amniocentesis performed in the area behind the fetal neck seemed to be associated with a higher rate of spontaneous premature rupture of the membranes [60]. In the performance of amniocentesis without ultrasound, the risk of injury to the fetus or to the umbilical cord can be reduced by using a short needle appropriate for intramuscular injections (21-gauge by 1.5 in.). A needle of this size, when introduced to the hub, is sufficient to reach the amniotic sac in most cases except over the placenta. If blood is obtained, which most likely will be from the intervillous space, the needle should be withdrawn and amniocentesis attempted with a new needle in a different site [66].

Amniocentesis With Ultrasound

Ultrasonic guidance in the performance of amniocentesis can be carried out at three levels of complexity: (1) localization of the placenta, (2) localization of the placenta and the pocket of amniotic fluid to be aspirated, and (3) continuous ultrasonic guidance of the needle during insertion.

Placental Localization

When static-image, bistable B-scan sonography became generally available more than a decade ago, the main use of ultrasound in amniocentesis was placental localization. Often the ultrasound examination was performed at a different time and location from the amniocentesis. The position of the fetus and of pockets of amniotic fluid could change during the interim, and even the location of the placenta could be substantially altered depending on whether or not the patient's bladder was full or empty and depending also on her position on the examining table. It is highly desirable that the ultrasound examination and the amniocentesis should take place together, and that the patient should not change her position nor relieve the fullness of her bladder between the time of the ultrasound examination and the performance of the amniocentesis. The widespread availability of portable real-time ultrasound scanners makes it feasible to perform ultrasonic examination and amniocentesis as a unified procedure in most clinical situations.

At the present time, the usual equipment for ultrasonic evaluation with amniocentesis is a real-time linear-array scanner. With this equipment the operator should be able to: (1) rule out multiple gestation, (2) locate accessible pockets of amniotic fluid, and (3) avoid injury to the placenta and to the fetus. Other ultrasound equipment, such as real-time sector-scanner or a stored-image compound scanner, may be used with equal effectiveness.

Localization of Site for Amniocentesis

With the use of a linear-array real-time scanner, the operator should first complete a thorough survey of the fetus and the placenta. He should identify the pocket of amniotic fluid best suited for amniocentesis. He can then insert a finger or a pencil under the transducer directly over a pocket of fluid. This will cast a sonic shadow into the pocket and identify the path of the needle. The operator should then rotate the transducer through 90° to demonstrate that the pocket is indeed a pocket and not a narrow slit. Once the exact spot for puncture has been marked on the maternal skin, the operator can use ultrasound to measure the exact depth to which the needle must penetrate to reach the center of the pocket and fix in his mind the proper angle for needle insertion.

Amniocentesis Under Continuous Ultrasonic Guidance

This technique is possible using special transducers with a hole or slot through which the needle is inserted, or "free-hand," using a standard transducer. The advantages of continuous guidance are: (1) it allows direct observation of the placement of the needle, and (2) it permits recognition of fetal movement during the placement of the needle and, thus, may reduce the risk of fetal injury. The disadvantages of this approach are: (1) the technique is slower and more cumbersome, (2) the cautious advancement of the needle causes the patient greater discomfort and/or requires the use of local anesthesia (usually with greater discomfort), (3) proper visualization of the needle often requires that it be of larger caliber than would otherwise be necessary, (4) maintenance of sterile technique, though not impossible, is rendered much more difficult, and (5) if special transducers are used, they add substantially to the cost of the procedure, especially if the transducer has no use except for amniocentesis. For amniocentesis insertion of the needle under direct guidance seems unnecessary, although it may be very helpful in other aspiration procedures. Percutaneous aspiration under direct ultrasonic guidance is described in detail in other publications, to which the reader is referred [67–70].

Equipment

Prepackaged, disposable amniocentesis trays are available on the market and are convenient to use. Most contain many items which are unnecessary, however, and very few contain all the essentials. These are the essentials: (1) sponge sticks and sponges for prepping the abdomen, (2) povidone–iodine solution, (3) a fenestrated drape, (4) a 3.5-in., 22-gauge spinal needle with a stylette, (5) an intravenous extension (a short length of clear plastic tubing fitted with adaptors for a needle hub at one end and a syringe at the other), (6) two or more 20-ml disposable syringes, (7) containers for fluid transport (these must be of blown glass if the fluid is to be analyzed for optical density of heme pigments), and (8) a centimeter ruler.

Procedure

Our procedure for amniocentesis is as follows: Unless the site for puncture is close to some natural marker such as the umbilicus or a skin blemish, it is marked with a drop of gentain violet dye. The skin is prepped three times with povidone-iodine solution and draped. The needle is measured with the centimeter ruler and is held at the required length from the tip. The patient is warned that there will be a sharp sensation as the needle goes in. No local anesthetic is used. The needle is then inserted at the proper angle and to the proper depth in a single quick thrust. The stylette is removed. Usually within a few seconds, the hub of the needle begins to fill with amniotic fluid. If no fluid appears, the needle is rotated and the interior of the hub is observed. If still no fluid appears, the needle is advanced an additional 1-2 cm, the needle is rotated if necessary, and the hub is again observed for fluid. When fluid appears, the needle is attached to the IV extension and the extension is attached to the syringe and the fluid is aspirated. Clear fluid should flow through the tubing into the syringe. When the appropriate amount (preferably 20-30 ml) of the fluid has been collected, the needle is withdrawn quickly without replacement of the stylette.

While most fetal maturity tests require considerably less than 20 ml of amniotic fluid for analysis, withdrawal of 20-30 ml of fluid has two distinct practical advantages over smaller samples. Most fetal maturity tests require centrifugation of the specimen and standard laboratory centrifuge tubes hold a maximum volume of 12-15 ml. Therefore, 20-30 ml of sample must be centrifuged in two separate tubes, whereas 10-15 ml of sample may be centrifuged in one tube. In the event that one tube is lost because of spillage or breakage, a second tube of sample will remain. This may prevent the very embarrassing situation of the necessity for a repeat amniocentesis because no laboratory result was obtained. Secondly, larger samples also provide additional fluid for repeat tests in cases in which equivocal results have been obtained.

The IV extension tubing has certain advantages over direct connection of the needle to the syringe. (1) It permits the needle to yield or pivot out of the way when the fetus bumps against it. This may reduce the risk of fetal puncture or laceration. (2) When the tap is done relatively high in the abdomen the needle attached to the tubing can seesaw back and forth in response to the mother's breathing efforts. This may reduce the likelihood of injury to maternal or placental vessels. (3) If the flow of fluid stops (perhaps because a flap of amnion has covered the bevel of the needle), or if none is obtained by the procedures described earlier, one can easily manipulate the needle by advancement, withdrawal, or rotation to achieve a free flow. The needle can be manipulated using one hand while the other maintains negative pressure on the syringe. (4) In the event that blood is aspirated after withdrawal of fluid has started, one can observe the blood in the tubing and disconnect the syringe from the tubing before the blood reaches it and, thus, avoid blood contamination of the fluid already collected in the syringe.

We recommend the use of a 22-gauge needle for second- and third-trimester amniocentesis. Needles of 18–20-gauge were formerly recommended [71,72]. The smaller needle requires more time for aspiration of the sample but is otherwise satisfactory. It is probably safer than larger, more rigid needles [41,73]. We have not had a problem from flecks of vernix obstructing these small needles.

E. Special Situations

Obesity

An occasional patient is so obese that at the chosen site for amniocentesis a 3.5-in. needle cannot reach the amniotic sac unless the hub forcibly indents the skin. Under these circumstances, it is probably better to delay the procedure and obtain a longer needle, even if it must be of somewhat larger caliber.

Multiple Gestation

When it is necessary to obtain fluid from each sac in a twin gestation it is usually possible to identify the membrane separating the sacs by ultrasound and to identify two sites through which the sacs can be tapped separately. After fluid has been aspirated from the first sac, the needle should be left in place temporarily and 1 ml of indigo carmine or methylene blue should be diluted with a few milliliters of amniotic fluid and then injected into the sac. The needle is then withdrawn, and amniocentesis of the second sac is attempted. If dye-free fluid is obtained, successful tap of both sacs has been accomplished. In triplet pregnancies, the dye injection is repeated for each sac except the last. In cases where the membranes separating the sacs cannot be identified, or where the anatomy is such that the second sac can be reached only by traversing the first sac, amniocentesis of each sac may be accomplished by the method of Picker [74]. Essentially, this method involves advancing the needle to the skin of the fetal thigh and then withdrawing the needle just sufficiently to obtain fluid in immediate proximity to the skin of the thigh.

The specimen from each sac must be separately labeled (right upper sac, anterior sac, etc.). A description of the procedure for tapping each sac must be recorded in sufficient detail so that if the laboratory reports for each sac lead to divergent results (i.e., as in optical density studies when one twin is Rh negative and the other is Rh positive), it will be possible later on to identify with maximum certainty which fetus was associated with which laboratory report.

Bloody Tap

Not infrequently, after the initial insertion of the amniocentesis needle and the withdrawal of the stylette, the hub of the needle fills with blood. Usually this indicates that the tip of the needle is in a maternal vessel or in the intervillous space. The best approach is to replace the stylette, advance the needle 1-2 cm, and observe the fluid that fills the hub when the stylette is removed. Often, the amniotic fluid will be bloody (initially) and will clear with aspiration. It is best to use a separate syringe to aspirate the bloody portion and then switch to a clean syringe as soon as clear fluid appears.

If the fluid continues to be bloody, one must assume that bleeding from an injured vessel has taken place into the amniotic fluid, and may be continuing. A sample of the fluid should be sent to the laboratory immediately to determine whether the bleeding is of maternal or fetal origin. If the blood is coming from the fetus, this is potentially very serious. Close observation for the effects of continued fetal hemorrhage is necessary and emergency termination of the pregnancy must be considered [75].

If the initial fluid is clear but later turns bloody, possibly the needle has injured an umbilical vessel, or the bevel of the needle may have retracted into the placenta and may be aspirating fetal blood from an injured fetal vessel or maternal blood from the intervillous space. Under these circumstances, identification of whose blood is in the syringe may be of critical importance.

The Rh-Negative Patient

The routine use of ultrasound in third-trimester amniocentesis appears to decrease the need for more than one attempt to obtain fluid and to decrease the incidence of bloody taps [76]. Nevertheless, clinically significant fetal-maternal hemorrhage is a frequent occurrence even with the use of ultrasound. Harrison and his colleagues [77] showed that there was evidence of fetal cells in the maternal circulation after aminocentesis in 36% of patients when the tap was done with ultrasound guidance and in 34% when it was done without. Picker and his colleagues [73] noted that in a series of 2003 third-trimester amniocentesis, there were 126 blood-stained specimens, of which only 108 could be related to an anterior placenta and transplacental insertion of the needle. It seems clear that the use of ultrasound to avoid the placenta and the collection of a specimen of clear amniotic fluid are inadequate assurances against passage of fetal cells into the maternal circulation after third-trimester amniocentesis. We recommend that all unsensitized Rh-negative patients receive a

300 μg dose of Rh-immune globulin after third-trimester amniocentesis. The one exception would be the Rh-negative patient in whom the known father of the child is also Rh-negative. Administration of this dose of immune globulin usually produces anit-D titers of 1:1 or 1:2. These levels are insufficient to cause evidence of fetal hemoloysis or anemia but should be sufficient to prevent sensitization where up to 15 ml of fetal red cells are released into the general circulation [78].

When transplacental amniocentesis is unavoidable, there is the risk that fetal-maternal hemorrhaging may be massive and may require multiples of the usual dose of Rh-immune globulin in order to prevent maternal isoimmunization [63,79]. Placental injury should be suspected whenever transplacental amniocentesis is performed, and in such cases, Kleihauer–Betke testing of the maternal blood should be carried out to measure the extent of fetal–maternal hemorrhage and adjust the Rh-immune globulin dosage accordingly. Furthermore, evidence of massive fetal–maternal hemorrhage may indicate impending fetal jeopardy and the need for emergency delivery [75].

F. Summary

Third-trimester amniocentesis is a relatively safe procedure, but it is not innocuous. Its performance should be limited to cases where the benefits of the information obtained through amniocentesis clearly outweigh the risks involved in obtaining the specimen. Careful attention to technique and the appropriate use of ultrasound guidance can substantially reduce, but not eliminate, the risk of injury to the fetus, placenta, or umbilical cord. Fetal–maternal hemorrhage leading to isoimmunization may occur despite ultrasound guidance and despite the collection of a sample of clear fluid. In unsensitized Rh-negative patients, Rh-immune globulin should be given routinely after third-trimester amniocentesis. If placental injury is suspected, tests for fetal cells in the maternal circulation should be carried out so that the dose of immune globulin can be adjusted accordingly.

References

1. Wilson, J., D. L. Levy, and P. L. Wilds, Premature rupture of membranes prior to term: Consequences of non-intervention, *Obstet. Gynecol.*, **60**: 601 (1982).
2. Andersen, H. F., T. R. B. Johnson, Jr., M. L. Barclay, and J. D. Flora, Jr., Gestational age assessment: I. Analysis of individual clinical observations, *Am. J. Obstet. Gynecol.*, **139**:173 (1981).
3. Treloar, A. E., B. G. Behn, and D. W. Cowan, Analysis of gestational interval, *Am. J. Obstet. Gynecol.*, **99**:34 (1967).

4. Nakano, R., Post-term pregnancy, *Acta Obstet. Gynecol. Scand.*, **51**:217 (1972).
5. Wenner, W. and Young, E. B., Non-specific date of last menstrual period. An indication of poor productive outcome, *Am. J. Obstet. Gynecol.*, **120**:1071 (1974).
6. Hertz, R. H., R. J. Sokol, J. D. Knoke, et al., Clinical estimation of gestational age: Rules for avoiding pre-term delivery, *Am. J. Obstet. Gynecol.*, **131**:395 (1978).
7. Zador, I. E., R. H. Hertz, R. J. Sokol, and V. J. Hirsch, Sources of error in the estimation of fetal gestational age, *Am. J. Obstet. Gynecol.*, **138**:344 (1980).
8. Kraus, G. W. and C. H. Hendricks, Significance of the quickening date in determining duration of pregnancy, *Obstet. Gynecol.*, **24**:178 (1964).
9. Beazley, J. M. and R. A. Underhill, Fallacy of the fundal height, *Br. Med. J.*, **4**:404 (1970).
10. Worthen, N. and M. Bustillo, Effect of urinary bladder fullness on fundal height measurements, *Am. J. Obstet. Gynecol.*, **138**:759 (1980).
11. Westin, B., Gravidogram and fetal growth, *Acta Obstet. Gynecol. Scand.*, **56**:273 (1977).
12. Belizan, J. M., J. Villar, J. C. Nardin, et al., Diagnosis of intrauterine growth retardation by a simple clinical method: Measurement of uterine height, *Am. J. Obstet. Gynecol.*, **131**:643 (1978).
13. Andersen, H. F., T. R. B. Johnson, Jr., J. D. Flora, and M. L. Barclay, Gestational age assessment. II. Prediction from combined clinical observations, *Am. J. Obstet. Gynecol.*, **140**:770 (1981).
14. Schreiber, M. H., M. M. Nichols, and W. J. McGanity, Epiphyseal ossification center visualization, *J.A.M.A.*, **184**:504 (1963).
15. Russell, J. G. R., Radiological assessment of fetal maturity, *J. Obstet. Gynaecol. Br. Cwlth.*, **76**:208 (1969).
16. Robinson, H. P., E. M. Sweet, and A. H. Adam, The accuracy of radiological estimates of gestational age using early fetal crown-rump length measurements by ultrasound as a basis for comparison, *Br. J. Obstet. Gynaecol.*, **86**:525 (1979).
17. Hellman, L. M., M. Kobayashi, L. Fillisti, and M. Lavenhar, Growth and development of the human fetus prior to the twentieth week of gestation, *Am. J. Obstet. Gynecol.*, **103**:789 (1969).
18. Bulic, M. and M. Vrtar, Ultrasonic planimetry of the gestation sac as a biometric method in early pregnancy, *J. Clin. Ultrasound*, **6**:228 (1978).
19. Robinson, H. P., Sonar measurement of fetal crown-rump length as means of assessing maturity in first trimester of pregnancy, *Br. Med. J.*, **4**:28 (1973).

20. Robinson, H. P. and J. E. E. Fleming, A critical evaluation of sonar "crown-rump length" measurements, *Br. J. Obstet. Gynaecol.*, **82**:702 (1975).
21. Nelson, L. H., Comparison of methods for determining crown-rump measurement by real-time ultrasound, *J. Clin. Ultrasound*, **9**:67 (1981).
22. Bovicelli, L., L. F. Orsini, N. Rizzo, et al., Estimation of gestational age during the first trimester by real-time measurement of fetal crown-rump length and biparietal diameter, *J. Clin. Ultrasound*, **9**:71 (1981).
23. Campbell, S., The prediction of fetal maturity by ultrasonic measurement of the biparietal diameter, *J. Obstet. Gynaecol., Br. Cwlth.*, **76**:603 (1969).
24. Campbell, S. and G. B. Newman, Growth of the fetal biparietal diameter during normal pregnancy, *J. Obstet. Gynaecol. Br. Cwlth.*, **78**:513 (1971).
25. Thompson, H. E. and E. L. Makowski, Estimation of birth weight and gestational age, *Obstet. Gynecol.*, **37**:44 (1971).
26. Sabbagha, R. E., J. H. Turner, H. Rockette, et al., Sonar BPD and fetal age: Definition of the relationship, *Obstet. Gynecol.*, **43**:7 (1974).
27. Weiner, S. N., M. J. Flynn, A. W. Kennedy, and F. Bonk., A composite curve of ultrasonic biparietal diameters for estimating gestational age, *Radiology*, **122**:781 (1977).
28. Sabbagha, R. E. and M. Hughey, Standardization of sonar cephalometry and gestational age, *Obstet. Gynecol.*, **52**:402 (1978).
29. Hadlock, F. P., R. L. Deter, R. J. Carpenter, and S. K. Park, Estimating fetal age: Effect of head shape on BPD, *Am. J. Radiol.*, **137**:83 (1981).
30. Osinusi, B. O., A. J. Hall, A. H. Adam, and J. E. E. Fleming, Reproducibility of biparietal diameter measurements obtained with a real-time scanner, *Br. J. Obstet. Gynaecol.*, **97**:467 (1980).
31. Kopta, M. M., P. G. Tomich, and J. P. Crane, Ultrasonic methods of predicting the estimated date of confinement, *Obstet. Gynecol.*, **57**:657 (1981).
32. Sabbagha, R. E., M. Hughey, and R. Depp, Growth adjusted sonographic age. A simplified method, *Obstet. Gynecol.*, **51**:383 (1978).
33. Grennert, L., P. H. Persson, and G. Gennser, Intrauterine growth of twins judged by BPD measurements, *Acta Obstet. Gynecol. Scand.* (Suppl.), **78**:28 (1978).
34. Queenan, J. T., G. D. O'Brien, and S. Campbell, Ultrasound measurement of fetal limb bones, *Am. J. Obstet. Gynecol.*, **138**:297 (1980).
35. O'Brien, G. D., J. T. Queenan, and S. Campbell, Assessment of gestational age in the second trimester by real-time ultrasound measurement of the femur length, *Am. J. Obstet. Gynecol.*, **139**:540 (1981).
36. O'Brien, G. D. and J. T. Queenan, Growth of the ultrasound fetal femur length during normal pregnancy: Part I, *Am. J. Obstet. Gynecol.*, **141**: 833 (1981).

37. Hohler, C. W. and T. A. Quetel, Comparison of ultrasound femur length and biparietal diameter in late pregnancy, *Am. J. Obstet. Gynecol.,* **141**: 759 (1981).
38. Menees, T. O., J. D. Miller, and L. E. Holly, Amniography: Preliminary report, *Am. J. Roentgenol.,* **24**:363 (1930).
39. Bevis, D. C. A., The antenatal prediction of haemolytic disease of the newborn, *Lancet,* **397** (1952).
40. Queenan, J. T., When and how to do amniocentesis, *Contemp. Ob/Gyn.,* **15**:61 (1980).
41. Picker, R. H., R. D. Robertson, J. C. Pennington, et al., A safe method of amniocentesis for lecithin/sphingomyelin determination in late pregnancy using ultrasound, *Obstet. Gynecol.,* **47**:722 (1976).
42. Simpson, N. E., L. Dallaire, J. R. Miller, et al., Prenatal diagnosis of genetic disease in Canada: Report of a collaborative study, *Can. Med. Assoc. J.,* **115**:739 (1976).
43. National Institute of Child Health and Human Development Study Group: Mid-trimester amniocentesis for prenatal diagnosis–Safety and accuracy, *J.A.M.A.,* **236**:1471 (1976).
44. An Assessment of the Hazards of Amniocentesis. Report to the medical research council by their working party on amniocentesis, *Br. J. Obstet. Gynecol.,* **85** (Suppl. 2) (1978).
45. Burnett, R. G. and W. R. Anderson, The hazards of amniocentesis, *J. Iowa Med. Soc.,* **58**:130 (1968).
46. Creasman, W. T., R. A. Lawrence, and H. A. Thiede, Fetal complications of amniocentesis, *J.A.M.A.,* **204**:91 (1968).
47. Rome, R. M., J. I. Glover, and S. C. Simmons, The benefits and risks of amniocentesis for the assessment of fetal lung maturity, *Br. J. Obstet. Gynecol.,* **82**:662 (1975).
48. Kirshen, E. J. and K. Benirschke, Fetal exsanguination after amniocentesis, *Obstet. Gynecol.,* **42**:615 (1973).
49. Schwarz, R. H., Amniocentesis, *Clin. Obstet. Gynecol.,* **18**: (1975).
50. Goodlin, R. C. and W. H. Clewell, Sudden fetal death following diagnostic amniocentesis, *Am. J. Obstet. Gynecol.,* **118**:285 (1974).
51. C. C. Egley, Laceration of fetal spleen during amniocentesis, *Am. J. Obstet. Gynecol.,* **116**:582 (1973).
52. Leake, R. D., C. J. Hobel, and R. S. Lachman, Neonatal pneumothorax and subcutaneous emphysema secondary to diagnostic amniocentesis, *Obstet. Gynecol.,* **43**:884 (1974).
53. C. J. Hyman, R. Depp, P. Pakravan, et al., Pneumothorax complicating amniocentesis, *Obstet. Gynecol.,* **41**:43 (1973).
54. Grove, C. S., C. G. Trombetta, and M. S. Amstey, Fetal complications of amniocentesis, *Am. J. Obstet. Gynecol.,* **115**:1154 (1973).

55. Berner, H. W., E. P. Seisler, and J. Barlow, Fetal cardiac tamponade, a complication of amniocentesis, *Obstet. Gynecol.*, **40**:599 (1972).
56. Portman, M. A. and R. T. Brouillette, Fetal intracranial hemorrhage complicating amniocentesis, *Am. J. Obstet. Gynecol.*, **144**:731 (1982).
57. Liley, A. W., The technique and complications of amniocentesis, *N.Z. Med. J.*, **59**:581 (1960).
58. Gordon, H. R. and A. G. Deukmedjian, Subrapubic vs. periumbilical amniocentesis, *Am. J. Obstet. Gynecol.*, **122**:287 (1975).
59. Leach, G., A. Chang, and J. Morrison, A controlled trial of puncture sites for amniocentesis, *Br. J. Obstet. Gynaecol.*, **85**:328 (1978).
60. Teramo, K. and S. Sipinen, Spontaneous rupture of fetal membranes after amniocentesis, *Obstet. Gynecol.*, **52**:272 (1978).
61. Bennett, M. J., The technique and complications of amniocentesis, *S. Afr. Med. J.*, **46**:1545 (1972).
62. Woo Wang, M. Y. F., E. McCutcheon, and J. F. Desforges, Fetomaternal hemorrhage from diagnostic transabdominal amniocentesis, *Am. J. Obstet. Gynecol.*, **97**:1123 (1967).
63. Curtis, J. D., W. N. Cohen, H. B. Richerson, et al., The importance of placental localization preceding amniocentesis, *Obstet. Gynecol.*, **40**:194 (1972).
64. Kochenour, N. K. and J. H. Beeson, The use of Rh-immune globulin, *Clin. Obstet. Gynecol.*, **25**:283 (1982).
65. Benzie, R. J., Amniocentesis, amnioscopy and fetoscopy, *Clin. Obstet. Gynaecol.*, **7**:439 (1980).
66. Jeffares, M. J., C. J. Orchard, and M. A. Tettenborn, Third-trimester aminocentesis using a short needle: An assessment of its safety and value in cases of doubtful dates, *J. R. Naval Med. Serv.*, **64**:10 (1978).
67. Sneider, P., Ultrasound aspiration-biopsy transducer amniocentesis, *S. Afr. Med. J.*, **55**:829 (1979).
68. Holm, H. H., J. F. Pedersen, J. K. Kristensen, et al., Ultrasonically-guided percutaneous puncture, *Radiol. Clin. North Am.*, **13**:493 (1975).
69. Goldberg, B. B., C. Cole-Beuglet, A. B. Kurtz, et al., Real-time aspiration-biopsy transducer, *J. Clin. Ultrasound*, **8**:107 (1980).
70. Bree, R. L., Use of a high-frequency aspiration-biopsy transducer for direct ultrasound-guided amniocentesis, *Obstet. Gynecol.*, **53**:523 (1979).
71. Werch, A., Amniocentesis: Indications, technique and complications, *South. Med. J.*, **69**:824 (1976).
72. Mellows, H. J., Practical procedures: How to do an amniocentesis, *Br. J. Hosp. Med.*, **24**:268 (1980).
73. Picker, R. H., D. H. Smith, D. M. Saunders, et al., A review of 2,003 consecutive amniocenteses performed under ultrasonic control in late pregnancy, *Aust. N.Z. J. Obstet. Gynaecol.*, **19**:83 (1979).

74. Picker, R. H., D. H. Smith, and D. M. Saunders, A new method of amniocentesis using ultrasound in multiple pregnancy to assess the second twin, *Obstet. Gynecol.,* **50**:489 (1977).
75. Ryan, G. T., R. Ivy, Jr., and J. W. Pearson, Fetal bleeding as a major hazard of amniocentesis, *Obstet. Gynecol.,* **40**:702 (1972).
76. Platt, L. D., F. A. Manning, and M. LeMay, Real-time B scan-directed amniocentesis, *Am. J. Obstet. Gynecol.,* **130**:700 (1978).
77. Harrison, R., S. Campbell, and I. Craft, Risks of feto-maternal hemorrhage resulting from amniocentesis with and without ultrasound placental localization, *Obstet. Gynecol.,* **46**:389 (1975).
78. Bowman, J. M., Suppression of Rh-isoimmunization, *Obstet. Gynecol.,* **52**:385 (1978).
79. Dubin, C. F. and K. J. Staisch, Amniocentesis and fetal–maternal blood transfusion. A review of the literature, *Obstet. Gynecol. Surv.* (Suppl.), **37**:272, 1982.

6

Methods of Amniotic Fluid Analysis for Evaluation of Fetal Maturity

GEORGE H. NELSON, HOSSAM E. FADEL, and JAMES C. McPHERSON, JR.

Medical College of Georgia
Augusta, Georgia

I. Introduction

The assessment of fetal lung maturity based on the examination of amniotic fluid is of relatively recent origin. However, there were many preceding observations that were essential to arrive at a state of the art that would not only permit assessment of fetal lung maturity but indicate its importance as well. Amniocentesis to obtain samples for evaluation was first reported in 1881 [1] and 71 years elapsed before its reintroduction in the 1950s [2] for the management of Rh incompatibility. In evaluation of this disease it became a routine procedure in the 1960s. Therefore not only were more samples available for study but of equal importance serial analyses on the same patient were possible.

Early investigations on amniotic fluid for evaluation of fetal maturity involved the measurements of nonsurfactant substances and these measurements were correlated with gestational age and/or fetal weight. Several centers in the mid to late 1960s reported a variety of correlations of this type.

The following observations were reported before investigators began examining amniotic fluid for evaluation of fetal lung maturity:

1. Mature fetal lungs had their alveoli lined with a surfactant film.
2. Surfactant was largely phospholipid with its chief component dipalmitoyl lecithin.
3. The surfactant film was deficient in hyaline membrane disease (HMD) of the newborn.
4. The occurrence of HMD was related to gestational age (i.e., related to the time when fetal lungs produced enough surfactant to prevent HMD).
5. The flow of alveolar fluid was from the lungs into the amniotic fluid.

These points were demonstrated by 1968, at which time we at the Medical College of Georgia began looking at amniotic fluid phospholipids. However, it was not until the early 1970s that amniocentesis became accepted for the prospective evaluation of fetal lung maturity.

In this chapter we will review the various amniotic fluid determinations which have been utilized for evaluation of fetal maturity, with emphasis on those which specifically evaluate fetal lung maturity. No attempt will be made to compare methods with respect to their accuracy of predictions. No systematic scientific study has been or will ever be carried out which will compare the various methods. The number of different methods and the number of variations of the same method are simply too great to allow any type of meaningful study to be initiated. We have expressed various views regarding several methods in other chapters throughout this book.

II. Amniotic Fluid Cytology

The first widely employed test to determine fetal maturity was based on the cytological examination of amniotic fluid. Fetal squamous cells had been described in amniotic fluid as early as 1904 [3] and their occurrence became clinically important to prove the diagnosis of amniotic fluid embolism in the maternal lungs in 1926 [4] and to diagnose premature rupture of the membranes (PROM) in 1942 [5] by examination of vaginal secretions. Blystad et al. in 1951 [6] in studies of respiratory distress syndrome (RDS) demonstrated that the number of squamous cells increased with gestational age of the fetus. Kittrich in 1963 [7] and Brosens and Gordon in 1966 [8] developed methods for estimating gestational age based on the percentage of fat-staining or orange-staining cells in amniotic fluid using Nile blue stain. These investigators and others have not only used this method to assess gestational age but also to predict that the infant will not develop HMD after birth. It is generally believed that the orange-staining cells are derived from the maturation of sebaceous glands and represent a generalized maturation of skin. This test is generally performed by placing one or two drops of amniotic fluid (taken from the junction of the supernatant and sediment of centrifuged specimens) on a microscope slide. To this are added one or two drops of 0.1% Nile blue sulfate, the slide is warmed gently, a coverslip is applied, and the sample is examined microscopically. The cells are either anucleated and stain orange or are nucleated and stain blue. Generally one counts from 500 to 1000 cells and the percentage of orange cells is determined. An orange cell count of 10% or more was indicative of a gestational age of 36 weeks or greater or a birth weight of 2500 g or more with about 90% accuracy in our laboratory.

III. Optical Density of Amniotic Fluid

A. Δ 450-mμ

Mandelbaum et al. [9] described the use of spectrophotometric analysis for estimation of gestational age. It had long been recognized by investigators following Rh-sensitized patients that the amniotic fluid Δ 450 mμ OD decreased with gestational age in the absence of an intrauterine hemolytic process. The Δ 450-mμ OD is an indirect measure of the concentration of bilirubin in the amniotic fluid and the reason for the decrease with gestational age is still a matter of debate. It probably reflects an increased placental clearance of bilirubin from fetus to mother with advancing gestation. In our laboratory we have used a value of 0.02 or less as indicative of a gestational age of 36 weeks or greater. This has about the same predictive accuracy as an orange cell count of 10% or more.

B. OD 650

The determination of the optical density of amniotic fluid at 650 mμ was first employed by Sbarra et al. [10] as a means of assessing fetal maturity. A value of 0.15 or above of centrifuged amniotic fluid correlated with fetal lung maturity and corresponded to an lecithin/sphingomyelin (L/S) ratio of 2.0 or greater. The principle of this technique has never been adequately explained and we have found that the optical density varies with the cloudiness of the sample which is a function of time of collection to time of analysis as well as several other variables.

IV. Amniotic Fluid Creatinine

Williams and Bargen in 1924 [11] reported that the creatinine level in amniotic fluid at term was 2 mg%. Its usefulness was not realized until the 1960s when Woyton [12] and Pitkin and Zwirek [13] reported that the creatinine levels were related to gestational age. The amniotic fluid creatinine level has been found to be directly related to fetal muscle mass and renal maturity, both of which increase with gestational age. We have used a concentration value of 1.8 mg% or more as indicative of a fetal weight of 2500 g or more with about the same accuracy as a mature orange cell count or Δ 450-mμ OD. Amniotic fluid urea and uric acid concentrations also rise with advancing gestational age and to some extent parallel the pattern seen with creatinine. However, these measurements have not received as much attention as a fetal maturity test as has the creatinine measurement.

V. Amniotic Fluid Osmolality

The osmolality of amniotic fluid is similar to that of maternal serum during the first half of pregnancy. However, during the last half of pregnancy it begins to decrease and begins to become hypotonic with respect to plasma. Lind and Hytten [14] have shown that the decrease in osmolality parallels a simultaneous decline in sodium concentration in amniotic fluid. This decline in osmolality and sodium concentration is generally thought to be the result of a progressive dilution by hypotonic fetal urine in late pregnancy. Miles and Pearson [15] proposed that a mature fetus was likely if the osmolality was 250 mOsm/liter or less. In the early 1970s we purchased an osmometer and attempted to determine its clinical usefulness in patient management. We eventually abandoned this technique because of the wide spread of values that we obtained.

VI. Amniotic Fluid Lung Surfactant

A. Introduction

Amniotic fluid for measurement of surfactant content or activity is usually collected by transabdominal amniocentesis. The techniques for measuring lung surfactant per se are technically very difficult; therefore, most studies have been based on the determination of the various phospholipid moieties of surfactant. Since dipalmitoyl lecithin is the most abundant surface-active component in surfactant, many methods have in a variety of ways centered on its measurement.

B. Effect of Storage of Amniotic Fluid

One of the technical problems in surfactant assay has been related to handling the collected sample. Ideally, the tube of amniotic fluid should be placed in an ice slush at the bedside, immediately transported to the laboratory, and immediately processed on arrival. This situation is rarely achieved. Some studies suggest little or no change occurs in surfactant concentration within a 24-hr storage period at room temperature, up to 10 days at 0-4°C, and almost indefinitely with storage at −20°C. We have analyzed centrifuged specimens on the day of collection and again at 1, 2, 3, and 4 days after collection. We have found the lecithin fraction to be stable at room temperature during this time period.

C. Methods and Effect of Centrifugation

The amount of centrifugation, i.e., g-force, rpm, time, and temperature, is probably the most diverse step in the analysis of lung surfactant. There is little agreement as to just which conditions of centrifugation are optimal. The goal of this step is to remove all of the vernix and cellular material without removing any of the surfactant. From our literature review and experience in our laboratory it appears that amniotic fluid samples should be centrifuged at 350 g for 10 min, preferably in a refrigerated centrifuge at 4°C. This step should be done prior to storage or shipment to a distant laboratory. For a lecithin analysis this can be accomplished by most ordinary table-top centrifuges.

D. Surfactant Extraction Methods

Most of the methods for measuring surfactant require extraction of the lipids from the amniotic fluid sample. In the most common technique for chemical determination, 1 vol of amniotic fluid is mixed with 1 vol of methanol followed by 2 vols of chloroform. This mixture separates into two layers and the lower chloroform is removed for analysis. For methods measuring ratios, i.e., lecithin/sphingomyelin (L/S) or palmitic acid/stearic acid (P/S) ratios, this cholorform extract is adequate; however,for other chemical methods a quantitative recovery of the lipid in the amniotic fluid requires further chloroform extractions of the aqueous phase. Several other extraction mixtures have been employed such as ethanol-chloroform, methanol-1-chlorobutane, ether-methanol, Freon 113-methanol-methylal. While some of these mixtures may give more quantitative extractions of surfactant lipids, their comparison with the methanol-chloroform extraction technique has rarely been reported. After extraction most procedures require evaporation of the lipid-containing layer (usually chloroform layer) to dryness.

E. Acetone Precipitation of Lung Surfactant

This step in the determination of lung surfactant is a most controversial one. Inclusion of this procedure in the determination is based on the observation that the solubility of saturated, long-chain fatty acid lecithins in cold acetone is negligible, while lecithins containing short-chain or unsaturated fatty acids are soluble in cold acetone. In theory, this acetone precipitation step should concentrate the surface-active lecithins (principally dipalmitoyl lecithin). However, it has been reported [16] with artificial mixtures and with phospholipid extracts of amniotic fluid that the amount of dipalmitoyl lecithin which is precipitated is influenced by the presence of other phospholipids in the mixture. The presence of water as a contaminant in the dried chloroform extract and the total amount of phospholipid in the extract have also been shown to alter the amount of lecithin precipitated by acetone. While many laboratories, including our own, employ this step in their surfactant determination, it has not been proven that it is necessary.

F. Phospholipid Measurements

Total Phospholipid

Many clinical laboratories routinely determine total serum phospholipid concentration. The transfer of these methods to amniotic fluid requires only minor modifications. We have reported [17] our results using a total phospholipid phosphorus (TPP) measurement in evaluation of fetal lung maturity. We reported a TPP concentration of 0.140 mg/dl correlated well with lung maturity. Several investigators [18,19] have reported total amniotic fluid phospholipid concentrations as a part of a battery of determinations on amniotic fluid. A total phospholipid measurement is technically easier to perform than individual phospholipid determinations because it does not require the use of thin-layer chromatography (TLC).

Lecithin

The measurement of the concentration of lecithin in amniotic fluid has been advocated as a fetal lung maturity test. We have measured the acetone precipitable fraction by thin-layer chromatography and our results are presented in Chapter 7. We have used a value of 0.100 mg/dl lec P as indicative of maturity. Bhagwanani and associates [20] do not include the acetone precipitation step in their determination and recommend a lecithin value of 3.5 mg/dl as suggestive of pulmonary maturity. Coverting this to lecithin phosphorus (lecithin is about 4% phosphorus), the value becomes 0.140 mg/dl lec P. Considering that about 65% of the lecithin in amniotic fluid is acetone precipitable, these two values are in very close agreement. Torday et al. [21] have suggested treatment of the anmiotic fluid sample with osmium tetroxide to separate the saturated lecithins (surfactant lecithins) from the unsaturated compounds. They report that 93% of the unsaturated lecithins are removed by this treatment, leaving a residue which is 97% saturated lecithin. Theoretically, addition of this step should improve the accuracy of RDS predictions. In addition, enzymatic methods to determine the lecithin concentration have been reported [22]. One such procedure is known as the button test. Amniotic fluid is mixed with phospholipase A and calcium ions to convert the lecithin to lysolecithin, which is a hemolytic agent. A known quantity of washed RBCs is added to the mixture and the fluid is centrifuged. The size of the button of unhemolyzed RBCs is inversely related to the concentration of lecithin in the original sample. The practicality of this principle needs further evaluation.

The lecithin content of amniotic fluid has also been assayed [23] by measuring the turbidity developed after the addition of a phenol solution.

Lecithin/Sphingomyelin Ratio

In 1971 Gluck et al. [24] suggested a method of assessing fetal lung maturity by comparing the amount of lecithin in amniotic fluid to the amount of sphingomyelin. Originally, lecithin and sphingomyelin were separated by thin-layer chromatography, identified by charring of the TLC plate, and estimated by comparing visually the size and density of the lecithin and sphingomyelin spots. An L/S ratio of 2.0 was correlated with fetal lung maturity. The quantitation step was later modified by comparing the density of the spots using a densitometer. Without a doubt this technique has received the most attention worldwide and has generated literally hundreds of articles in the literature concerned with modifications of the TLC solid support and solvent system, the acetone-precipitation step, detection of the spots, and the quantitation procedures. Despite the various modifications, most laboratories have used a L/S of 2.0 to predict the absence of RDS. However, other numbers have been suggested and numbers as high as 3.5 have been used in diabetic pregnancies. We think it is important for the reader to understand that by this technique the *relative* concentrations of lecithin and sphingomyelin are determined and that the concentration of sphingomyelin (a nonsurfactant phospholipid) influences the final answer just as much as the lecithin concentration does. However, despite this fact, this procedure has been the most widely used technique over the years to monitor fetal lung maturity and many clinical laboratories have had reasonably good results in their accuracy of predictions. The usefulness of the L/S ratio in diabetic pregnancies is discussed elsewhere in this book.

Phosphatidylglycerol

Hallman et al. [25] studied two additional phospholipids in amniotic fluid as to their relationship to fetal lung maturity. They found that the percentage (% of total phospholipid phosphorus) of phosphatidylinositol (PI) increased from about 28 weeks to 35 weeks and then decreased to term. On the contrary, the percentage of phosphatidylglycerol (PG) began to increase at 36 weeks and continued to term. Numerous reports concerning PG have since been published and most investigators agree that the appearance of PG in surfactant is a late event and signifies a mature type of surfactant. There is no consensus as to what constitutes a "mature" level of PG. Values have been expressed both as a percentage of total phospholipid and as a concentration measurement. Recently a kit (Amniostat-FLM, Hana Biologics Incorporated) has been released for PG determination. It is an immunological test and one reagent contains antibodies specific for PG-containing particles. The presence of PG in the specimen results in the agglutination (clumping) of the particles by the antibodies. The results are semiquantitative in that a negative result indicates a PG concentration of < 0.002 mg/ml; a positive result 0.002-0.003; and a strong positive result 0.004 or $>$. Our experience with this test is that it yields an inordinate amount of falsely negative tests. It may prove to be of particular use in vaginally obtained specimens from patients with premature rupture of the membranes.

Palmitic Acid/Stearic Acid Ratio

Andrews et al. [26] measured the palmitic acid/stearic acid ratio in the acetone precipitable fraction of the amniotic fluid lipid extract. They feel that this test is superior to other tests in predicting fetal lung maturity in the presence of diabetes mellitus. Determination of individual fatty acids requires the use of gas chromatography, which is a cumbersome technique for routine clinical laboratories at the present time.

G. Physical Measurements of Lung Surfactant

Introduction

As the amount of fetal lung surfactant increases in amniotic fluid, the physical characteristics of the fluid change. Two notable changes which accompany an accumulation of surfactant are decreases in surface tension and microviscosity. The following methods measure these characteristics and have been used in fetal lung maturity evaluation.

Wilhelmy Balance

The Wilhelmy balance measures the surface tension of the amniotic fluid in relation to the area of the water-air interface using a movable barrier. As the area decreases, the surfactant molecules on the surface become more tightly packed and the surface tension at the interface falls to a minimum value. Amniotic fluid from fetuses with mature lungs has a minimum surface tension of 17 dynes/cm^2 or less [27]. This method of quantitation is very accurate; however, it suffers because of the lack of availability of the instrument and the technical difficulties of the procedure. Nevertheless, this could emerge as a practical method in the future.

Du Nouy Tensiometry

Du Nouy tensiometers accurately measure the surface tension of amniotic fluid and are equivalent in accuracy to the Wilhelmy balance methods. This method differs from the Wilhelmy balance methods in that it measures the surface tension of the fluid without packing the surfactant molecules at the surface. It has been reported [28] that amniotic fluid from fetuses with mature lungs has a surface tension of < 48 dynes/cm^2, while lipid extracts have a surface tension of < 56 dynes/cm^2. These instruments have not received as much attention in the clinical setting as they have in industrial laboratories.

Shake Test

The shake test is also referred to as the bubble stability test, foam test, and the SF-50 test. This test was first described in 1972 by Clements et al. [29], as a bedside method to evaluate fetal lung maturity using uncentrifuged amniotic fluid. In this test, serial dilutions of amniotic fluid are mixed with ethanol, final concentration 47.5%, the mixture shaken vigorously and observed for the amount of bubbles remaining on the surface at 15 min. The stability of the bubbles depends upon the concentration of the surface-active material in the final mixture. The results generally are reported as positive, intermediate, or negative. Edwards and Baillie [30] modified this method using a 50% final concentration of ethanol (the SF-50 test). With a positive test we, as well as others, have found that the incidence of RDS is very low. A further modification of this test has recently appeared on the market as the Lumadex-FSI fetal lung maturity test (Beckman Instruments, Inc.). With this test six concentrations of ethanol are used and the volumes are all premeasured, thereby simplifying the technique.

The Tap Test

Socol et al. [31] recently described the tap test for evaluation of fetal lung maturity. Acidified amniotic fluid is added to diethyl ether and the tube is briskly tapped three or four times, which creates an estimated 200–300 bubbles in the ether layer. In amniotic fluid from a mature fetus the bubbles quickly rise to the surface and break down; in amniotic fluid from an immature fetus the bubbles are stable or break down slowly. It is interesting that the presence or absence of stable bubbles has opposite interpretations in the tap test and the shake test. The reason for this is not readily apparent from the report. At any rate, the authors feel that the tap test shows promise and should be evaluated by other laboratories.

Fluorescence Polarization

Some time ago it was observed [32] that certain chemicals (probes) quantitatively fluoresce in polarized light in relation to the viscosity of the mineral oil in which they are dissolved. The change in fluorescence polarization of a probe in a fluid measures the microviscosity of the fluid. This principle has been applied to measure amniotic fluid microviscosity. As lung surfactant accumulates in amniotic fluid, the microviscosity of the fluid decreases which results in a decreased fluorescence polarization. This method was first applied to amniotic fluid by Shinitzky et al. [33] to assess fetal lung maturity. Elrad et al. [34] reported that a fluorescence polarization (FP) value of <0.345 correlated with a mature L/S ratio and resulted in no cases of RDS in their study. This principle has resulted in the development of a commercially available instrument known as the FELMA (Fetal Lung Maturity) analyzer. This method is rapid; however, the cost of the instrument has prevented widespread use of this technique, even though it is theoretically one of the most desirable methods of analysis.

Other Methods

Pattle's bubble stability method [35], maximum bubble pressure measurement [36] and the bubble clicking method [37] have also been reported to measure amniotic fluid lung surfactant activity. However, they have been employed predominately in research settings and their applicability for clinical use has not been demonstrated.

VII. Amniotic Fluid Hormones

A. Cortisol

Glucocorticoids have been shown to be important in the synthesis of fetal lung surfactant. In addition, it is generally accepted that amniotic fluid cortisol is of fetal origin. Consequently, many investigators have assayed cortisol in amniotic fluid. It has been shown to increase with gestational age [38]; however, the spread of values for any specific gestational age has been so wide that there has been no real concensus as to its value as a fetal lung maturity test.

B. Estriol

Bacigalupo et al. [39] have reported on estriol (E_3) levels of amniotic fluid as have several others. Estriol levels tend to increase with gestational age but the spread of values is as great as with cortisol. They also calculated the unconjugated/total E_3 ratio and found a significant negative correlation with gestational age. However, no specific level was reported which indicated maturity. Little interest has subsequently been shown in amniotic fluid E_3 as a fetal maturity test.

VIII. Amniotic Fluid Enzymes

A. Phosphatidic Acid Phosphohydrolase

Phosphatidic acid phosphohydrolase (PAPase) catalyzes the hydrolysis of phosphatidic acid to diglyceride, the cosubstrate for lecithin biosynthesis, as well as the hydrolysis of phosphatidylglycerophosphate in the synthesis of phosphatidylglycerol. Amniotic fluid PAPase originates in the fetal lungs and its concentration increases with gestational age. This increase was reported to parallel the rise in L/S ratio and to precede it by approximately 1 week [40]. On a theoretical basis this enzyme should herald fetal lung surfactant synthesis and further studies are indicated.

B. Alkaline Phosphatase

Alkaline phosphatase (ALP) is found in lamellar bodies of fetal pneumocytes where it is thought to be directly involved in surfactant biosynthesis. Amniotic fluid ALP activity peaks in midpregnancy (19–21 weeks), falls to a nadir at 28-30 weeks, and then rises again to another peak at term [41]. This increase is mostly in the heat-labile fraction thought to represent fetal sources (bone, kidney, liver), and its continued rise suggests fetal maturity.

C. Amylase

Amylase is present primarily in the saliva and urine. Because these fluids contribute significantly to amniotic fluid (AF) it was speculated that amylase will be present in AF. Indeed, amylase activity was detected in AF as early as 16–18 weeks and was reported to increase sharply after 34 weeks [42]. Because of the wide range of values the test was not considered useful in fetal maturity assessment. However, a more recent study renewed interest in the use of AF amylase determinations for that purpose [43]. An amylase concentration > 300 U/liter was found to correlate significantly with gestational age of > 37 weeks, and an L/S ratio > 2.0; whereas, amylase concentration < 200 U/liter was found to correlate significantly with gestational age < 37 weeks and L/S ratio < 2.0. The test is very simple, cheap, and rapid, and it should be investigated further.

D. Other

Armstrong et al. [44] reported that AF peroxidase was detectable in early pregnancy with a gradual increase till 34 weeks. During the final 6 weeks of normal pregnancy, peroxidase activity rises sharply. Acid phosphatase and hexosaminidase activities were reported to increase with gestational age. However, the variation in activity was too great to be useful in predicting gestational age [45]. Gamma-glutamyl transaminase and 5′-nucleotidase have also been assayed in amniotic fluid in relation to gestational age [41] and appear to be of little value as a fetal maturity test.

IX. Miscellaneous

The amniocrit [46] utilizes an ordinary centrifuge and a special centrifuge tube to measure the sediment in amniotic fluid (similar to a hematocrit test), which correlates well with gestational age. The amniocrit is read in a similar fashion as an hematocrit. This test is based on the fact that cellular debris and vernix increases with advancing fetal maturity and is a very simple test to perform. The squalene content of the centrifuged pellet of amniotic fluid, assayed by gas chromatography, has been found to also be related to gestational age [47].

Antibodies to the protein moiety of lung surfactant have been made using material isolated from adult lungs and these antibodies have been employed to measure surfactant in amniotic fluid [48]. Surfactant protein first appears at 30 weeks' gestation and reaches a maximum at 37 weeks. It is unclear whether the apoprotein of lung surfactant appears free in amniotic fluid or occurs only bound to the lipid moiety. Theoretically, this may be the most important method for assaying fetal lung maturity, since it presumably measures true lung surfactant activity. The difficulty with this assay currently is the unavailability of the antibodies commercially.

X. Summary

There are a variety of tests available to clinical laboratories to evaluate fetal maturity. Since the lungs are generally the last organ system to mature in the developing fetus and since RDS is the most feared disease in the premature infant, those tests that evaluate fetal lung maturity are the most widely utilized. The fundamental principles upon which all fetal lung maturity tests are based are that the production of lung surfactant increases with advancing pulmonary maturity and the surfactant gains entrance into the amniotic cavity aided by fetal respiratory movements. The surfactant concentration or activity is generally measured by one of two means: (1) determination of one or more of its phospholipid moieties, or (2) determination of the physical properties of the amniotic fluid, i.e., surface tension or microviscosity.

Fetal maturity tests, in general, vary considerably in overall cost, technical expertise required, necessary equipment, technician time, and accuracy of prediction. Regarding the latter, most fetal lung maturity tests will fairly accurately predict the absence of RDS, i.e., few false positive results; however, no test or battery of tests will consistently predict that an infant will develop RDS, i.e., a high percentage of false negative results. For this reason we feel that values below the "mature" cut-off point should be viewed as representing a certain degree of risk of RDS should delivery occur, with the general concept that the lower the value the higher the risk.

It would seem reasonable that a combination of several tests would increase the accuracy of prediction; however, the greater the number of tests, the larger is the overall expense. The tests selected to be performed by a clinical laboratory are generally determined by the overall demand, the hospital budget, the interest of the laboratory director, and previous experience with particular tests. Regardless of which tests are selected, we think it is of utmost importance for laboratories to establish their own cut-off points for maturity and to monitor their accuracy of predictions through neonatal follow-up. The only way obstetricians, pediatricians, and laboratory directors can get a feel for the predictive accuracy of a particular test is for there to be a concerted, joint effort in providing neonatal follow-up.

References

1. Lambl, D., Ein seltener Fall von Hydramnios, *Centralbl. f. Gynakol.*, **5**:329 (1881).
2. Bevis, D. C. A., The antenatal prediction of haemolytic disease of the newborn, *Lancet,* **i**:395 (1952).
3. Daniel, M., Recherches sur la cytologie du liquide amniotique, *Ann. de Gynec. et d'Obst.,* Paris, 2nd Ser., **1**:466 (1904).
4. Meyer, J. R., Embolia pulmonar amnio-caseosa, *Bra. Med.,* **2**:301 (1926).
5. Bourgeois, G. A., The identification of fetal squames and the diagnosis of ruptured membranes by vaginal smear, *Am. J. Obstet. Gynecol.,* **44**:80 (1942).
6. Blystad, W., B. H. Landing, and C. A. Smith, Pulmonary hyaline membranes in newborn infants. Statistical, morphologic and experimental study of their nature, occurrence and significance, *Pediatrics,* **8**:5 (1951).
7. Kittrich, M., Zytodiagnostik des Fruchtwasserabflusses mit Hilfe von Nilblau, *Geburtshilfe, Frauenheilkd.,* **23**:156 (1963).
8. Brosens, I., and H. Gordon, The estimation of maturity by cytological examination of the liquor amnii, *J. Obstet. Gynaecol. Br. Cwlth.,* **73**:88 (1966).
9. Mandelbaum, B., G. C. LaCroix, and A. R. Robinson, Determination of fetal maturity by spectrophotometric analysis of amniotic fluid, *Obstet. Gynecol.,* **29**:471 (1967).
10. Sbarra, A. J., H. Michlewitz, R. J. Selvaraj, G. W. Mitchell, Jr., C. L. Detrulo, E. C. Kelley, Jr., J. L. Kennedy, Jr., M. J. Merschel, B. B. Paul, and F. Louis, Correlation between amniotic fluid optical density and L/S ratio, *Obstet. Gynecol.,* **48**:613 (1976).
11. Williams, J. L., and J. A. Bargen, The uric acid content of human amniotic fluid, *Am. J. Obstet. Gynecol.,* **7**:406 (1924).

12. Woyton, J., Die Beurteilung des Reifegrades der Frucht aug grund der Fruchtwasseruntersuchung. II. Bestimmung des Kreatinin- und Fettgehaltes sowie der Fruchtwassertrubung, *Zentralbl. Gynakol.,* **85**:552 (1963).
13. Pitkin, R. M., and S. J. Zwirek, Amniotic fluid creatinine, *Am. J. Obstet. Gynecol.,* **98**:1135 (1967).
14. Lind, T., and F. E. Hytten, Fetal control of fetal fluids. In *Physiological Biochemistry of the Fetus.* Edited by A. A. Hodari and F. G. Mariona. Springfield, Illinois, Charles C. Thomas, 1972, pp. 54-65.
15. Miles, P. A., and J. W. Pearson, Amniotic fluid osmolality in assessing fetal maturity, *Obstet. Gynecol.,* **34**:701 (1969).
16. Penny, L. L., D. D. Hagerman, and C. A. Sei, Specificity and reproducibility of acetone precipitation in identifying surface-active phosphatidylcholine in amniotic fluid, *Clin. Chem.,* **22**:681 (1976).
17. Nelson, G. H., Determination of amniotic fluid total phospholipid phosphorus as a test for fetal lung maturity, *Am. J. Obstet. Gynecol.,* **115**:933 (1973).
18. Schreyer, P., I. Tamir, I. Bukovsky, Z. Weinraub, and E. Caspi, Amniotic fluid total phospholipids versus lecithin/sphingomyelin ratio in the evaluation of fetal lung maturity, *Am. J. Obstet. Gynecol.,* **120**:909 (1974).
19. Fairbrother, P. F., V. Baynham, and D. A. Davey, A comparative clinical evaluation of the foam test and phospholipid assay of amniotic fluid, *Br. J. Obstet. Gynaecol.,* **82**:187 (1975).
20. Bhagwanani, S. G., D. Fahmy, and A. C. Turnbull, Prediction of neonatal respiratory distress by estimation of amniotic fluid lecithin, *Lancet,* **i**:159 (1972).
21. Torday, J., L. Carson, and E. E. Lawson, Saturated phosphatidyl choline in amniotic fluid and prediction of the respiratory distress syndrome, *New Engl. J. Med.,* **301**:1013 (1979).
22. Sbarra, A. J., R. J. Selvaraj, J. L. Kennedy, Jr., G. W. Mitchell, Jr., and B. B. Paul, A new amniotic fluid lecithin button test, *Obstets. Gynecol.,* **44**:500 (1974).
23. Tatsumi, H., N. Shimada, R. Kuramoto, Y. Mochizuki, M. Nishizima, M. Arai, K. Osanai, K. Ishihara, K. Goso, and K. Hotta, The phenol trubidity test for measurement of pulmonary surfactants in aminiotic fluid. Rapid test for fetal lung maturity, *Acta Obstet. Gynaecol. Jpn.,* **33**:643 (1981).
24. Gluck, L., M. V. Kulovich, R. C. Borer, Jr., P. H. Brenner, G. G. Anderson, and W. M. Spellacy, Diagnosis of the respiratory distress syndrome by amniocentesis, *Am. J. Obstet. Gynecol.,* **109**:440 (1971).
25. Hallman, M., M. Kulovich, E. Kirkpatrick, R. G. Sugarman, and L. Gluck, Phosphatidylinositol and phosphatidylglycerol in amniotic fluid: Indices of lung maturity, *Am. J. Obstet. Gynecol.,* **125**:613 (1976).
26. Andrews, A. G., J. B. Brown, P. E. Jeffery, and I. Horacek, Amniotic fluid palmitic acid/stearic acid ratios, lecithin/spingomyelin ratios and palmitic

acid concentrations in the assessment of fetal lung maturity in diabetic pregnancies, *Br. J. Obstet. Gynaecol.,* **86**:959 (1979).
27. Muller-Tyl, E., and J. Lempert, The prediction of fetal lung maturity from the surface tension characteristics of amniotic fluid, *J. Perinat. Med.,* **3**:47 (1975).
28. Rubaltelli, F. F., M. Rondinelli, C. Zorzi, and O. S. Saia, Amniotic fluid surface tension during pregnancy, *Biol. Neonate,* **29**:112 (1976).
29. Clements, J. A., A. C. G. Platzker, D. F. Tierney, C. J. Hobel, R. K. Creasy, A. J. Margolis, D. W. Thibeault, W. H. Tooley, and W. Oh, Assessment of the risk of the respiratory distress syndrome by a rapid test for surfactant in amniotic fluid, *New Engl. J. Med.,* **286**:1077 (1972).
30. Edwards, J., and P. Baillie, A simple method of detecting pulmonary surfactant activity in amniotic fluid. *S. Afr. Med. J.,* **47**:2070 (1973).
31. Socol, M. L., E. Sing, and O. R. Depp, The tap test: A rapid indication of fetal pulmonary maturity, *Am. J. Obstet. Gynecol.,* **148**:445 (1984).
32. Shinitzky, M., A. C. Dianoux, C. Gitler, and G. Weber, Microviscosity and order in the hydrocarbon region of miscelles and membranes determined with fluorescent probes. I. Synthetic miscelles, *Biochemistry,* **10**:2106 (1971).
33. Shinitzky, M., A. Goldfisher, A. Bruck, B. Goldman, E. Stern, G. Barkai, S. Mashiach, and D. M. Serr, A new method of assessment of fetal lung maturity, *Br. J. Obstet. Gynaecol.,* **83**:838 (1976).
34. Elrad, H., S. N. Beydoun, J. H. Hagen, M. T. Cabalum, and R. H. Aubry, Fetal pulmonary maturity as determined by fluorescent polarization of amniotic fluid, *Am. J. Obstet. Gynecol.,* **132**:681 (1978).
35. Pattle, R. E., G. J. Robards, and P. D. Sutherland, Stability of very small bubbles in human amniotic fluid, *J. Physiol.,* (Lond.) **259**:60P (1976).
36. Enhorning, G., and T. H. Kirschbaum, Surface tension of the respiratory tract fluid in fetal guinea pigs, *Am. J. Obstet. Gynecol.,* **90**:537 (1964).
37. Parkinson, C. E., D. Harvey, and D. Talbert, Bubble clicking in amniotic fluid, *Lancet,* **i**:1264 (1973).
38. Sivakumaran, T., M. L. Duncan, S. B. Effer, and E. V. Younglai, Relationship between cortisol and lecithin/sphingomyelin ratios in human amniotic fluid, *Am. J. Obstet. Gynecol.,* **122**:291 (1975).
39. Bacigalupo, G., E. Z. Saling, and J. W. Dudenhausen, Unconjugated and total estriol in human amniotic fluid-changes in the ratios between the two estriol levels with advancing gestational age, *J. Perinat. Med.,* **7**:262 (1979).
40. Jimenez, J. M., F. M. Schultz, and J. M. Johnston, Fetal lung maturation. III. Amniotic fluid phosphatidic acid phosphohydrolase (PAPase) and its relation to the lecithin/sphingomyelin ratio, *Obstet. Gynecol.,* **46**:588 (1975).

41. Brocklehurst, D., and C. E. Wilde, Amniotic fluid alkaline phosphatase, gamma-glutamyltransferase, and 5′-nucleotidase activity from 13 to 40 weeks' gestation, and alkaline phosphatase as an index of fetal lung maturity, *Clin. Chem.,* **26/5**:588 (1980).
42. Wolf, R. O., and L. M. Taussig, Human amniotic fluid isoamylases: Functional development of fetal pancreas and salivary glands, *Gynecol. Obstet.,* **41**:337 (1973).
43. De Grandi, P., M. Ramzin, A. Luthi, and M. Hinselmann, Relationship between amylase concentration, L/S ratio and lecithin concentrations in amniotic fluid, *Obstet. Gynecol. Invest.,* **10**:23 (1979).
44. Armstrong, D., D. E. Van Wormer, S. Dimmitt, P. May, and W. P. Gideon, The determination of peroxidase in amniotic fluid, *Obstet. Gynecol.,* **47**: 593 (1976).
45. Sutcliffe, R. G., D. J. H. Brock, H. G. Robertson, et al., Enzymes in amniotic fluid: A study of specific activity patterns during pregnancy, *J. Obstet. Gynaec. Br. Commwlth.,* **79**:895 (1972).
46. Ver-Medrano, C., J. Ramirez, G. Canovas, G. Aguad, S. Zuleta, S. Pescio, C. Weber, R. Gonzalez, and F. Zapata, Determination of fetal maturity from the measurement of the sedimentary fraction of the amniotic fluid (amniocrit), *J. Perinat., Med.,* **6**:28 (1978).
47. Wysocki, S. J., R. Hahnel, M. J. Millward, and D. T. Jenkins, Amniotic fluid squalene and fetal maturity, *Br. J. Obstet. Gynaecol.,* **86**:854 (1979).
48. King, R. J., J. Ruch, E. G. Gikas, A. C. G. Platzker, and R. K. Creasy, Appearance of apoproteins of pulmonary surfactant in human amniotic fluid, *J. Appl. Physiol.,* **39**:735 (1975).

7

Amniotic Fluid Lecithin Concentration as a Fetal Lung Maturity Test

GEORGE H. NELSON and HOSSAM E. FADEL

Medical College of Georgia
Augusta, Georgia

I. Introduction

We began examining phospholipids in amniotic fluid in the late 1960s following reports which suggested that lecithin-rich surfactant might be present in amniotic fluid associated with mature infants, while it might be deficient in cases in which the infant might develop hyaline membrane disease (HMD). Klaus et al. [1] had identified lecithin as the major component of surfactant. Also Chu et al. [2] and Adams et al. [3] had reported a significant decrease in the lecithin content of the lungs of infants dying of HMD. Several investigators [4,5] as well as Reynolds in 1953 [6] had already suggested that fetal alveolar fluid contributed to the formation of amniotic fluid. In addition, Ross [4] and Setniker et al. [5] felt that the outward flow of alveolar fluid toward the amniotic fluid was aided by respiratory movements. Therefore, these investigators had already planted the seeds for a study of phospholipids (particularly lecithin) in amniotic fluid collected from pregnancies in which the infants did or did not develop respiratory distress syndrome (RDS).

At the time we were investigating placental phospholipid patterns by thin-layer chromatography [7]. Therefore, it was relatively easy to modify our tissue technique to determine the phospholipids in amniotic fluid. In order to correlate the amniotic fluid phospholipid patterns with the development of RDS, we realized two things from the beginning: (1) the amniotic fluid had to be collected within a reasonable time of delivery (we later defined this as 72 hr); and (2) the amniotic fluid had to be relatively blood-free, since plasma was known to be rich in phospholipids. Since amniocentesis at that time was a procedure virtually limited to patients with Rh incompatibility, sample collection was initially done at the time of artificial rupture of membranes. Another point which was not known at the time was whether or not the fluid should be centrifuged prior to phospholipid determination. Initially, we ran fluids both ways and finally determined it was better to centrifuge the fluids. By the end of 1968 we had analyzed 10 control fluids (infants did not develop RDS) and three fluids from infants who did develop RDS, one of whom died from HMD. These data were published in 1969; Table 1 shows the lecithin phosphorus concentration data. Initially we thought that an expression of lecithin as a percentage of total phospholipid might be the best way to evaluate fetal lung maturity; however, it soon became apparent that a concentration measurement was probably the best way. Despite the fact that these data supported the concept that amniotic fluid lecithin analysis might be employed prospectively as a fetal lung maturity test, amniocentesis for evaluation of fetal lung maturity was very slow to come. Therefore, we continued to collect samples at the time of artificial rupture of membranes in an attempt to enlarge our series of fluids collected near delivery from

Table 1 Lecithin Concentration in Amniotic Fluid from RDS and Control Infants

			Amniotic fluid lecithin phosphorus (mg/dl)	
Patient	Diagnosis	AF centrifuged	Patient	Control
S.W.	Eclampsia	No	0.035 (HMD, died)	0.445[a]
T.W.	Severe preeclampsia	Yes	0.031 (RDS, lived)	0.318[b]
M.D.	Diabetes	Yes	0.075 (RDS, lived)	0.318

[a]Mean of 10 uncentrifuged amniotic fluid samples.
[b]Mean of 10 centrifuged amniotic fluid samples.
Source: Nelson, G. H., Amniotic fluid phospholipid patterns in normal and abnormal pregnancies. *Am. J. Obstet. Gynecol.*, **105**:1072 (1969).

pregnancies whose infants developed RDS. It was not until 1971 that we had accumulated an additional 10 patients who developed RDS. These data along with 89 control patients were presented at the Sixth Rochester Trophoblast Conference in Rochester, N.Y., in 1971, and were published in the transcript of that meeting [8] and in the *American Journal of Obstetrics and Gynecology* in 1972 [9]. It was in early 1971 that a few obstetricians in our area began to perform amniocentesis prospectively for fetal lung maturity evaluation. The first obstetrician to utilize our lecithin test for patient management was G. Pat Williams, a private practitioner in Augusta, Georgia. He was followed by O. Eduardo Talledo at the Medical College of Georgia and then other faculty, residents, and private Augusta obstetricians followed. At about this time Micki Souma and Cecil Whitaker in Columbus, Georgia, Thom Gailey in Greenville, South Carolina, and Hugh Gibson and Harvey Roddenberry in Macon, Georgia, began to do amniocentesis in their local hospitals and send the fluid to us by mail. Of the first 13 fluids we analyzed from pregnancies in which the infants developed RDS, 12 had lecithin P concentrations < 0.050 mg/dl and all 13 had values < 0.100. Therefore, the figure of 0.100 was chosen as being indicative of fetal lung maturity because: (1) most samples associated with RDS were less than half this figure and all were below this; and (2) it represented a round figure. However, the concept of having a "mature" and "immature" cut-off point never really appealed to us because it seemed clear from the very beginning that we were dealing with a risk of RDS and the lower the lecithin P value, the higher the risk. By approximately the end of 1973 we had accumulated 25 cases of RDS in which the lecithin P values were < 0.100. After grouping these values and plotting on semilog graph paper the mean values in each group against the risk of RDS in each group, a remarkable correlation was found. These data were submitted to the American Association of Obstetricians and Gynecologists for their 1974 Foundation Prize, which was subsequently awarded. The data are shown in Figure 1 and Table 2. As can be seen in Figure 1, the regression line extrapolates almost exactly through a lecithin P concentration value of 0.100 at 0% risk of RDS. Therefore, this mathematical equation verified our selection of 0.100 as the lecithin P value above which RDS should be rare indeed. Between 1972 and 1974, because of the national interest in the lecithin/sphingomyelin (L/S) ratio determination, we performed several hundred measurements of lecithin P concentration and L/S ratio on the same amniotic fluid samples. Most of the time the two measurements agreed; however, sometimes the L/S ratio would be high, while the lecithin P value was not. In those cases, the L/S ratio was falsely elevated because of an unusually low sphingomyelin level. To this date no one knows what controls the sphingomyelin level in amniotic fluid. We strongly suspect that many cases of RDS associated with "mature" L/S ratios are the result of falsely elevated values because of low sphingomyelin levels. This seems to be particularly true in diabetic pregnancies. We feel that it was an unfortunate occurrence that most of the investigators chose to monitor fetal lung maturity with L/S ratios rather than a quantitative lecithin measurement. In our institution we have not done an L/S ratio since 1974 and the L/S ratio has never been utilized in patient management.

After following a number of patients with serial lecithin phosphorus measurements, we made another interesting observation. The amniotic fluid lecithin P concentrations remain below 0.050 mg/dl until some point in time when they rise, sometimes rise quite abruptly. The lecithin P values usually did not remain in the 0.050–0.099 zone longer than 1 week. Some typical serial lecithin assays are illustrated in Figure 2. This prompted us to manage many patients whose values were in the 0.050–0.099 zone by not repeating the amniocentesis but instead delaying delivery by at least a week. Therefore, these general guidelines have been in effect since approximately 1973: (1) If the lecithin P concentration is < 0.050 mg/dl, repeat the amniocentesis in 1–2 weeks;

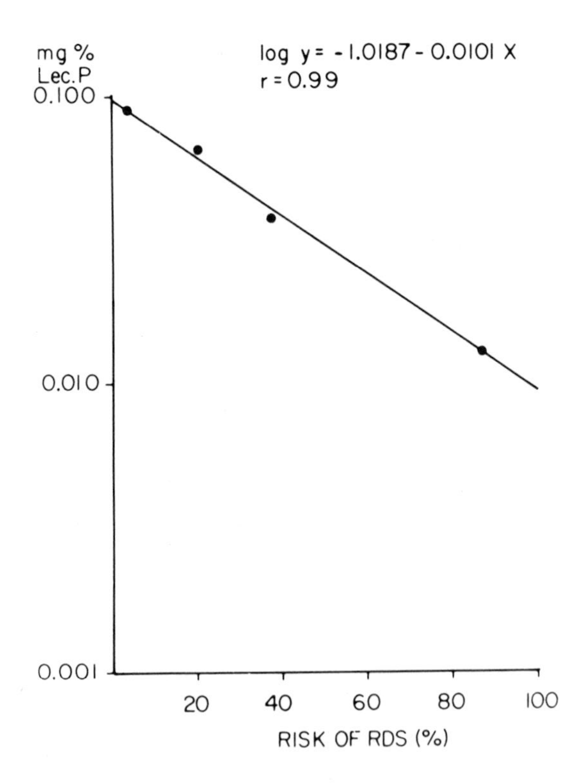

Figure 1 Relationship between amniotic fluid lecithin concentration and risk of RDS. (From Nelson, G. H., Risk of respiratory distress syndrome as determined by amniotic fluid lecithin concentration. *Am. J. Obstet. Gynecol.*, **121**:753 [1975].)

Table 2 Relationship Between Amniotic Fluid Lecithin Concentration and Risk of RDS

Lec P conc. (mg/dl)	Risk of RDS (%)
< 0.025	60 - 100
0.025-0.049	30 - 60
0.050-0.074	10 - 30
0.075-0.099	1 - 10
0.100 or greater	< 1

Source: Nelson, G. H., Risk of respiratory distress syndrome as determined by amniotic fluid lecithin concentration, *Am. J. Obstet. Gynecol.*, **121**:753 (1975).

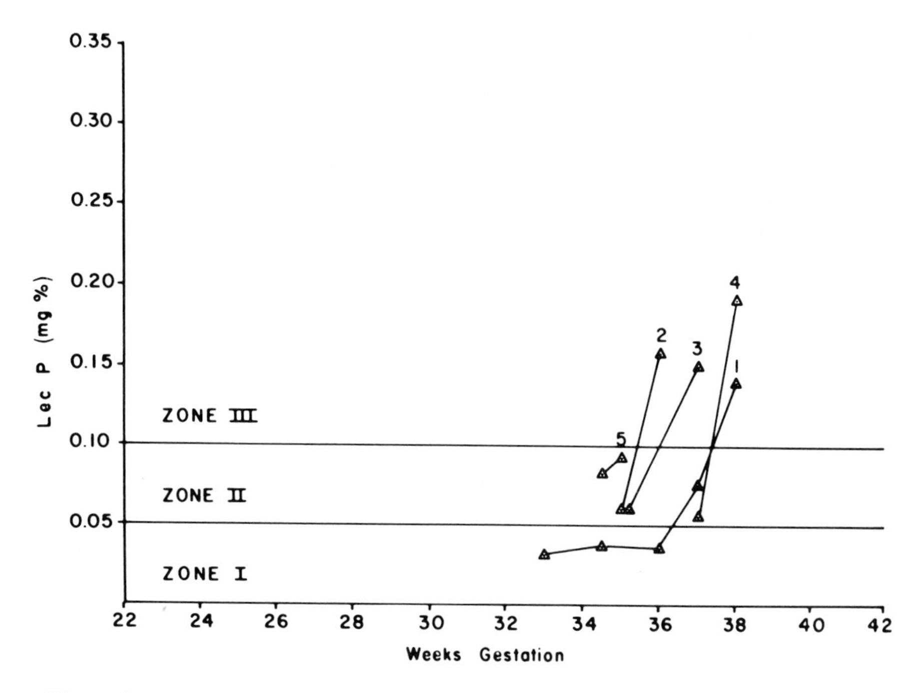

Figure 2 Serial analyses of amniotic fluid lecithin concentration in five patients. (From Nelson, G. H., Lecithin concentration of amniotic fluid as an index of fetal maturity. In *Amniotic Fluid Physiology, Biochemistry, and Clinical Chemistry*. Edited by S. Natelson, A. Scommegna, and M. B. Opstein. New York, Wiley, 1974, pp. 221–246.)

(2) if the lecithin value is between 0.050 and 0.099, delay delivery at least 1 week, then proceed with delivery if indicated; and (3) if the lecithin value is 0.100 or greater, proceed with delivery if indicated.

II. Data Collected at the Medical College of Georgia from 1970-1983

We have recently reviewed our data with the lecithin concentration measurement from amniocentesis specimens from 1970 through 1983. Table 3 shows that we have done 4635 measurements on 3720 patients. By one of the two methods described above we have made a prediction of mature fetal lungs and have neonatal follow-ups in 2673 patients. Neonatal follow-up was obtained in one of two ways. First, the neonatal records of infants delivered at the Medical College of Georgia were reviewed and the discharge diagnoses were obtained. Secondly, for deliveries occuring outside the Medical College of Georgia the attending obstetrician was mailed a follow-up sheet, which contained questions concerning the date and method of delivery and the development of RDS. In all cases, a diagnosis of transient tachypnea of the newborn was not considered to be RDS. In cases where the diagnosis was pneumonia vs. RDS, the latter was considered to be the diagnosis. In cases where the severity of RDS was in doubt, the more severe diagnosis was recorded. We fully realize that there were no uniform criteria applied to either the diagnosis of RDS or its various degrees of severity in the many institutions involved and during the time span covered in this report. Despite these shortcomings, this concerted attempt at follow-up has confirmed the accuracy of this method of predicting fetal lung maturity. It should be emphasized that the procedural aspect of lecithin P determination has not changed during this time period (1970-1983).

Table 3 Amniotic Fluid Lecithin[a] Concentration

No. of amniocentesis samples analyzed	4635
No. of patients studied	3720
No. of patients with lecithin 0.100 or greater prior to delivery with neonatal follow-up	2136
No. of patients with last lecithin 0.050-0.099 at least 1 week prior to delivery with neonatal follow-up	537
No. of patients with last lecithin < 0.050 or last lecithin 0.050-0.099 < 1 week prior to delivery or no neonatal follow-up available	1047

[a]Expressed as mg/dl lec P.

Table 4 Source of Study Patients

Amniocentesis performed at	No.	%
A. Medical College of Georgia	1381	37.1
B. Greenville, South Carolina	503	13.5
C. Columbus, Georgia	413	11.1
D. Macon, Georgia	394	10.6
E. Other[a]	1029	27.7
Total	3720	100.0

[a]Approximately 20 hospitals throughout Georgia and South Carolina.

Table 4 illustrates the distribution of patients which we have studied. It can be seen that 37% of the patients are from the Medical College of Georgia (MCG), while 63% have been outside patients, the majority of whom have been from outside Augusta with Greenville, South Carolina, Columbus, Georgia, and Macon, Georgia, being the most frequent cities from which we have received amniotic fluid samples. Our general policy for processing fluids from outside Augusta has been for the referring laboratory to centrifuge the fluid soon after collection (approximately 1200 rpm for 10 min). The supernatant is placed in a brown bottle and mailed by ordinary mail. Amniotic fluid lecithin is stable for at least 4 days when the fluid is shipped in this manner. If the fluids are sent uncentrifuged and then are centrifuged 3 days after collection, falsely low lecithin values may be obtained. Table 5 shows that we have had 20 possible cases of RDS associated with a lecithin P concentration of 0.100 or greater. Table 6 describes these 20 patients. In four of the patients there was evidence of old blood in the amniotic fluid on collection. This means that the fluids were brown in color, had no intact RBCs present on centrifugation, and had a 410 nm hemoglobin peak on spectral scan. While hemoglobin per se does not elevate a

Table 5 RDS in All Patients Lecithin[a] Concentration

0.100 or greater prior to delivery	
Total	2136
RDS	20 (0.9%)

[a]Expressed as mg/dl lec P.

Table 6 20 Patients with Lecithin[a] Value 0.100 or Greater Prior to Delivery Whose Infants Developed RDS

Reason for amniocentesis	Vaginal delivery (V) or cesarean section (CS)	EOB[b]	Severity of RDS
1. Hypertension	CS	Yes	Severe
2. Hypertension	CS	Yes	Severe
3. Diabetes	CS	No	Severe
4. Repeat CS	CS	No	Severe
1. Diabetes	CS	No	Moderate
2. Repeat CS	CS	No	Moderate
3. Repeat CS	CS	No	Moderate
4. RH disease	CS	No	Moderate
5. Premature labor	V	?	Moderate
1. Diabetes	?	Yes	Unknown
1. Diabetes	CS	No	Mild
2. Diabetes	CS	No	Mild
3. RH disease	V	No	Mild
4. RH disease, twins	V	No	Mild
5. Repeat CS	CS	No	Mild
6. Repeat CS	CS	No	Mild
7. Repeat CS	CS	No	Mild
8. Repeat CS	CS	No	Mild
9. Repeat CS	CS	No	Mild
10. Sickle cell disease, twins	CS	Yes	Mild

[a]Expressed as mg/dl lec P.
[b]EOB = Evidence of old blood in amniotic fluid on spectral scan.

lecithin P determination, contamination with plasma would increase the value. Following a bleed into the amniotic fluid we have always assumed that a subsequent tap would yield accurate results if the fluid showed no evidence of hemoglobin contamination. However, we might logically reason that the fluid contains residual plasma contamination if it shows evidence of hemoglobin contamination. Table 7 illustrates the risk of "serious" RDS associated with a lecithin value of 0.100 or greater. We have defined "serious" as being severe or moderate

Table 7 Risk of Serious (Severe, Moderate, Unknown) RDS With Lecithin[a] 0.100 or Greater Prior to Delivery

		Risk (%)
1. All patients including those with EOB[b]	10/2136	0.5
2. All patients excluding those with EOB[b]	7/2133	0.3

[a]Expressed as mg/dl lec P.
[b]EOB = Evidence of old blood in amniotic fluid on spectral scan.

RDS or RDS of unknown severity. As can be seen, if we exclude the three cases which exhibited evidence of contamination of the amniotic fluid with old blood, the number of false positive predictions was seven out of 2133 or 0.3%. In Table 8 we see the false positive prediction rate when the last lec P concentration obtained was between 0.050 and 0.099 mg/dl at least 1 week prior to delivery. There were 12 possible cases of RDS and these are detailed in Table 9. Of these 12, four were severe or moderate and two of these also showed evidence of old blood in the amniotic fluid. Therefore, as seen in Table 10, the risk of serious RDS associated with a last lecithin value of 0.050-0.099 at least 1 week prior to delivery was two out of 535 or 0.4%, excluding those with evidence of old blood in the fluid.

Tables 11-13 summarize the data obtained from Medical College of Georgia patients. As can be seen, we have studied 1381 patients and made a prediction of fetal lung maturity antepartum and have a neonatal follow-up in 1093 patients. In these patients there were seven possible cases of RDS (Tables 12 and 13), three of which were serious. Of these three cases, the final diagnosis in one was moderate RDS vs. neonatal pneumonia, and in another the infant had severe RDS and septicemia and died at 2 days of age. It is of interest that we have not had a case of RDS, that we are aware of, in an infant of a diabetic mother

Table 8 RDS in All Patients Lecithin[a] Concentration

0.050-0.099	
At least 1 week prior to delivery	
Total	537
RDS	12 (2.2%)

[a]Expressed as mg/dl lec P.

Table 9 12 Patients With Last Lecithin[a] Value 0.050-0.099 at Least 1 Week Prior to Delivery Whose Infants Developed RDS

Reason for amniocentesis	Vaginal delivery (V) or cesarean section (CS)	EOB[b]	Severity of RDS
1. Placenta previa	CS	Yes	Severe
1. Hypertension Abruptio placentae	CS	Yes	Moderate
2. Hypertension, twins	V	No	Moderate
3. Repeat CS	CS	No	Moderate
1. Repeat CS	CS	No	Mild
2. Repeat CS	CS	No	Mild
3. Repeat CS	CS	No	Mild
4. Hypertension	V	No	Mild
5. Diabetes	CS	No	Mild
6. Diabetes	CS	No	Mild
7. Unsure dates	V	No	Mild
8. Unsure dates	V	No	Mild

[a]Expressed as mg/dl lec P.
[b]EOB = Evidence of old blood in amniotic fluid on spectral scan.

Table 10 Risk of Serious (Severe, Moderate, or Unknown) RDS With Last Lecithin[a] Value 0.050-0.099 At Least 1 Week Prior to Delivery

		Risk (%)
1. All patients including those with EOB[b]	4/537	0.7
2. All patients excluding those with EOB[b]	2/535	0.4

[a]Expressed as mg/dl lec P.
[b]EOB = Evidence of old blood in amniotic fluid on spectral scan.

Table 11 Amniotic Fluid Lecithin[a] Concentration in MCG Patients

No. of MCG patients studied	1381
No. of patients with lecithin 0.100 or greater prior to delivery with neonatal follow-up	937
No. of patients with last lecithin 0.050-0.099 at least 1 week prior to delivery with neonatal follow-up	156
No. of patients with last lecithin < 0.050 or last lecithin 0.050-0.099 < 1 week prior to delivery or no neonatal follow-up available	288

[a]Expressed as mg/dl lec P.

delivering at MCG in whom we made an antepartum prediction of mature fetal lungs. Fadel and Hammond [10] reviewed the management of 107 diabetics between July 1976 and December 1978 and reported this observation. As noted in Tables 6 and 9 we have had false positive predictions in diabetic patients from outside hospitals.

Table 12 RDS in MCG Patients—5 Patients with Lecithin[a] Value 0.100 or Greater Prior to Delivery Whose Infants Developed RDS

Total 937–5 RDS (0.5%)

Reason for amniocentesis	Vaginal delivery (V) or cesarean section (CS)	EOB[b]	Severity of RDS
1. Hypertension	CS	Yes	Severe
1. Premature labor	V	?	Moderate
2. Repeat CS	CS	No	Moderate
1. Repeat CS	CS	No	Mild
2. Sickle cell disease, twins	CS	Yes	Mild

[a]Expressed as mg/dl lec P.
[b]EOB = Evidence of old blood in amniotic fluid on spectral scan.

Table 13 RDS in MCG Patients–2 Patients with Last Lecithin[a] Value 0.050-0.099 at Least 1 Week Prior to Delivery Whose Infants Developed RDS

Total 156–2 RDS (1.3%)			
Reason for amniocentesis	Vaginal delivery (V) or cesarean section (CS)	EOB[b]	Severity of RDS
1. Repeat CS	CS	No	Mild
2. Unsure dates	V	No	Mild

[a]Expressed as mg/dl lec P.
[b]EOB = Evidence of old blood in amniotic fluid on spectral scan.

III. Discussion

Over the years we have been very satisfied with this method of predicting fetal lung maturity. It is quite apparent that these data support the hypothesis that a concentration measurement of lecithin (or surfactant) accurately predicts fetal lung development. Concentration measurements were originally criticized because it was believed that they would be significantly influenced by variations in amniotic fluid volume. We have recent data which show that, overall, amniotic fluid volume changes have minimal effects on concentration measurements [11]. Surely the effects are far less than are generally believed by many perinatologists. At any rate, we feel strongly that future research toward surfactant determinations should utilize concentration measurements.

We feel that the best way of considering any test for predicting fetal lung maturation is to consider a cut-off point above which the risk of RDS is minimal if the fetus is delivered (0.100 mg/dl lec P, by our method). In considering values below this cut-off point, it is best to consider the fetus as being at various degrees of risk. We should not expect that the neonate will always develop RDS if delivery occurs with a lecithin value below this point. The physiology of the situation prohibits such a conclusion. The fetal lungs must mature to the point that RDS will not occur *before* this is reflected in the amniotic fluid. We have previously shown [12] in the rat that amniotic fluid lecithin concentration lags about 1 day behind the concentration in fetal lung tissue. In human pregnancies this lag time is unknown, is possibly of a week or so in duration, and probably varies significantly from one subject to another. There are two factors operating when we observe a rise in amniotic fluid lecithin levels during serial analyses. One is an increased production of surfactant in the fetal lungs and the second is the rate at which surfactant-rich fluid is delivered to the amniotic fluid. We have seen amniotic fluid levels change abruptly from low to high values in as little time as a week. How long the high level had been present in the lungs prior to its manifestation in the amniotic fluid is not known.

By this method plasma contamination of the amniotic fluid will falsely elevate the lecithin concentration. The degree of blood contamination following a bloody tap can be estimated by measuring the volume of RBC after centrifugation. Small amounts of blood contamination (up to 0.1–0.2 ml RBC/9 ml of amniotic fluid) can be corrected for. However, when fresh blood contamination exceeds this or when the RBCs have hemolyzed and the reddish hemoglobin pigment has been changed to a brown color, it is not possible to correct for the degree of plasma contamination; hence, falsely high values may be obtained. We feel that old blood contamination probably contributed to some of our false predictions of mature fetal lungs in the past.

IV. Summary

1. A historical review of the development of the evaluation of fetal lung maturity by amniotic fluid analysis at the Medical College of Georgia has been presented.
2. The measurement of the concentration of lecithin phosphorus has been and continues to be the primary means of evaluating fetal lung maturity at this institution.

Acknowledgments

The senior author (G. H. N.) gratefully recognizes the many obstetricians throughout Georgia and South Carolina who diligently completed and returned the neonatal follow-up sheets after delivery so that he could record the neonatal outcome, without which this report would have been impossible. In addition to those previously cited the following are acknowledged: Drs. Inman, George, and Middleton in Albany, Georgia; Dr. Dixon in Greenville, South Carolina, and Tifton, Georgia, and Dr. Hester in Macon, Georgia, and Tifton, Georgia; Drs. Amos, Roberts, Ward, Stamey, Dashiell, Everidge, Flanagen, and Lawler in Columbus, Georgia; Drs. Coppage, Hanberry, Herring, May, Souma, Schuessler, and Browne in Macon, Georgia; Drs. Cook, Hearin, Puckett, Ellison, House, Easley, Quattlebaum, Kellett, and Kellett, and the Smith Clinic in Greenville, South Carolina; Dr. Goodrich in Milledgeville, Georgia; Drs. Ramsey, Bodziner, and Bodziner in Savannah, Georgia; Drs. Wages and Gregory in Dalton, Georgia; Drs. Barfield, Daitch, Freedman, Owen, Bruns, Servy, Thaxton, and Mitchell in Augusta, Georgia; the numerous physicians who have had temporary assignments at Fort Gordon, Georgia, and Fort Benning, Georgia; plus the many obstetrical residents who trained over the years at the Medical Center of Central Georgia in Macon, Georgia and the Greenville General Hospital in Greenville, South Carolina.

References

1. Klaus, M. H., J. A. Clements, and R. J. Havel, Composition of surface-active material isolated from beef lung, *Proc. Natl. Acad. Sci.,* **47**:1858 (1961).
2. Chu, J., J. Clements, E. Cotton, M. Klaus, A. Sweet, M. Thomas, and W. Tooley, Preliminary report, The pulmonary hypoperfusion syndrome. *Pediatrics,* **35**:733 (1965).
3. Adams, F. H., T. Fujiwara, M. D. Emmanouilides, and A. Scudder, Surface properties and lipids from lungs of infants with hyaline membrane disease, *J. Pediatr.,* **66**:357 (1965).
4. Ross, B. B., Comparison of foetal pulmonary fluid with foetal plasma and amniotic fluid, *Nature,* **199**:1100 (1963).
5. Setniker, I., E. Agostoni, and A. Taglietti, The fetal lung, a source of amniotic fluid, *Proc. Soc. Exper. Biol Med.,* **101**:842 (1959).
6. Reynolds, S. R. M., A source of amniotic fluid in the lamb: The nasopharyngeal and buccal cavities, *Nature,* **172**:307 (1953).
7. Nelson, G. H., B. Kenimer, and A. Jones, Thin layer chromatography of placental phospholipids, *Am. J. Obstet Gynecol.,* **99**:262 (1967).
8. Nelson, G. H., Relationship between respiratory distress syndrome and amniotic fluid lecithin concentration. In *Trans. Sixth. Roch. Troph. Conf.* Edited by C. J. Lund and J. W. Choate. University of Rochester School of Medicine and Dentistry, **185**:217 (1971).
9. Nelson, G. H., Relationship between amniotic fluid lecithin concentration and respiratory distress syndrome, *Am. J. Obstet. Gynecol.,* **112**:827 (1972).
10. Fadel, H. E., and S. D. Hammond, Diabetes mellitus and pregnancy – Management and results, *J. Reprod. Med.,* **27**:56 (1982).
11. Nelson, G. H., and S. J. Nelson, Effect of amniotic fluid volume changes on surfactant concentration measurements, submitted for publication.
12. Nelson, G. H., K. Eguchi, and J. C. McPherson, Effects of gestational age, dexamethasone, and metopirone on lecithin concentration in fetal lung tissue and amniotic fluid, *Gynecol. Invest.,* **7**:337 (1976).

Part Three

INFLUENCING FACTORS

8

Respiratory Distress Syndrome in Various Cultures and a Possible Role of Diet

GEORGE H. NELSON and JAMES C. McPHERSON, JR.

Medical College of Georgia
Augusta, Georgia

I. Introduction

The attempt to determine the influence of culture and/or diet on the incidence of respiratory distress syndrome (RDS) and/or hyaline membrane disease (HMD) is a most difficult task. A major problem lies in the diagnosis. Much of the world literature fails to distinguish pulmonary surfactant deficiency (PSD) from other etiologies as a cause of respiratory distress. This is understandable because even now in many instances it is not possible to know with certainty whether PSD is or is not the reason for the respiratory problem. Also, earlier investigators did not appreciate the multiplicity of etiological factors in the development of respiratory distress. Another problem is that the role of heredity in the development of RDS has never been adequately studied. Also, there is not a single controlled study of the effect of diet on fetal pulmonary maturation in human subjects in the world literature. At least if such a study exists, the authors have been unable to locate it. Therefore, the only way one can attempt to relate diet and RDS in human subjects is to look at dietary patterns in various groups of women or in women in various parts of the world and the occurrence of RDS in these groups. Even this type of study is fraught with serious scientific deficiencies. Accurate dietary histories are almost impossible to obtain. Even if one could determine that some dietary pattern differed between two groups, it is impossible to control for the many other variables involved. Also, it is difficult for one to know if a certain dietary variable had a direct effect on surfactant production or an indirect effect on pulmonary maturation by modifying the incidence of premature deliveries.

Despite the problems and inaccuracies involved, we will review in this chapter the incidence of RDS in various parts of the world. We will not attempt to review the serious adverse effects of severe maternal malnutrition on the fetus. Rather, we have attempted to look at dietary patterns to see if diet could be a possible etiological factor. As a result, we have stumbled across one peculiar dietary item which has intrigued us immensely. While the evidence at this point in time is circumstantial at best, we will suggest – we repeat suggest – a hypothesis. The hypothesis is that a deficiency of dietary palmitic acid may be associated with an increased incidence of this disease. The corollary is that adequate maternal dietary consumption of palmitic acid may protect against the disease. We will attempt to defend this hypothesis as scientifically as possible while at the same time we fully realize that future research may completely refute the theory. However, we feel the concept has such medical significance that we would rather present it and be wrong than not to present it at all. The idea of being able to influence fetal lung maturation in a mother at risk of a premature delivery by modifying her dietary habits is so appealing to us that we embark upon this venture at this time.

II. Worldwide Occurrence of RDS

Data on perinatal morbidity and mortality have been reported from virtually every part of the world. Many of these reports have contained information concerning the respiratory distress syndrome. Many variables exist which influence the incidence of RDS or HMD in worldwide reports. Some of these are listed in Table 1. It is obvious, therefore, that one must be extremely cautious in attempting to compare data from different parts of the world.

The most frequent ways in which investigators have reported their RDS data are as follows: (1) percentage of live births; (2) percentage of live premature births, either < 2500 g or < 37 weeks' gestation; (3) percentage of neonatal deaths; or (4) percentage of neonatal autopsies. Some of the reports from various parts of the world are listed in Tables 2 through 5. It would appear that the incidence of RDS worldwide is approximately as follows: (1) 1% of all live births; (2) 10–15% of all live premature births; and (3) 20–30% of all neonatal deaths and/or autopsies.

Table 1 Variables that Influence the Incidence of RDS or HMD in Worldwide Reports

1. Variations in criteria for making the diagnosis – clinical and/or pathological.
2. Variations in methods for reporting percentage data, such as percentage of RDS deaths may mean as percentage of live births or percentage of neonatal deaths.
3. Variations in incidences of other diseases influencing percentage data, such as increased percentage of infants with infections or trauma will automatically decrease the percentage of RDS (death data).
4. Variations in inclusion or exclusion of certain conditions in percentage data, such as deaths due to congenital anomalies.
5. Variations in the quality of neonatal care, such as postdelivery chilling.
6. Coding of infants by another disease, such as a neonatal RDS death may be coded as intraventricular hemorrhage.
7. Variations in normal birth weights, such as a definition of prematurity as $<$ 2500 g may be appropriate in some parts of the world but not in others.
8. Variations in true incidences in prematurity, such as multiple gestations are more common in some parts of the world or diseases endemic to some parts of the world may predispose to prematurity.
9. Introduction of new diagnoses, such as transient tachypnea of newborn or wet lung syndrome.
10. Introduction of new techniques to determine fetal maturity prenatally, such as ultrasound and amniotic fluid fetal lung maturity tests.
11. Introduction of pharmacological agents to induce fetal lung maturation, such as betamethasone.

One country from which many statistical reports have come is India. The incidence of RDS does appear to vary in different parts of India; however, our attempt to determine if this was in any way diet related was futile. However, another country from which unusual reports have consistently come is Nigeria. We do have some evidence, meager as it may be, that the incidence of RDS in Nigeria may be influenced by their dietary customs. Azubuike and Izuora [12], reporting from the University of Nigeria Teaching Hospital in Enugu, found six cases of RDS among 4296 live births between December 1973 and November 1975. In this group there were 235 deliveries $<$ 37 weeks' gestation, 230 of which weighed $<$ 2500 g. Of the six infants who developed RDS, four were between 30 and 34 weeks' gestation, weighing between 1200 and 1500 g, while

Table 2 Incidence of RDS in Various Parts of the World (Percentage of Live Births)

Author	Ref. no.	Country	Year	Incidence (%)
Farrell and Avery	1	U.S.A.	1968-1973	1.1
Usher et al.	2	Canada	1961-1963	1.7
Chalmers et al.	3	Great Britain	1965-1972	1.5
			1972-1975	0.77
Amiel-Tison et al.	4	France	1968-1969	1.0
			1972-1973	0.5
			1975-1977	0.5
Fanconi et al.	5	Switzerland	1974	0.67
Reed et al.	6	Norway	1967-1973	0.27
Ziai	7	Iran	1971-1973	0.27
Bhakoo et al.	8	India	1971-1973	0.7
Pai	9	India	1975	0.23
Thomas	10	India	1979-1980	0.7
Teck	11	Singapore	1964-1965	0.64
Azubuike and Izuora	12	Nigeria	1973-1975	0.14
Olowe and Akinkugbe	13	Nigeria	1973-1976	0.09
Chintu and Sukhani	14	Zambia	1976	1.04
Malan et al.	15	South Africa	1972-1973	1.11
		blacks,		1.06
		coloureds,		1.06
		and whites		1.35

two were infants of diabetic mothers and were 36 weeks' gestation, weighing 3500 and 3600 g. Therefore, the incidence of RDS in this report is 0.14% of all live births, 2.6% of live births < 37 weeks, and 1.7% of live births < 2500 g, all of which are low compared to other studies throughout the world. In addition, Olowe and Akinkugbe [13], reporting from the Lagos University Teaching Hospital, diagnosed only nine cases of RDS in 10,435 live births in a 4-year period from 1973 through 1976. Although these workers [13] did not report on the number of live premature births during this time, they comment as follows: "In Nigeria, the incidence of prematurity, whether defined by birth weight or gestational age, is high; but the experience of neonatologists all over the country shows that RDS is rarely encountered among the premature babies." Although not presenting any definitive data, Effiong [35], writing from the University College Hospital (UCH) in Ibadan, reviews the management and care of low birth weight infants. While discussing his experience concerning the respiratory problems of Nigerian low birth infants, he comments as follows about RDS, "We have seen only 2 or 3 cases during the last 12 months in UCH Ibadan."

In attempting to compare Azubuike and Izuora's [12] and Olowe and Akinkugbe's [13] data with comparable studies in other parts of Africa, the reports of Chintu and Sukhani [14] and Malan et al. [15] were selected for comparison. Chintu and Sukhani [14], reporting from the University Teaching Hospital in Lusaka, Zambia (formally Northern Rhodesia), admitted 171 hospital-born neonates with RDS to the special neonatal unit in 1976 from 16,454 live hospital-born infants. In addition to the 171 babies with RDS, 128 with aspiration pneumonia and 203 with bacterial pneumonia were admitted. Therefore, the 171 cases of RDS would appear to be a reasonably accurate number representing true RDS. Malan et al. [15], reporting on all live births during 1972 and 1973 in the Peninsula Maternity Service of the University of Cape Town Teaching Units at Groote Schuur Maternity, Mowbray Maternity, and Peninsula Maternity Hospitals, found 29 cases of RDS among 2730 black live births, 143 cases among 13,464 coloured live births, and 44 cases among 3248 white live

Table 3 Incidence of RDS in Various Parts of the World (Percentage of Live Premature Births)

Author	Ref. no.	Country	Year	Incidence (%)
Farrell and Avery	1	U.S.A.	1968–1973	14.0 (< 2500 g)
Amiel-Tison et al.	4	France	1975–1977	5.2 (< 2500 g) 11.0 (< 35 weeks)
Ziai	7	Iran	1971–1973	7.1 (< 2500 g)
Teck	11	Singapore	1964–1965	11.8 (< 2500 g)
Lowry	16	Jamaica	1974–1976	32.0 (< 37 weeks)
Azubuike and Izuora	12	Nigeria	1973–1975	2.6 (< 37 weeks) 1.7 (< 2500 g)
Malan et al.	15	South Africa blacks, coloureds, and whites	1972–1973	12.0 (< 37 weeks) 14.1 (< 37 weeks) 10.5 (< 37 weeks) 25.3 (< 37 weeks)

Table 4 Incidence of RDS in Various Parts of the World (Percentage of Neonatal Deaths)

Author	Ref. no.	Country	Year	Incidence (%)
Farrell and Wood	17	U.S.A.	1968-1973	20.0
Scott et al.	18	Northern Ireland	1974-1975	20.3
Registrar General	19	England and Wales	1972	18.9
Heetai and Roopnarinesingh	20	Trinidad	1973-1975	40.2
Bhakoo et al.	8	India	1971-1973	12.6
Tan and Boo	21	Singapore	1971-1973	30.1
Teck	11	Singapore	1964-1965	23.5
Chintu and Sukhani	14	Zambia	1976	17.0

births. These data are presented in Table 6. There is no significant difference between the two Nigerian studies nor between the Zambian and South African studies; however, both Nigerian studies show significantly less RDS than the Zambian and South African reports. In addition, Azubuike and Izuora [12] and Malan et al. [15] reported on the number of cases of RDS among their premature deliveries (< 37 weeks' gestation). These data are shown in Table 7. Again, the incidence of RDS is less in the Nigerian newborns. While the overall incidence of RDS was not significantly different among the three groups in the study of Malan et al. [15], the incidence was significantly higher among the white premature babies than among the blacks or the coloureds. While Olowe and Akinkugbe's report [13] didn't subdivide their 10,435 deliveries into premature and mature groups, Lesi [36] reported a prematurity rate of 13.9% (< 2500 g) from the same hospital in Nigeria in 1967. If we assume that Olowe and Akinkugbe's [13] nine cases of RDS came from their premature group and we assume a modest 10% premature rate, then the incidence of RDS in their premature deliveries was less than 1%, which is obviously a very low rate. These workers [13], suspecting that fetal pulmonary maturation occurred earlier in Nigerian pregnancies, determined L/S ratios in normal pregnant Nigerian women and compared the results with ratios reported from San Diego. They found significantly higher L/S ratios at 24, 26, 29, 30, 32, 33, 34, 35, 36, 37, and 39 weeks' gestation compared to the San Diego experience.

All these data definitely suggest that fetal lung maturation is accelerated and the incidence of neonatal RDS is low in Nigerian pregnancies. If we accept this hypothesis, let us examine some possible etiological factors. First, it seems reasonable to exclude race as a factor, since the Nigerian, Zambian, and black South African newborns have the same racial background, while the incidence of RDS is less in Nigerian than in Zambian and black South African infants. In searching for some other etiological factor let us look briefly at the country of Nigeria.

Table 5 Incidence of RDS in Various Parts of the World (Percentage of Neonatal Autopsies)

Author	Ref. no.	Country	Year	Incidence (%)
Fujikura and Froehlich	22	U.S.A.	1966	30.2
British P.M. Survey	23	Great Britain	1958	24.7
British P.M. Survey	24	Great Britain	1970	31.7
Brown and Sandhu	25	Uganda	1953-1964	10.9
Sivanesan	26	Malaya	1960	29.8
			1962	18.2
			1965	28.4
			1966	35.8
			1971	32.3
Sparke and Lowry	27	Jamaica	1974-1977	15.3
Teck	11	Singapore	1964-1965	27.3
Chuang	28	Hawaii	1958-1960	32.1
Rosahn and Sheanaku	29	Thailand	1959	15.0
Bhakoo et al.	8	India	1971-1973	11.9
Webb et al.	30	India	1959-1961	19.4
Banerjee et al.	31	India	1971-1974	9.6
Maheshwari et al.	32	India	1970	7.4
Pahimtoola et al.	33	India	1973	9.4
Shnier and Isaacson	34	South Africa	1965	13.0

Table 6 Incidence of RDS in Nigeria, Zambia, and South Africa (Percentage of Live Births)

Study	Country	Ref. no.	Year	No. of live births	No. of cases of RDS	% RDS	Significance[a] p value
A	Nigeria	12	1973–1975	4296	6	0.14	A vs. B NS[b]
B	Nigeria	13	1973–1976	10435	9	0.09	A vs. C < 0.001
C	Zambia	14	1976	16454	171	1.04	A vs. D_1 < 0.001
D_1	South Africa	15	1972–1973	2730	29	1.06	A vs. D_2 < 0.001
D_2	South Africa	15	1972–1973	13464	143	1.06	A vs. D_3 < 0.001
D_3	South Africa	15	1972–1973	3248	44	1.35	B vs. C < 0.001
							B vs. D_1 < 0.001
							B vs. D_2 < 0.001
							B vs. D_3 < 0.001
							C vs. D_1 NS
							C vs. D_2 NS
							C vs. D_3 NS
							D_1 vs. D_2 NS
							D_1 vs. D_3 NS
							D_2 vs. D_3 NS

Study D_1 = Blacks; D_2 = Coloureds; D_3 = Whites.
[a]Statistical analyses were done using the Chi square test by Mr. Harry C. Davis, Consulting Statistician, Medical College of Georgia, Augusta, Georgia.
[b]NS = Not Significant.

Table 7 Incidence of RDS in Nigeria, Zambia, and South Africa (Percentage of Live Premature Births)

Study	Definition of prematurity	No. of premature births	No. of cases of RDS	% RDS	Significance[a] p value
A	< 37 weeks	235	6	2.55	A vs. D_1 < 0.001
D_1	< 37 weeks	198	28	14.14	A vs. D_2 < 0.001
D_2	< 37 weeks	1244	131	10.53	A vs. D_3 < 0.001
D_3	< 37 weeks	107	27	25.25	D_1 vs. D_2 NS
					D_1 vs. D_3 < 0.001
					D_2 vs. D_3 < 0.001

Studies A, D_1, D_2, D_3 are same as in Table 6.
[a]Same as Table 6.

III. Nigeria

Nigeria is located in West Africa on the Gulf of Guinea, approximately 5°–15° North of the Equator. The cities of Lagos, Ibadan, and Enugu are all located in Southern Nigeria, approximately 7° North of the Equator; Lagos is a port city, while Ibadan and Enugu are approximately 100 miles inland. Nigeria is located in the heart of that area of Africa in which the oil palm, the common name for the African trees of the genus *Elaesis*, flourishes. The more widely known species, *E. guineensis*, is confined mainly to a 300-mile wide region along the coast of West Africa from Gambia to Angola (approximately 15° North to 15° South of the Equator) [37]. The fruit of the oil palm produces two kinds of oil. The oil from the fleshy pulp of the fruit is known as palm oil, or palm butter, and is particularly rich in triglycerides containing palmitic acid. The fatty acid composition of palm oil is compared to other edible oils and fats in Table 8. It can be seen that palm oil contains from two and one-half to five times as much palmitic acid as other edible oils and about twice as much as other solid edible fats. Palm oil is actually a solid at room temperature (mp 27–42°C) and has a dirty reddish-yellow color with a faint, slightly sweet odor. The seed of the fruit yields an oil known as palm kernel oil, or palm nut oil, which has a distinctly different fatty acid composition compared to palm oil.

In 1979 Okoh et al. [38] commented on the high content of palm oil in the Nigerian diet and performed gas chromatographic analysis of the palm oil

Table 8 Fatty Acid Composition of Various Edible Oils and Fats Used Worldwide

	Fatty acid % composition							
	Lauric (12:0)	Myristic (14:0)	Palmitic (16:0)	Stearic (18:0)	Oleic (18:1)	Linoleic (18:2)	Other	Total
Palm oil	–	1	46	5	38	9	1	100
Palm-kernel oil	50	16	8	3	15	2	6	100
Peanut oil	–	–	10	4	53	30	3	100
Corn oil	–	–	10	3	30	57	0	100
Cotton seed oil	–	1	21	2	18	53	5	100
Olive oil	–	–	6	4	83	7	0	100
Coconut oil	48	16	9	2	7	3	15	100
Safflower oil	–	–	6	3	13	78	0	100
Butter	4	10	25	11	39	5	5	100
Lard	–	2	23	15	47	9	4	100
Beef tallow	–	3	24	21	43	5	4	100
Mutton tallow	–	1	21	30	43	5	0	100

Source: PVO International Inc, *Composition and Physical Properties of Oils and Fats.* St. Louis, Missouri, PVO International Inc.

used domestically in Nigeria. They found a palmitic acid content of 47%, virtually identical to that reported in Table 8. In addition, they injected radiolabeled palmitic acid intravenously into mother rabbits and measured the incorporation rate into the lecithin of various fetal organs. The radiochromatograms showed a high incorporation rate into the lecithin of the fetal lungs and placenta. In their summary Okoh et al. [38] state that palm oil in Nigerian meals might be partly responsible for the low incidence of RDS in Nigerian premature infants. The 1982 *Encyclopedia Americana* states that palm oil is valued in cooking in Nigeria and no such mention is made concerning Zambia or South Africa [39].

IV. Animal Experiments and Other Supporting Data

In 1979 we began experiments in animals to test the hypothesis that maternal dietary intake of palmitic acid might influence fetal lung maturation. We fed pregnant rats one of three diets: fat free (FF); 10% corn oil (CO); or 10% palm oil (PO). We determined the concentration of acetone-precipitable lecithin (APL) in fetal lung tissue on gestational days 18, 20, and 21. The results are illustrated in Table 9. As can be seen, the increase in APL concentration is less during the last 3 days of gestation in the absence of maternal dietary fat than in the fat-containing diets. In addition, there was a significantly increased APL on gestational days 20 and 21 when the animals were on the PO diet as compared to the CO diet. Therefore, these data supported the hypothesis that high maternal dietary palmitate could promote fetal lung maturation.

In 1982 we reported further experimental data supporting this hypothesis. Pregnant rats were maintained on one of the following dietary regimens: (1) Low fat (LF = 1% corn oil) diet throughout gestation; (2) LF diet to gestational day 15, then to a palmitic acid-rich (PAR = 10% palm oil) diet until term; or (3) PAR diet throughout gestation. APL concentration was determined on day 21 and the results are shown in Figure 1. We concluded that fetal lung maturation was accelerated on a PAR diet, was intermediate in the group on the LF diet switched to the PAR diet, and was delayed on the LF diet.

In order for the hypothesis to be reasonable that an increased amount of palmitate in the maternal diet improves fetal lung maturation, there must be evidence that maternal dietary fat enters the fetal compartment. In addition to the experiments previously alluded to, other authors have published supporting data. Whaley et al. [40] reported a positive correlation between maternal and fetal plasma levels of free fatty acids in normal human pregnancy. This supports the concept of passage of free fatty acids across the human placenta. Other studies [41] have confirmed this finding. More recently, Elphick et al. [42] injected an emulsion (Intralipid) into mothers intravenously a few hours before

Table 9 Concentration of Acetone-Precipitable Lecithin in Fetal Lung Tissue from Rats on Fat Free (FF), Corn Oil (CO), or Palm Oil (PO) Diets

Gestational day	Diet	mg Lec P per 100 g tissue mean + SD of 6–9 analyses (pooled samples)	Significance
18	FF	11.9 ± 3.0	
	CO	13.3 ± 1.2	CO vs. FF, NS[a]
	PO	13.6 ± 1.7	PO vs. FF, NS
			PO vs. CO, NS
20	FF	14.8 ± 1.6	
	CO	17.1 ± 3.4	CO vs. FF, NS
	PO	21.0 ± 1.8	PO vs. FF, $p < 0.05$
			PO vs. CO, $p < 0.05$
21	FF	14.9 ± 2.2	
	CO	19.3 ± 1.3	CO vs. FF, $p < 0.05$
	PO	25.0 ± 3.3	PO vs. FF, $p < 0.05$
			PO vs. CO, $p < 0.05$

[a]NS = Not Significant.
Source: Nelson, G. H., J. C. McPherson, L. Perling, and R. Ciechan, The effect of maternal dietary fat on fetal pulmonary maturation in rats. *Am. J. Obstet. Gynecol.*, **138**:466 (1980).

normal delivery or cesarean section. At delivery they measured the cord blood arterial-venous difference and the fatty acid composition of the free fatty acid and triglyceride fractions. They found the following results: There was a positive cord blood venous to arterial difference of free fatty acid and triglyceride concentrations in the patients in whom the Intralipid was given; no such difference was seen in control infants. Moreover, the fatty acids that had the largest triglyceride venous-arterial differences were the predominant fatty acids in the Intralipid triglyceride. These authors [42] conclude that the amount of fatty acid being supplied to the fetal free fatty acid and triglyceride blood fractions by direct transfer of the Intralipid across the placenta is significant. If the transfer rates attained in these experiments were maintained for 24 hr, this would supply more than 115 g of fatty acids per day to the fetus, which is many times the fetus's requirement.

Several reports in animals indicate that the fatty acid composition of fetal tissues is modified by the fatty acid composition of the maternal diet. Satonera and Soderhjelm [43] supplemented the diets of maternal guinea pigs with either safflower oil (high in linoleic acid) or olive oil (high in oleic acid) and found correspondingly increased concentrations of the respective fatty acids in the whole carcass and many organs, including the lungs, of the newborn guinea pigs. In similar experiments, Pavey and Widdowson [44] fed pregnant guinea pigs diets containing either corn oil or beef tallow as their sole source of fat. The fetuses of the corn oil-fed mothers had a significantly increased percentage of linoleic acid

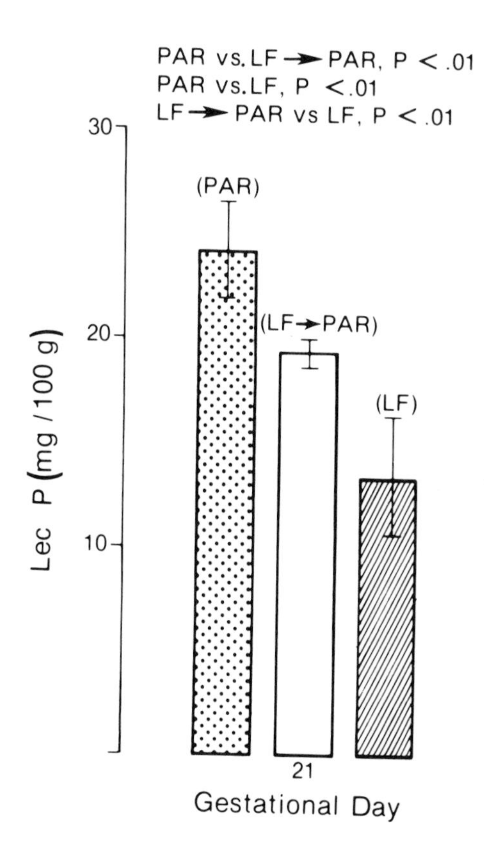

Figure 1 Concentration of acetone-precipitable lecithin in fetal lung tissue in rats fed a palmitic acid-rich (PAR) diet throughout gestation; low-fat (LF) diet for 15 days, then switched to a PAR diet; or LF diet throughout gestation. Fetal lungs were removed from all animals on gestational day 21. (From Nelson, G. H., J. C. McPherson, and L. Perling, Observations on maternal dietary fat intake and fetal pulmonary maturation in rats, *J. Repro. Med.*, 27:331 [1982].)

and decreased percentage of palmitic acid compared to the beef tallow-fed mothers. Widdowson et al. [45] also reported that the fatty acid composition of the body fat of newborn infants can be markedly influenced by the fatty acid composition of the milk fat in the diet. They analyzed body fat in British and Dutch infants at birth and at varying intervals up to 9 months of age. At birth, both British and Dutch infants had $< 3\%$ linoleic acid in the body fat. The British infants were fed milk containing fat which had 2% linoleic acid, while the Dutch infants received milk whose fat contained 58% linoleic acid. In 18 samples of body fat analyzed from 4 to 20 weeks after birth the linoleic acid content was $< 3\%$ in all British infants. In 25 samples from Dutch infants during this same period of time the linoleic acid content was approximately 10% at 4 weeks; 22% at 8 weeks; 26% at 12 weeks; 30% at 16 weeks; and 38% at 20 weeks. One Dutch infant had body fat with 46% linoleic acid at 40 weeks. These data prove conclusively that the fatty acid composition of newborn lipids can be markedly influenced by the fatty acid composition of the diet. Since the "diet" of the fetus is received by placental transport, it seems logical to assume that fetal lipid fatty acid composition would respond in a like manner and reflect the type of fatty acids being transported.

Therefore, the available data support a concept that a maternal diet rich in palmitic acid would modify the fatty acid composition of maternal blood lipids crossing the placenta and should provide the fetus with a rich supply of palmitic acid from which to synthesize essential fetal lipids such as dipalmitoyl lecithin in pulmonary surfactant.

However, in order for this concept to be viable there must be evidence that an increased supply of palmitic acid to the fetus will promote surfactant synthesis. Wolfe et al. [46] tested the influence of palmitic acid on the rate of pulmonary surfactant synthesis in the isolated (in situ), perfused rat lung. They found that an increase in the palmitic acid concentration from 0.5 to 1.5 mM doubled the rate of surfactant synthesis. Likewise, Shaw and Rhoades [47] showed that the incorporation of H^3 palmitate into pulmonary phospholipids in perfused rat lungs was directly related to the concentration of palmitate in the perfusate. These experiments are consistent with the belief that human fetal lungs will synthesize surfactant in utero in direct proportion to the palmitic acid concentration of the fetal blood perfusing the lungs.

Another substrate which may be important in surfactant synthesis is glycerol. Mims et al. [48] perfused the pulmonary artery in situ in term New Zealand newborn rabbits with two concentrations of glycerol. They found a twofold increase in lecithin synthesis when the higher concentration of glycerol was used. The role of circulating glycerol in human fetal pulmonary surfactant synthesis is completely unknown; however, placental transfer of triglycerides containing large amounts of palmitic acid, such as is found in palm oil, would present to the fetus adequate supplies of both glycerol and palmitic acid with which to synthesize surfactant.

V. Other Possible Substrate-Related Conditions

Some other conditions in obstetrics may also have substrate availability as an etiological factor in either predisposing to or protecting against RDS. These conditions include diabetes, fetal stress, and preeclampsia.

A. Diabetes

As mentioned elsewhere in this volume, fetal hyperglycemia resulting in fetal hyperinsulinemia would tend to promote lipogenesis and the deposit of palmitic acid and glycerol into fetal fat stores, thereby inducing a deficiency state in the lung for surfactant synthesis. Wolfe et al. [46] feel strongly that hyperinsulinemia per se does not directly inhibit surfactant synthesis. If this is true, then the infant of the diabetic mother, with its hyperglycemia, hyperinsulinemia, and hypopalmitic acidemia, is born surfactant deficient, possibly because its lungs have been perfused in vivo with a substrate (palmitic acid)–deficient fluid. Several pediatricians have recognized this possibility and have attempted to treat RDS with intravenous lipid therapy. Gunn et al. [49] did not have much success with Intralipid. Since the primary fatty acid in Intralipid is linoleic acid, it is possible the lungs were still receiving a palmitic acid–deficient perfusate. Another possibility is that in the face of a palmitic acid deficiency and an abundance of other fatty acids, the type II cells may divert from the synthesis of dipalmitoyl lecithin to a lecithin containing other fatty acids which may function very poorly as a surfactant material.

B. Fetal Stress

Stress is generally accompanied by an increase in the secretion of glucocorticoids and epinephrine, both of which tend to promote lipolysis and release of palmitic acid and glycerol into the blood which could be utilized as substrate by the fetal lungs for surfactant synthesis.

C. Preeclampsia

It is thought that infants of mothers with preeclampsia have a lower incidence of RDS than controls. This subject is covered in Chapter 10 of this volume. While the relationship of diet and preeclampsia is much less clear, there are data which indicate that patients who develop preeclampsia tend to consume high-fat diets [50]. In addition, Mitchell et al. [51] took careful dietary histories from 33 severely preeclamptic patients in Tuskegee City, Alabama. The diets of the preeclamptics contained an average of 148 g of fat, and fat calories represented 58% of the total calories. This is in contrast to an optimal diet recommended by the Food and Nutrition Board of the National Research Council containing approximately 100 g of fat with fat calories representing 36% of the total calories.

While the factors which predispose to preeclampsia are indeed complex, the concensus in medical centers in the South in years past has been that these patients tended to be young, primigravid, black, and from a low socioeconomic status. As a growing boy in a Southern U.S. town, one of us (GHN) worked many long hours in his father's meat market. I wish I had a nickel (that happened to be the price) for every large grocery bag of "scrap meat" that I sold to the downtown poor black population of Charleston, South Carolina. Scrap meat consisted mainly of bones and tallow (beef, lamb, and pork trimmings). There is no doubt in my mind that the diets of my young black pregnant customers were rich in saturated fat, containing considerable palmitic acid. I am equally confident that the obstetrical residents at the Medical College of South Carolina (now MUSC) saw many of my customers with the fullblown "triad." I am disappointed that some astute Charleston pediatrician did not wonder why my customer's premature baby breathed normally in the newborn nursery, while his colleague's affluent, below Broad Street, private patient's premature baby gasped, grunted, and retracted. I wonder now, was I hurting the mother, or was I helping the baby for a nickel a bag.

VI. Summary

1. RDS is found in various cultures throughout the world.
2. A multitude of variables exist which affect the true incidence of the disease worldwide and, equally important, influence the data reported in the literature from around the world.
3. One country of the world which seems to have a low incidence of RDS is Nigeria.
4. There is evidence that the diet of Nigerians may contain significant quantities of palm oil, a fat rich in palmitic acid.
5. Animal and human studies support the hypothesis that a diet high in palmitic acid could enhance the amount of palmitic acid crossing the human placenta, which could result in high levels of palmitic acid in the blood perfusing the fetal lungs which could promote surfactant synthesis.

6. Whether the low incidence of RDS in Nigeria is related to the dietary habits of Nigerians is unknown; however, it is definitely a viable possibility.
7. Certainly the thought of being able to accelerate fetal lung maturation by increasing the palmitic acid content of the maternal diet has enormous medical potential.
8. It is hoped that this chapter will induce the combined efforts of a team of nutritionists, epidemiologists, obstetricians, and neonatologists to investigate this matter further.

References

1. Farrell, P. M., and M. E. Avery, Hyaline membrane disease, *Am. Rev. Resp. Dis.,* **111**:657 (1975).
2. Usher, R. H., A. C. Allen, and F. H. McLean, Risk of respiratory distress syndrome related to gestational age, route of delivery, and maternal diabetes, *Am. J. Obstet. Gynecol.,* **111**:826 (1971).
3. Chalmers, I., M. E. Duancey, E. R. Verrier-Jones, J. A. Dodge, and O. P. Gray, Respiratory distress syndrome in infants of Cardiff residents during 1965–75, *Br. Med. J.,* **2**:1119 (1978).
4. Amiel-Tison, C., M. Barbiani, H. Hornych, C. Tchobroutsky, and R. Henrion, Incidence of idiopathic respiratory distress syndrome during the last ten years, *Eur. J. Obstet. Gynecol., Reprod. Biol.,* **11**:263 (1981).
5. Fanconi, A., W. Stoll, G. Duc, E. Bossi, and S. Prod'hom, Das Atemnotsyndrome des Neugeborenen in der Schweiz, *Schweiz. Med. Wochenschr.,* **106**: 1426 (1976).
6. Reed, D. M., L. S. Bakketeig, and R. P. Nugent, The epidemiology of respiratory distress syndrome in Norway, *Am. J. Epidemiol.,* **107**(4):299 (1978).
7. Ziai, M., Hyaline membrane disease in Iran, *South. Med. J.,* **68**(9):1062 (1975).
8. Bhakoo, N. O., A. Narang, N. K. Kulkarni, A. S. Patil, C. K. Banerjee, and B. N. S. Walia, Neonatal morbidity and mortality in hospital-born babies, *Indian Pediatr.,* 7(6):433 (1975).
9. Pai, P. M., N. W. Tibrewala, and S. R. Engineer, *Indian Pediatr.,* **12**:229 (1975). Cited in Coulter, J. B. S., Review: The incidence of the respiratory distress syndrome: With particular reference to developing countries, *Trop. Geogr. Med.,* **32**:277 (1980).
10. Thomas, S., I. C. Verma, M. Singh, and P. S. N. Menon, Spectrum of respiratory distress syndrome in the newborn in north India: A prospective study, *Indian J. Pediatr.,* **48**:61 (1981).

11. Teck, T. W. T., Respiratory distress syndrome of the newborn in Kandang Kerbau hospital, *J. Singapore Pediatr. Soc.,* **7**(2):44 (1965).
12. Azubuike, J. C., and G. I. Izuora, Incidence of idiopathic respiratory distress syndrome (IRDS) among neonates in Enugu, *Niger. J. Paediatr.,* **4**(2):24 (1977).
13. Olowe, S. A., and A. Akinkugbe, Amniotic fluid lecithin/sphingomyelin ratio: Comparison between an African and a North American community, *Pediatrics,* **62**(1):38 (1978).
14. Chintu, C., and S. Sukhani, Perinatal and neonatal mortality and morbidity in Lusaka, 1976, *Med. J. Zambia,* **12**(5):110 (1978).
15. Malan, A. F., C. Vader, and P. F. Fairbrother, Hyaline membrane disease: Incidence in Cape Town, 1974, *S. Afr. Med. J.,* **48**(53):2226 (1974).
16. Lowry, M. F., Respiratory distress syndrome in Jamaica, *West Indian Med. J.,* **23**:87 (1979).
17. Farrell, P. M., and R. E. Wood, Epidemiology of hyaline membrane disease in the United States: Analysis of national mortality statistics, *Pediatrics,* **58**(2):167 (1976).
18. Scott, M. J., G. R. McClure, M. McC. Reid, J. W. K. Ritchie, and S. R. Keilty, Neonatal death in Northern Ireland, *Br. Med. J.,* **2**:987 (1978).
19. Registrar General's Statistical Review of England and Wales, Part I. London, Her Majesty's Stationery Office, 1972, p. 378.
20. Heetai, R., and S. Roopnarinesingh, Perinatal mortality at the Port-of-Spain General Hospital, Trinidad, *West Indian Med. J.,* **37**:24 (1979).
21. Tan, K. L., and P. K. Boo, Perinatal mortality, *J. Singapore Pediatr. Soc.,* **16**(2):95 (1974).
22. Fujikura, T., and L. A. Froehlich, The influence of race and other factors on pulmonary hyaline membranes, *Am. J. Obstet. Gynecol.,* **95**:572 (1966).
23. Fredrick, J., and N. R. Butler, Certain causes of neonatal death. I. Hyaline membranes, *Biol. Neonate,* **15**:229 (1970).
24. Claireaux, A. E., *The First Week of Life.* London, Heinemann, 1974, p. 234.
25. Brown, R. E., and T. S. Sandhu, An autopsy survey of perinatal deaths in Uganda, *Trop. Georgr. Med.,* **18**:292 (1966).
26. Sivanesan, S., Mortality in hyaline membrane disease, *Med. J. Malaysia,* **27**(3):207 (1973).
27. Sparke, B., and M. F. Lowry, Neonatal death at the University Hospital of the West Indies, *West Indian Med. J.,* **27**:130 (1978).
28. Chuang, K. A., Pulmonary hyaline membrane disease in Hawaii, *Am. J. Dis. Child.,* **103**:718 (1962).
29. Rosahn, P. D., and C. Sheanaku, Hyaline membrane disease of the lung in Thailand, *Am. J. Dis. Child,* **102**:236 (1961).

30. Webb, J. K. G., T. J. John, M. Jadhav, M. D. Graham, and A. Walter, The incidence of hyaline membrane syndrome in south India, *J. Indian Pediatr. Soc.,* **1**(6):193 (1962).
31. Banerjee, C. K., A. Narang, O. N. Bhakoo, and B. K. Aikat, *Indian Pediatr.,* **12**:1247 (1975). Cited in Coulter, J. B. S., Review: The incidence of the respiratory distress syndrome: With particular reference to developing countries, *Trop. Geogr. Med.,* **32**:277 (1980).
32. Maheshwari, H. B., K. Teja, S. Rani, and S. Kumar, Causes of late fetal and neonatal death (an autopsy study), *Indian Pediatr.,* **8**(9):417 (1971).
33. Pahimtoola, R. J., A. F. Qureshi, and M. Ramzan, *J. P. M. A.,* **27**:258 (1977). Cited in Coulter, J. B. S.: Review: The incidence of the respiratory distress syndrome: With particular reference to developing countries, *Trop. Geogr. Med.,* **32**:277 (1980).
34. Shnier, M. H., and C. Isaacson, Perinatal mortality in the Bantu, *S. Afr. Med. J.,* **39**(30):676 (1965).
35. Effiong, G. E., Case of the low birthweight infant in Nigeria, *Trop. Dis.,* **8**:141 (1978).
36. Lesi, F. E. A., The incidence of prematurity in Lagos, Nigeria, *West Afr. Med. J.,* **16**:132 (1967).
37. *Encyclopedia Britannica,* **16**:902 (1972).
38. Okoh, O., R. Grosspietzsch, and L. von Klitzing, Hat die Ernahrungsgewohnheit mit hohem Anteil an Palmol (Palmitinsaure) Einfluss auf die niedrige Atemnotsyndromrate in Nigeria? *Monatsschr. Kinderheilkd.,* **127**:669 (1979).
39. *Encyclopedia Americana,* **20**:337 (1982).
40. Whaley, W. H., F. Z. Zuspan, and G. H. Nelson, Correlation between maternal and fetal plasma levels of glucose and free fatty acids, *Am. J. Obstet. Gynecol.,* **94**:419 (1966).
41. Elphick, M. C., D. Hull, and R. R. Sanders, Concentrations of free fatty acids in maternal and umbilical cord blood during elective cesarean section, *Br. J. Obstet. Gynecol.,* **83**:539 (1976).
42. Elphick, M. C., G. M. Filshie, and D. Hull, The passage of fat emulsion across the human placenta, *Br. J. Obstet. Gynecol.,* **85**:610 (1978).
43. Satonera, K., and L. Soderhjelm, Deposition of fatty acids in the newborn in relation to the diet of pregnant guinea pigs: A preliminary report, *Tex. Rep. Biol. Med.,* **20**:671 (1962).
44. Pavey, D. E., and E. M. Widdowson, Influence of dietary fat intake of the mother on composition of body fat of newborn guinea pigs, *Proc. Nutr. Soc.,* **34**:107A (1975).
45. Widdowson, E. M., M. J. Dauncey, D. M. T. Gairdner, J. H. P. Jonxis, and M. Pelikan-Filipkova, Body fat of British and Dutch infants, *Br. Med. J.,* **1**:653 (1975).

46. Wolfe, R. R., J. M. Snowden, and J. F. Burke, Influence of insulin and palmitic acid concentration on pulmonary surfactant synthesis, *J. Surg. Res.,* **27**:262 (1979).
47. Shaw, M. E., and R. A. Rhoades, Substrate metabolism in the perfused lung: Response to change in circulating glucose and palmitate levels, *Lipids,* **12**:930 (1977).
48. Mims, L. C., L. F. Mazzuckelli, and R. V. Kotas, The significance of circulating glycerol as a precursor of pulmonary phosphatidyl choline in the developing mammalian lung, *Pediatr. Res.,* **9**:165 (1975).
49. Gunn, T., G. Reaman, E. W. Outebridge, and E. Colle, Peripheral total parenteral nutrition for premature infants with respiratory distress syndrome: A controlled study, *J. Pediatr.,* **92**:608 (1978).
50. Chung, R., H. Davis, Y. Ma, O. Naivikue, C. Williams, and K. Wilson, Diet-related toxemia in pregnancy. *Am. J. Clin. Nutr.,* **32**:1902 (1979).
51. Mitchell, J. R., J. Morehead, and I. R. Brooks, Dietary habits of a group of severe preeclamptics in Alabama, *J. Natl. Med. Assoc.,* **41**:122 (1949).

9

Effects of Maternal Drugs on Fetal Pulmonary Maturity

WILLIAM E. ROBERTS and JOHN C. MORRISON

University of Mississippi Medical Center
Jackson, Mississippi

I. Introduction

The respiratory distress syndrome (RDS) is a physiological manifestation of neonatal pulmonary immaturity. It is still the most common cause of neonatal morbidity and mortality, and it accounts for 8000 to 10,000 deaths annually in this country alone. Attempts at altering the consequences of this disease have progressed along three separate avenues. First, great strides have been made in the care of the high-risk parturient and improved neonatal care has resulted in an increased number of surviving infants. For example, a 62% neonatal survival was reported in one study of infants weighing 750-1500 g at birth [1]. Of significant importance is the finding that most survivors do not suffer from major neurological handicaps. Secondly, methods to prevent or inhibit premature labor have been developed. Several pharmacological agents have been found to be effective tocolytic agents, and some success in prolonging these gestations has been reported. Lastly, a number of drugs have been shown to promote early fetal lung maturity when a preterm delivery is anticipated.

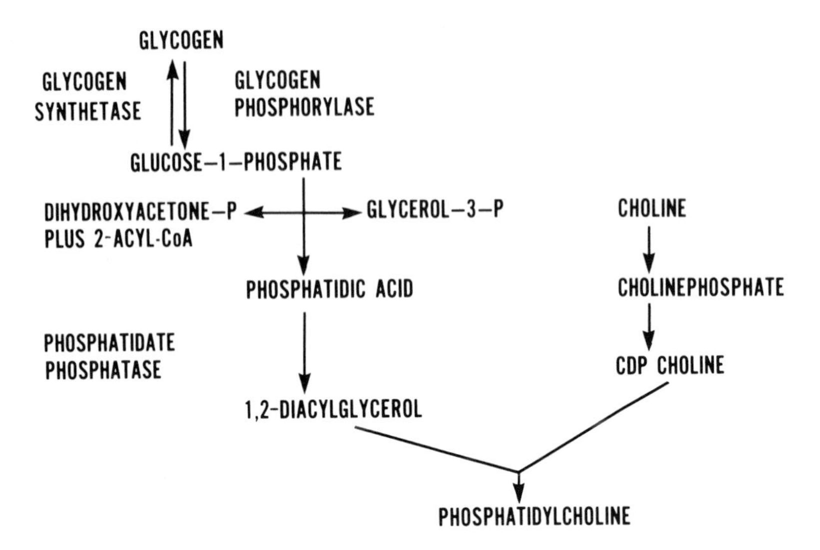

Figure 1 The basic biosynthetic pathway for the synthesis of phosphatidylcholine.

RDS occurs secondary to a deficiency of pulmonary surfactant, a surface-active material necessary for alveolar stability in extrauterine life. The majority of this phospholipid is in the form of phosphatidylcholine. The biochemical formulation and synthesis of phosphatidylcholine have been reviewed in Chapter 3. The basic biosynthetic pathway, including the requisite substances, is shown in Figure 1. Numerous experiments, both in animals and in humans, have demonstrated the ability of certain hormones and medications to modify the rate of phosphatidylcholine synthesis or secretion. This pharmacological effect occurs by enzyme induction and is limited by substrate availability. The ability to reliably accelerate phospholipid synthesis in a preterm gestation would decrease the overall incidence as well as the morbidity and mortality associated with RDS. If an adequate production of phosphatidylcholine is responsible for the reduction in RDS, clinical verification should be reflected by a measurement of mature fetal pulmonary assessment. The mechanism of drug interaction with the biosynthetic pathway of phospholipid synthesis, the result of that interaction upon the incidence of RDS, and the future prospects of pharmacological manipulation will form the basis of this chapter. Drugs which delay normal pulmonary maturation are also included.

II. Pharmacological Agents

A. Ethanol

After Fuchs and coworkers [2] in 1967 demonstrated that intravenous ethyl alcohol could inhibit premature labor, the use of this agent became commonplace in many hospitals. Because ethyl alcohol is associated with enzyme induction in adults and since it crosses the placenta, studies were conducted to determine whether its use would accelerate pulmonary maturity. In a prospective study using alcohol in the 28-32-week gestation period, Barrada and associates [3] showed a statistically significant decrease in neonatal RDS. No laboratory assessment of pulmonary maturity was performed and no mechanism of action was proposed. However, because there was no difference in the incidence of RDS between the treated and control groups when delivery occurred < 48 hr following the initiation of therapy, it is possible that direct or indirect induction of enzyme systems could explain these findings.

Studies comparing ethanol with other tocolytic agents have demonstrated newer pharmacological drugs to be more effective inhibitors of preterm labor [4-6]. Moreover, there appears to be an increase in the incidence of RDS in the preterm neonate when ethanol utilization is not effective in arresting labor. The probable mechanism is respiratory depression with resultant asphyxia. Thus, due to the potential of birth asphyxia as well as an increase in RDS and because more effective tocolytic agents are presently available, ethanol now is used infrequently as a first-line drug for the treatment of idiopathic premature labor.

B. Smoking

Cigarette smoking has been called the greatest health problem in the United States. Numerous studies have documented the deleterious effects of smoking during pregnancy. Smoking has been associated with an increase in spontaneous abortion, congenital abnormalities, placental lesions, lower birth weight, and perinatal mortality [7-10]. Low birth weight and some placental abnormalities have been shown independently to be associated with accelerated pulmonary maturity. A recent study compared the incidence of neonatal RDS in smoking and nonsmoking parturients and found a significant decrease in the incidence of RDS among the offspring of the smoking mothers [11]. The lower incidence of RDS among the neonates of smoking mothers was not associated with a difference in the L/S ratios. Whether this outcome was secondary to one of the more than 200 compounds contained in cigarette smoke or specifically related to a compromised intrauterine environment is unknown.

C. Heroin

The opiate drugs have been shown to induce hepatic enzyme systems in humans and laboratory animals. They also have been found to be associated with an increased level of cortisol during drug withdrawal [12]. Among human subjects addicted to heroin there is a virtual absence of RDS in preterm births unless growth retardation and/or birth asphyxia are present [13]. In rabbits, using a drug dosage schedule less than that required for addiction, Taeusch and associates were able to prematurely induce fetal lung maturity [14]. These authors postulated a stimulatory action of heroin upon enzymes necessary for the production of surfactant, although no L/S ratios were performed.

D. Aminophylline and Methylxanthine

Hallman [15] was able to induce pulmonary maturity in fetal rabbits with the administration of cyclic adenosine monophosphate (AMP). This lead to the hypothesis that the synthesis of phosphatidylcholine could be mediated through the cyclic AMP system within the fetal alveolar cell. Aminophylline and compounds that contain methylxanthines are known to increase tissue levels of cyclic AMP through the inhibition of cyclic AMP phosphodiesterase, the principal degrading enzyme of cyclic AMP. Barrett and coworkers [16] were able to accelerate maturation of the pulmonary system of fetal rabbits by injecting aminophylline into pregnant does. They also found depressed levels of cyclic AMP phosphodiesterase, increased levels of cyclic AMP, and higher amounts of saturated phosphatidylcholine in the fetal lung preparations of treated vs. control animals. In a recent report regarding maternal administration of aminophylline during preterm labor, Hadjigeorgiou demonstrated a threefold reduction in the incidence of neonatal RDS compared with matched controls [17]. Further evidence that cyclic AMP may be important in surfactant synthesis was provided by Liu, who observed a decreased incidence of neonatal RDS following the administration of a methylxanthine as a tocolytic agent to pregnant women at risk for preterm delivery [18].

A naturally occurring xanthine derivative which is widely distributed in food substances is caffeine. It is present in substantial amounts in coffee, tea, cola beverages, and over-the-counter medications used as treatment for headache as well as obesity. Caffeine is similar structurally to theophylline and it is possible that it could lead to early maturation of the fetal lung. Although caffeine usage in pregnancy has received considerable adverse publicity recently [19-22] (which led the FDS to remove it from the "safe to use during pregnancy" list), no human studies have been performed relating caffeine ingestion during pregnancy to untoward neonatal outcome, to indicators of fetal pulmonary maturity (L/S ratios), or to the incidence of RDS.

Another interesting possibility is the role of cyclic AMP on fetal pulmonary maturity via glycogen metabolism [23]. Glycogen breakdown may provide the necessary substrate, glucose-1-phosphate, for phospholipid synthesis and thereby enhance the synthesis of phosphatidylcholine. Because this pathway would not involve induction of enzyme systems, one would expect a more rapid formation of phosphatidylcholine than that observed with agents classified as enzyme inducers. Aminophylline injected into fetal rabbits was shown to effect a demonstrable decrease in surface tension and augmented surfactant secretion within a interval of 2.5 hr. The phospholipid content of fetal lung tissue in the group of animals receiving dexamethasone was not increased significantly after a similar period of time [24]. Whether these two modes of accelerated surfactant production work synergistically is not known presently. To date, no studies using aminophylline or the methylxanthine derivatives have been reported to show either short- or long-term adverse effects upon exposed infants.

E. β-Sympathomimetic Agents

The family of drugs termed β-sympathomimetics exhibit β-receptor stimulation and varying degrees of α-receptor stimulation. They have been used in obstetrical patients because of their tocolytic action upon the gravid uterus. Data from several retrospective human studies have shown a reduced incidence of RDS when these agents were utilized in attempts to arrest preterm labor [25-28]. The β-mimetic agents increase tissue levels of cyclic AMP through stimulation of adenyl cyclase and probably exert their effect by a mechanism similar to that of xanthine derivatives. In a prospective, placebo-controlled, double-blind study utilizing one of these agents, hexoprenaline, Lipshitz et al. demonstrated a significant improvement in fetal lung pressure/volume relationships as well as an increase in the L/S ratios among treated rabbits compared with control animals [29]. Significantly, this effect was observed as early as 3 hr following administration of hexoprenaline. Such a finding is inconsistent with the mechanism of enzyme induction, but rather implicates a facilitated early release of phospholipid from the fetal alveolar cells.

It has been demonstrated in the human that as early as 30 weeks' gestation there is sufficient surfactant present to avoid RDS [30]. Thus, some investigators feel that RDS may represent a deficiency in the release system rather than an absolute deficiency of surfactant. The mechanism by which some pharmacological agents accelerate fetal lung maturity may be secondary to more efficient release of available surfactant rather than enzyme induction and increased production. Which of these mechanisms are responsible for the acceleration in pulmonary maturity seen with the sympathomimetics is not known. The ability to enhance pulmonary maturity appears to be a property of all drugs in this group, since it has been observed with ritodrine, hexoprenaline, salbutamol, and isoxsuprine [25-28].

A retrospective, controlled human study demonstrated that hypotension, hypoglycemia, hypocalcemia, ileus, and death occurred more commonly in infants exposed to maternal isoxsuprine than controls [31]. Hypotension and death were associated with altered maternal circulatory homeostasis or with a short loading dose of isoxsuprine to delivery time. These two conditions could be minimized with careful titration of the tocolytic agent and close monitoring of changes in maternal pulse and blood pressure as well as the avoidance of its usage in patients with advanced cervical dilatation. Hypoglycemia, hypocalcemia, and ileus probably occur secondary to β-receptor stimulation in the fetus. Although these conditions are potentially dangerous if unrecognized, they are amenable to treatment if anticipated and diagnosed.

III. Hormones

A. Thyroxine

Thyroxine is a hormone essential to normal phospholipid metabolism. It has been suggested that thyroxine may have a major influence upon the synthesis of surfactant in the type II pneumocyte. Redding and associates demonstrated morpholigical changes in the type II pneumocytes following exposure to L-thyroxine which were interpreted to reflect augmented storage and production of surfactant [32]. Cuestas et al. detected low levels of T_3 and T_4 with elevated TSH levels in association with RDS in newborns [33]. This finding could be secondary to RDS itself rather than a thyroid hormone deficiency per se, since RDS is not encountered more frequently in infants with congenital hypothyroidism. Maschiach and associates, however, following intra-amniotic instillation of thyroxine in eight parturients before preterm delivery, demonstrated mature pulmonary values in the amniotic fluid after treatment and none of the infants had RDS [34]. Whether the use of thyroxine is indeed efficacious and without possible deleterious effects upon the fetus is unknown, since there are no published, controlled studies in humans.

B. Prolactin

During pregnancy there is a steady rise in maternal serum prolactin levels [35-36]. Fetal serum levels of prolactin remain relatively stable until about 30 weeks' gestation, after which there is a rapid rise to approximately 350-375 ng/ml at birth [37]. Since the rise in prolactin is abrupt and precedes the increase in pulmonary surfactant, the hormone may have a role in the maturation of the fetal pulmonary system (see Fig. 2). Following the injection of prolactin into fetal rabbits, Hamosh demonstrated a 67% increase in phosphatidylcholine

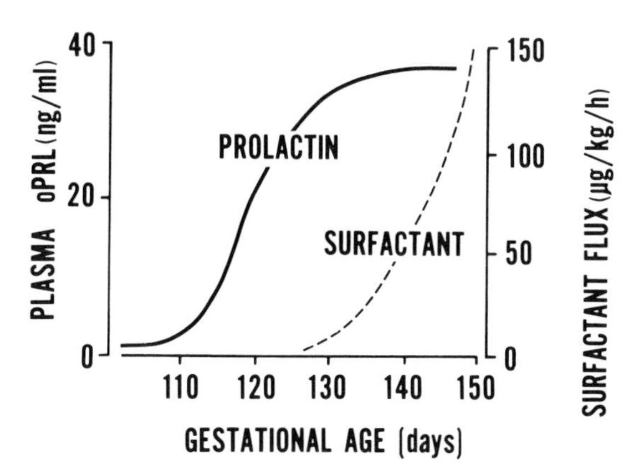

Figure 2 Normal developmental pattern of plasma PRL and trachea fluid surfactant in fetal sheep.

in the fetal lung preparations of the treated does [38]. Other investigators, however, have not been able to reproduce these findings [39]. Indirect evidence that prolactin is a stimulant to surfactant production is suggested by the fact that depressed cord blood levels of prolactin have been detected in infants who developed RDS [40]. In a recent report, however, Hatjis found no correlation between amniotic fluid prolactin levels and L/S ratios, gestational age, or birth weight [41]. In view of these conflicting findings, the role of prolactin in surfactant production cannot be stated until further research is undertaken.

C. Estrogen

The amount of estrogen excreted in the maternal urine late in pregnancy exceeds 25 mg/day [42]. This represents a 1000-fold increase over prepregnancy levels. There is a sharp increase in serum estrogen levels at about 32 weeks' gestation, which precedes the rapid rise of surfactant levels that occurs at about 35 weeks' gestation. This correlation between estrogen and surfactant indicates a possible effect of estrogen upon phospholipid synthesis in the maturing fetal lung. This hypothesis received further indirect support with the observation that infants with RDS have low estrogen levels [43]. Following intramuscular injections of 17-β-estradiol into pregnant rabbits at 25 and 26 days' gestation, Khosla and Rooney found evidence to suggest early lung maturation [44]. Specifically, they found that: (1) the 17-β-estradiol–treated group had three to four times more phospholipid and phosphatidycholine in lung lavages; (2) the L/S ratios were significantly higher in the treated group; and (3) the lung tissues of the treated group had almost twice as much phospholipid and phosphatidylcholine as did control animals. The time from administration of 17-β-estradiol until lipid extraction of the lung preparations was 24–48 hr, a time interval consistent with enzyme induction as the probable mechanism.

Administering conjugated estrogens (Premarin) antenatally to women in preterm labor, Dickey et al. [45] failed to demonstrate any benefit of estrogen upon the development of RDS. The time from administration to delivery averaged only 1 hr, so that if surfactant synthesis by enzyme induction was involved, it would not have been detected. Spellacy and associates administered conjugated estrogens (Premarin) orally for 2 weeks to women between 28 and 32 weeks' gestation and found an improvement in the L/S ratio [46]. The increase was not statistically significant, probably due to the small number of patients in the treated group (n = 9). Owing to the proven relationship between intrauterine exposure to diethylstilbesterol and the development of genital abnormalities in male and female fetuses, investigators have been reluctant to conduct the large study which would be necessary to prove any benefit of estrogen treatment upon the subsequent development of RDS.

D. Progesterone

Animal studies offer indirect evidence that progesterone inhibits uterine contractility, and labor in several species is preceded by a fall in progesterone. Although this relationship has not been demonstrated in humans, Johnson et al. have shown in some high-risk parturients that progestin administration can be associated with a lower incidence of preterm birth [47–48]. Using the premise that falling progesterone levels might be a factor in pulmonary maturation, Pulkkinen and Kero injected near-term rabbit fetuses with progesterone [49]. The treated animals had clinical and pathological evidence of RDS when compared to the controls. These investigators postulated that progesterone could act as an intermediary in the maturation of the fetal lung, particularly if cortisol increases progesterone catabolism. Whether this indeed explains the association of RDS with the elevated levels of progesterone and whether there is any such correlation in the human is unknown.

E. Insulin

Glucose crosses the placenta by facilitated diffusion, whereas maternal insulin does not cross at all. Hyperglycemia in the mother, therefore, exposes the fetus to elevated levels of glucose and fetal hyperinsulinism develops. This process has been thought to have an inhibitory effect upon surfactant production, since RDS is five times more common in the infant of a diabetic mother, regardless of gestational age or mode of delivery [50]. Smith and associates using monolayer cell cultures from fetal rabbit lung found that the addition of insulin abolished the stimulatory effect of cortisol upon lecithin synthesis [51]. Major actions of insulin include the inhibition of gluconeogenesis as well as the stimulation of glycogen formation. Secondary to these actions of insulin would be lower levels of glucose-1-phosphate and glycerol-3-phosphate, compounds which are necessary for the formation of complex lipids, including surfactant. If this is the mechanism responsible for the higher incidence of RDS in diabetic parturients, it emphasizes the need to attempt to achieve euglycemia in the pregnant diabetic. Moreover, the glucocorticoids with their known stimulatory action upon surfactant synthesis are potent "anti-insulin" agents. Their possible mechanism of action may be secondary to an antagonism of insulin's inhibitory effect at the cellular level of the type II pneumocyte.

F. Glucocorticoids

More basic research and clinical studies utilizing various glucocorticoids to stimulate fetal lung maturity have been performed than with any of the previously described pharmacological agents or hormones. The very early animal studies as well as prospective human studies have become an important aspect of perinatal research. There continues to be great optimism that some hormone and/or pharmacological agent can be administered to women destined to deliver premature neonates which will prevent RDS without exerting any deleterious effects upon the fetus. Evidence is present to suggest that the glucocorticoids represent the best pharmacological agent to fulfill these requirements.

Buckingham and colleagues in 1968 were the first to suggest that glucocorticoids could stimulate fetal lung maturity [52]. Data to support this hypothesis came from studies indicating that a stimulation of alkaline phosphatase in the gut of suckling mice occurred after glucocorticoid administration. Since the primitive gut and lung arise from the same embryonic analog, it was concluded that glucocorticoids might have similar effect upon other organs, including the lung. Liggins lent experimental support to this hypothesis when he noted that fetal lambs to which he had administered maternal glucocorticoids failed to have evidence of pulmonary immaturity after preterm delivery [53]. He postulated that enzymatic induction of surfactant formation occurred secondary to glucocorticoid administration. His initial prospective study of similarly treated preterm human gestations correlated well with the animal data [54]. RDS was significantly decreased to 4.3% in the betamethasone-treated infants compared with 24.0% in the control group. The incidence of RDS was not reduced if delivery occurred < 24 hr after treatment. This time interval appears to be the shortest period necessary for enzyme induction. Since Liggins' initial report in 1972, more than 30 studies investigating the maternal administration of steroids have been published. All have demonstrated a reduced incidence of RDS following exogenous glucocorticoid administration.

The mode of action of glucocorticoids was demonstrated by deLemos and associates in vitro to be a lowering of the surface tension of fetal lamb lungs

[55] . This is one of the basic functions of surfactant, a deficiency of which is pivotal in the development of RDS. Electron microscopy studies have verified that glucocorticoids stimulate the formation of lamellar inclusion bodies in the type II pneumocyte [56,57] .

Presently available data indicate that normal pulmonary maturation in the human may be mediated through glucocorticoid systems. Ballard and Ballard have demonstrated the presence of glucocorticoid-binding sites in the fetal lung [58] . Also, decreased lung phosphatidylcholine levels and increased pressure/ volume curves have been produced experimentally in laboratory animals by the administration of metyrapone (Metopirone) [59] , an agent which inhibits cortisol synthesis. Therefore, it seems that endogenous cortisol is vitally important for normal pulmonary maturation.

In the adult organism, cortisol has a number of functions in several different organ systems. It is reasonable to postulate that cortisol probably has a similar spectrum of functions in the fetus. Investigators have begun to look at organ systems other than the lung to determine whether glucocorticoids have physiological importance. Rats treated with pharmacological but not physiological doses of cortisol acetate were found to have decreased deoxyribonucleic acid (DNA) synthesis and retarded cell replication [60] . The finding of retardation in the development of motor skills in offspring (rats and mice) who received corticosteroids suggests that the effects are not temporary [61,62] . Also, in a human study in which methyl prednisolone was administered to infants 1 month or older as adjunctive therapy for bacterial meningitis, there was residual neurological damage reported to occur in 42% of the treated group as compared to 20% of the controls [63] . These studies suggest that glucocorticoids, as expected, have effects upon developing organ systems other than the lung and that some of these effects may be deleterious to the fetus. It is important to emphasize that the amount of exogenously administered corticosteroids necessary to accelerate pulmonary maturity is within the physiological range for the fetus during labor [64] .

The above studies [60-64] have been criticized because large pharmacological doses of steroids were used. Using doses of betamethasone comparable to that used in humans clinically, Johnson et al. investigated the drug effect upon pulmonary function in the *Rhesus* monkey [65] . They found, as expected, an increase in peak lung volumes in the treated animals as compared to controls. The lung volume increase between saline filling and air filling in the treated animals were comparable. Von Neergaard previously had correlated an increase in air filling to surfactant and tissue elasticity, whereas saline filling correlates with tissue elasticity [66] . The data of Johnson et al. therefore suggest that the increase in lung volume after glucocorticoid administration may be due to a change in the connective tissue of the lung rather than alveolar surfactant production [65] . Whether this finding indicates that steroid therapy will have long-term pulmonary sequelae is unknown. It is reassuring that Liggins has found no pulmonary dysfunction in the betamethasone-treated infants [67]. Furthermore, he has found no differences in IQ scores, vocabulary style, or visual perception between the infants of steroid-treated parturients and the control group at 4.5 years of age [67].

Since small numbers of patients and lack of controls have hindered interpretation of many steroid studies, the Division of Lung Diseases, National Heart, Lung, and Blood Institute and the National Institute of Child Health and Human Development jointly sponsored a workshop in 1974 to review all data relevant to the pharmacological enhancement of fetal lung maturation. The participants recommended that a double-blind, collaborative, randomized trial be performed to determine the efficacy of antenatal steroid administration in preventing RDS and to determine whether there might be significant short- or long-term adverse effects associated with such administration. The study was begun in 1976 and the preliminary data were published in 1981 [68].

The five clinical centers participating in the collaborative study randomized patients at risk for premature delivery into two groups, one receiving dexamethasone (5 mg IM q 12 hr for four doses) and the other, a placebo. The incidence of RDS among the offspring was reduced from 18.0% in the placebo group to 12.6% in the treated group ($P = 0.05$). Many criteria, however, had to be fulfilled to obtain this benefit. The principal advantage of glucocorticoid therapy appeared to be present only for those patients treated between 30 and 34 weeks' gestation. The group < 30 weeks' gestation had too few patients to allow any valid conclusions. Delay from the institution of therapy to delivery of at least 24 hr but < 7 days was necessary to achieve maximum benefit. Also, there was no reduction in the incidence of RDS among those with multiple gestations, but the numbers were small. Also of interest was the finding that females were found to have a higher incidence of RDS than males (18.8 vs. 14.1%), a finding at variance with previously published studies. Females, however, were noted to experience a more marked reduction in the incidence of RDS following dexamethasone therapy (18.8 to 4.8%), while male infants had no reduction at all (14.1 to 14.9%). In addition, black infants had a greater reduction in RDS (9.8 to 4.3%) after dexamethasone administration than did caucasian infants (19.7 to 16.7%). In summary, premature females had a reduction in RDS after dexamethasone therapy regardless of race, there was no reduction among caucasian male infants after treatment, and only a slight reduction of RDS was observed in male infants of other ethnic groups.

With regard to adverse outcome, there was no observed difference in the Prechtl neurological examination performed at 40 weeks between infants from the dexamethasone and placebo groups in the large collaborative study. Likewise, there was no apparent increase in infectious morbidity in the parturients or neonates. Although the study demonstrated no short-term effects of

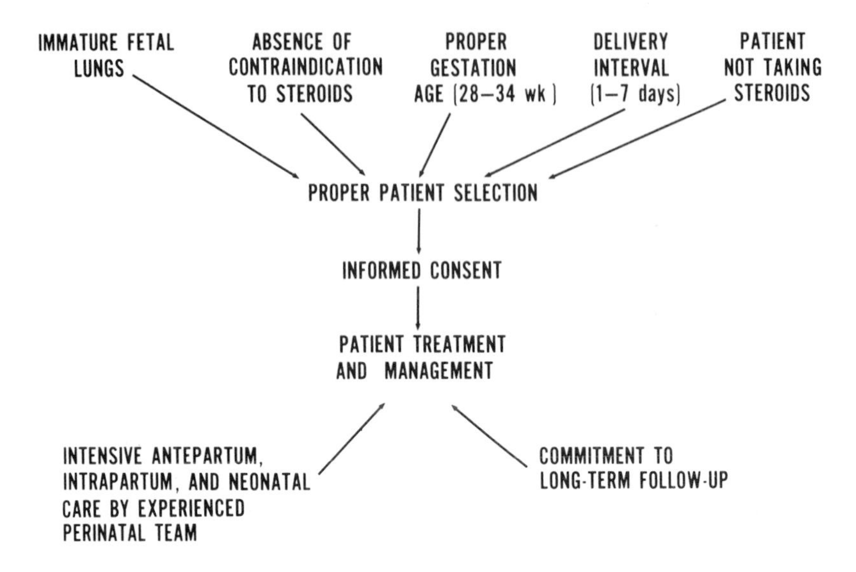

Figure 3 Patient selection for steroids.

glucocorticoid administration, the long-term effects are still unknown. Additional examinations are planned at 9, 18, and 36 months.

The general consensus of most participants of the collaborative project was that proper patient selection is critically important (Fig. 3). Since up to 25% of fetuses < 32 weeks' gestation have L/S ratios > 2.0, amniotic fluid assessment prior to initiation of glucocorticoid therapy is imperative. In addition, because a minimum of 24 hr is needed before any reduction in neonatal RDS is seen, those in whom early delivery is suspected or necessary should not receive glucocorticoids. Furthermore, one must be cognizant of the standard contraindications to glucocorticoid administration, i.e., active tuberculosis, viral keratitis, active peptic ulcer disease, and allergy to such agents. Persons already receiving glucocorticoids for other diseases do not derive an additional benefit from further glucocorticoid therapy and, therefore, its use should not be considered. Using this approach with intensive antepartum, intrapartum, and neonatal care by an experienced perinatal team, one can hope to achieve the greatest reduction in RDS and the greatest likelihood of improved survival with minimal risk.

IV. Summary

RDS is a significant health problem. It is the consequence of preterm birth and usually not due to a developmental abnormality. Affected infants are usually completely normal aside from their untimely premature birth. Because RDS is still the most common cause of neonatal morbidity and mortality, great emphasis has been placed upon its treatment and possible prevention. Normal pulmonary maturation is regulated by several hormonal factors. There appears to be little doubt that antenatal administration of some pharmacological agents or hormones can accelerate fetal lung maturation. The mechanisms effecting accelerated maturation involve either induction of enzyme systems, increased availability of needed substrates for phospholipid synthesis, the release of previously synthesized surfactant, and/or a change in lung compliance.

What remains to be clarified is the determination of risk vs. benefit of such therapy. Clearly, the fetus most likely to benefit is between the twenty-eighth and thirty-fourth week of gestation with an immature L/S ratio and in whom delivery can be postponed for at least 24 hr but < 7 days. Also of paramount importance is the realization that the long-term effects of these pharmacological agents upon the fetus are unknown.

A commitment for long-term postnatal surveillance of "treated infants" is a serious responsibility of the individual administering these compounds to enhance pulmonary maturity. Future prospective studies and research hopefully can determine whether administration of other medications may be associated with a greater reduction of RDS as well as fewer side effects. Perhaps the greatest breakthrough would be the final elucidation of the physiological mechanisms intrinsic to the initiation of parturition and, conversely, the prevention of preterm labor.

References

1. Hirata, T., and W. G. Peacock, Outcome in low-birth-weight infants (750 to 1,500 grams): A report on 164 cases managed at Children's Hospital, San Francisco, California, *Am. J. Obstet. Gynecol.,* **140**:165 (1981).
2. Fuchs, F., A. Fuchs, V. F. Poblete, and A. Risk, Effect of alcohol on threatened labor, *Am. J. Obstet. Gynecol.,* **99**:627 (1967).
3. Barrada, M. I., N. L. Virnig, L. E. Edwards, and E. Y. Hakanson, Maternal intravenous ethanol in the prevention of respiratory distress syndrome, *Am. J. Obstet. Gynecol.,* **129**:25 (1977).

4. Lauersen, N. H., I. R. Merkatz, N. Tejani, et al., Inhibition of premature labor: A multicenter comparison of ritodrine and ethanol, *Am. J. Obstet. Gynecol.,* **127**:837 (1977).
5. Steer, C. M., and R. H. Petrie, A comparison of magnesium sulfate and alcohol for the prevention of premature labor, *Am. J. Obstet. Gynecol.,* **129**:1 (1977).
6. Sims, C. D., G. V. P. Chamberlain, I. E. Boyd, and P. J. Lewis, A comparison of salbutamol and ethanol in the treatment of preterm labor, *Br. J. Obstet. Gynaecol.,* **85**:761 (1978).
7. Kline, J., Z. A. Stein, M. Susser, and D. Warburton, Smoking: A risk for spontaneous abortion, *N. Engl. J. Med.,* **297**:793 (1977).
8. Naeye, R. L., Relationship of cigarette smoking to congenital anomalies and perinatal death, *Am. J. Pathol.,* **90**:289 (1978).
9. Meyer, M. B., and J. A. Tonascia, Maternal smoking, pregnancy complications, and perinatal mortality, *Am. J. Obstet. Gynecol.,* **128**:494 (1977).
10. Hickey, R. J., R. C. Clelland, and E. J. Bowers, Maternal smoking, birth weight, infant death, and the self-selection problem, *Am. J. Obstet. Gynecol.,* **131**:805 (1978).
11. Curet, L. B., R. D. Zachman, P. M. Farrell, et al., Maternal smoking and respiratory distress syndrome, *Am. J. Obstet. Gynecol.,* **147**:446 (1983).
12. Eisenman, A., H. M. Fraser, and J. Brooks, Urinary excretion and plasma levels of 17-hydroxycorticosteroids during a cycle of addiction to morphine, *J. Pharmacol. Exp. Ther.,* **132**:226 (1961).
13. Glass, L., B. Rajegowda, and H. Evans, Absence of respiratory distress syndrome in premature infants of heroin-addicted mothers, *Lancet,* **ii**:685 (1971).
14. Taeusch, W., Jr., S. H. Carson, N. S. Wang, and M. E. A. Avery, Heroin induction of lung maturation and growth retardation in fetal rabbits, *J. Pediatr.,* **82**:869 (1973).
15. Hallman, M., Induction of surfactant phosphatidylglycerol in the lung of fetal and newborn rabbits by dibutryl adenosil 3′, 5′ monophosphate, *Biochem. Biophys. Res. Commun.,* **77**:1094 (1977).
16. Barrett, C. T., A. Sevanian, N. Lavin, and S. A. Kaplan, Role of adenosine 3′, 5′-monophosphate in maturation of fetal lungs, *Pediatr. Res.,* **10**:621 (1976).
17. Hadjigeorgiou, E., S. Kitsiou, A. Psaroudakis, et al., Antepartum aminophylline treatment for prevention of the respiratory distress syndrome in premature infants, *Am. J. Obstet. Gynecol.,* **135**:257 (1979).
18. Liu, D. T. Y., Phosphodiesterase inhibition and respiratory distress syndrome, *Lancet,* **ii**:378 (1973).

19. Weathersbee, P. S., L. K. Olsen, and J. R. Lodge, Caffeine and pregnancy, *Postgrad. Med.,* **62**:64 (1977).
20. Vaughan R., Coffee in pregnancy, *Lancet,* **i**:554 (1981).
21. Morris, M. B., and L. Weinstein, Caffeine and the fetus: Is trouble brewing?, *Am. J. Obstet. Gynecol.,* **140**:607 (1981).
22. Soyks, L. F., Caffeine ingestion during pregnancy: In utero exposure and possible effects, *Semin. Perinatol.,* **5**:305 (1981).
23. Maniscalco, W. M., C. M. Wilson, and I. Gross, The influence of aminophylline and cyclic AMP on glycogen metabolism in fetal rat lung in organ culture, *Pediatr. Res.,* **13**:1319 (1979).
24. Corbet, A. J., P. Flax, C. Alston, and A. J. Rudolph, Effect of aminophylline and dexamethasone on secretion of pulmonary surfactant in fetal rabbits, *Pediatr. Res.,* **12**:797 (1978).
25. Kero, P., T. Kirvonen, and I. Valimaki, Prenatal and postnatal isoxsuprine and respiratory distress syndrome, *Lancet,* **ii**:198 (1973).
26. Hastwell, G., Salbutamol and respiratory distress syndrome, *Lancet,* **ii**:354 (1977).
27. Boog, G., B. Brahim, and R. Gandar, Beta-mimetic drugs and possible prevention of respiratory distress syndrome, *Br. J. Obstet. Gynaecol.,* **82**:285 (1975).
28. Bergman, B., and T. Hedner, Antepartum administration of terbutaline and the incidence of hyaline membrane disease in preterm infants, *Acta Obstet. Gynecol. Scand.,* **57**:217 (1978).
29. Lipshitz, J., K. Broyles, J. R. Hessler, et al., Effects of hexoprenaline on the lecithin/sphingomyelin ratio and pressure-volume relationships in fetal rabbits, *Am. J. Obstet. Gynecol.,* **139**:726 (1981).
30. Platzker, A., J. A. Clements, and W. Tooley, Surfactant development in the human fetal lung, *Clin. Res.,* **19**:232 (1971).
31. Bruszy, J. E., and M. J. Pupkin, Effects of maternal isoxsuprine administration on preterm infants, *J. Pediatr.,* **94**:444 (1979).
32. Redding, R. A., W. H. J. Douglas, and M. Stein, Thyroid hormone influence upon lung surfactant metabolism, *Science,* **175**:994 (1972).
33. Cuestas, R. A., A. Lindall, and R. R. Engel, Low thyroid hormones and respiratory distress syndrome of the newborn, *N. Engl. J. Med.,* **295**:297 (1976).
34. Mashiach, S., G. Barkai, J. Sack, et al., Enhancement of fetal lung maturity by intra-amniotic administration of thyroid hormone, *Am. J. Obstet. Gynecol.,* **130**:289 (1978).
35. Jaffe, R. B., B. H. Yuen, W. R. Keye, Jr., and A. R. Midley, Jr., Physiologic and pathologic profiles of circulating human prolactin, *Am. J. Obstet. Gynecol.,* **117**:757 (1973).

36. Tyson, J. E., P. Hwang, H. Guyda, and H. G. Friesen, Studies of prolactin secretion in human pregnancy, *Am. J. Obstet Gynecol.,* **113**:14 (1972).
37. Schenker, J. G., M. Ben-David, and W. Z. Polishuk, Prolactin in normal pregnancy: Relationship of maternal, fetal, and amniotic fluid levels, *Am. J. Obstet. Gynecol.,* **123**:834 (1975).
38. Hamosh, M., and P. Hamosh, The effect of prolactin on the lecithin content of fetal rabbit lung, *J. Clin. Invest.,* **59**:1002 (1977).
39. Ballard, P. L., P. D. Gluckman, A. Brehier, et al., Failure to detect an effect of prolactin on pulmonary surfactant and adrenal steroids in fetal sheep and rabbits, *J. Clin. Invest.,* **62**:879 (1978).
40. Hauth, J. C., C. R. Parker, P. C. MacDonald, et al., A role of fetal prolactin in lung maturation, *Obstet. Gynecol.,* **51**:81 (1978).
41. Hatjis, C. G., C. H. Wu, and S. G. Gabbe, Amniotic fluid prolactin levels and lecithin/spingomyelin ratios during the third trimester of human gestation, *Am. J. Obstet. Gynecol.,* **139**:435 (1981).
42. Adlercreutz, H., and T. Luukkainen, Identification and determination of oestrogens in various biological materials in pregnancy, *Ann. Clin. Res.,* 2:365 (1970).
43. Dickey, R. P., and A. F. Roberson, Newborn estrogen excretion. Its relationship to sex, birth weight, maternal complications, and idiopathic respiratory distress syndrome, *Am. J. Obstet. Gynecol.,* **104**:551 (1969).
44. Khosla, S. S., and S. A. Rooney, Stimulation of fetal lung surfactant production by administration of 17 beta-estradiol to the maternal rabbit, *Am. J. Obstet. Gynecol.,* **133**:213 (1979).
45. Dickey, R. P., D. L. Vaughn, and J. R. Mourer, Effect of estrogen administration during labor on the incidence of hyaline membrane disease in premature infants, *J. Reprod. Med.,* **111**:204 (1969).
46. Spellacy, W. N., W. C. Buhl, F. C. Riggall, and K. L. Holsinger, Human amniotic fluid lecithin/sphingomyelin ratio changes with estrogen or glucocorticoid treatment, *Am. J. Obstet. Gynecol.,* **115**:216 (1973).
47. Johnson, J. W. C., K. L. Austin, G. S. Jones, et al., Efficacy of 17 alphahydroxyprogresterone caproate in the prevention of premature labor, *N. Engl. J. Med.,* **293**:675 (1975).
48. Johnson, J. W. C., P. A. Lee, A. S. Zachary, et al., High-risk prematurity—Progestin treatment and steroid studies, *Obstet. Gynecol.,* **54**:412 (1979).
49. Pulkkinen, M. O., and P. Kero, Effect of progesterone on the initiation of respiration of the newborn, *Biol. Neonate,* **32**:218 (1977).
50. Robert, M. F., J. P. Hubbell, H. W. Taeusch, and M. E. Avery, The association between maternal diabetes and the respiratory distress syndrome, *Pediatr. Res.,* **9**:370 (1975).

51. Smith, B. T., C. J. P. Giroud, M. Robert, and M. E. Avery, Insulin antagonism of cortisol action on lecithin synthesis by cultured fetal cells, *J. Pediatr.*, **87**:953 (1975).
52. Buckinham, S., W. F. McNary, S. C. Sommers, et al., Is lung an analog of Mogg's intestine? Phosphatase and pulmonary alveolar differentiation in fetal rabbits, *Fed. Proc.*, **27**:328 (1968).
53. Liggins, G. C., Premature delivery of foetal lambs infused with glucocorticoids, *J. Endrocrinol.*, **45**:515 (1969).
54. Liggins, G. C., and R. N. Howie, A controlled trial of antepartum glucocorticoid treatment for prevention of the respiratory distress syndrome in premature infants, *Pediatrics*, **50**:515 (1972).
55. deLemos, R. A., D. Shermeta, J. Knelson, et al., Acceleration of pulmonary surfactant in the fetal lamb by administration of corticosteroids, *Am. Rev. Resp. Dis.*, **102**:59 (1970).
56. Wang, N. S., R. V. Kotas, M. E. Avery, et al., Accelerated appearance of osmiophilic bodies in fetal lungs following steroid injection, *J. Appl. Physiol.*, **30**:362 (1971).
57. Motoyama, E. K., M. M. Orzalesi, Y. Kikkawa, et al., Effects of cortisol on the maturation of fetal rabbit lungs, *Pediatrics*, **48**:547 (1971).
58. Ballard, P. L., and R. A. Ballard, Cytoplasmic receptor for glucocorticoids in lungs of human fetus and neonate, *J. Clin. Invest.*, **53**:447 (1974).
59. Vidyasagar, D., and V. Chernick, Effect of Metopirone on the synthesis of lung surfactant in does and fetal rabbits, *Biol. Neonate*, **27**:1 (1975).
60. Cotterrell, M., R. Balazs, and A. L. Johnson, Effects of corticosteroids on the biochemical maturation of rat brain: Postnatal cell formation, *J. Neurochem.*, **19**:2151 (1972).
61. Shapiro, S., M. Salas, and K. Vikovich, Hormonal effects on ontogeny of swimming ability in the rat: Assessment of central nervous system development, *Science*, **168**:147 (1970).
62. Howard, E., and D. M. Granoff, Increased voluntary running and decreased motor coordination in mice after neonatal corticosterone implantation, *Exp. Neurol.*, **22**:661 (1968).
63. deLemos, R. A., and R. J. Haggerty, Corticosteroids as an adjunct to treatment in bacterial meningitis, *Pediatrics*, **44**:210 (1969).
64. Ballard, P. L., P. Granberg, and R. A. Ballard, Glucocorticoid levels in maternal and cord serum after prenatal betamethasone therapy to prevent respiratory distress syndrome, *J. Clin. Invest.*, **56**:1548 (1975).
65. Johnson, J. W. C., W. Mitzner, and W. T. London, Glucocorticoids and the Rhesus fetal lung, *Am. J. Obstet. Gynecol.*, **130**:5 (1978).

66. Von Neergaard, K., Neue auffassungen uber einen gruudbegriff der attemmechanik, *Z. Ges. Exp. Med.,* **66**:373 (1929).
67. Liggins, G. C., The prevention of RDS by maternal betamethasone administration. 70th Ross Conference Report. *Lung Maturation and the Prevention of Hyaline Membrane Disease.* Ross Lab., Columbus, Ohio, Dec., 1975, pp. 189–198.
68. Collaborative group on antenatal steroid therapy: Effect of antenatal dexamethasone administration on the prevention of respiratory distress syndrome, *Am. J. Obstet. Gynecol.,* **141**:276 (1981).

10

Effect of Maternal-Fetal Disorders on Fetal Pulmonary Maturation

HOSSAM E. FADEL and GEORGE H. NELSON

Medical College of Georgia
Augusta, Georgia

I. Introduction

Respiratory distress syndrome (RDS) is the major cause of neonatal deaths in many parts of the world. The great majority of the neonates who suffer from RDS are the products of preterm deliveries (< 37 weeks). In most of these the onset of preterm labor was spontaneous, and the process—for one reason or another—was not or could not be halted. However, there is a growing number of patients who are delivered prior to term because of various maternal and/or fetal disorders, and their neonates may suffer from RDS. In these situations the obstetrician decides that the risk of the disorder to the mother and/or fetus outweighs the risk of developing RDS or at least of dying from RDS or its complications. In these difficult situations an estimate of the risk of development of RDS becomes an invaluable guide to the obstetrician.

Fetal lung maturity is a term used to indicate that production of surfactant by the fetal lungs has reached a level that will protect the neonate from the development of RDS. In normal pregnancy this is usually achieved by the thirty-seventh week. Clinical experience has been that certain maternal and/or fetal disorders appear to be associated with a decreased and others with an increased incidence of RDS in the neonate compared to neonates of similar gestational age delivered of healthy pregnancies. This led to the concept that some maternal and/or fetal disorders will accelerate and others will delay fetal lung maturation.

Amniotic fluid (AF) surfactant levels closely reflect fetal pulmonary maturity and the various tests available for determining pulmonary maturity are outlined in Chapter 6. The predictive ability of these tests in normal pregnancy is generally good. However, their predictive accuracy in certain high-risk pregnancies is less well documented.

In this chapter the current literature will be reviewed and information about the effect of several maternal and/or fetal disorders on fetal lung maturation will be presented. Also, the question of whether the results of AF studies are equally predictive of fetal lung maturity in abnormal as they are in normal pregnancies will be addressed.

II. Accelerated and Delayed Fetal Pulmonary Maturation

A. Definition

Authors have used a variety of methods to investigate whether a certain disease or condition may be associated with accelerated or delayed fetal pulmonary maturation. In general, authors have attempted to establish a control relationship between gestational age and an AF surfactant measurement and then to compare values obtained in a particular disease or condition with the control. These comparisons are generally made as mean values at various gestational ages or as a percentage of mature and immature values at a specific gestational age. Therefore, a condition which accelerates fetal lung maturation would have either higher mean values or a greater percentage of mature values at corresponding gestational ages than the control group. Likewise, a condition which delays fetal lung maturation would have lower values.

Another method that has been used is to determine the incidence of RDS in a disease or condition at a certain time in gestation and compare this with that of a control population. Obviously in a condition with accelerated fetal lung maturation there will be a lower incidence of RDS and vice versa for delayed lung maturation.

B. Possible Mechanisms

It is difficult to understand how maternal and/or fetal disorders accelerate or delay fetal pulmonary maturity because of our incomplete knowledge of all the factors that influence normal fetal maturation. The physiological processes involved in fetal lung maturation have been reviewed elsewhere in this volume. While it seems that cortisol is a very important hormone for the induction of the enzymes for surfactant synthesis, it also would appear that catecholamines, prolactin, thyroxine, and insulin may be involved. AF cortisol was found to correlate with L/S ratios [1,2], and a positive correlation between AF cortisol and phosphatidylglycerol (PG) has been reported [3]. Also, metyrapone (Metopirone) administration to pregnant rats significantly delayed fetal pulmonary maturation, while dexamethasone accelerated it [4].

It has been proposed that fetal stress (unfavorable intrauterine environment, placental insufficiency) is the underlying mechanism for acceleration of pulmonary maturation. The stress could lead to increased production and/or release of cortisol. However, catecholamines may also be involved. Divers et al. [3] found a positive correlation between the levels of AF 3,4-dihydroxphenylglycerol (DOPEG), norepinephrine, and epinephrine and the level of PG in both normal and complicated pregnancies. As mentioned elsewhere in this volume, a possible mechanism of catecholamine action may be its effect on lipoprotein lipase with elevation of the plasma free fatty acid (particularly palmitic acid) levels and, thereby, providing additional substrate to the fetal lungs for lecithin biosynthesis. Also, the catecholamines may act by releasing surfactant from the type II pneumocytes. In addition, they may act by modulating either the secretion or, more likely, the action of other hormones. Epinephrine infusion in the fetal lamb has been shown to result in elevated adrenocorticotropin (ACTH) levels that may trigger increased cortisol production, which may by a direct effect on the pancreatic B cells inhibit insulin secretion. Insulin is thought to have a suppressive effect on lecithin biosynthesis.

In support of the role of intrauterine fetal stress in accelerated pulmonary maturation was the finding of accelerated neurological maturation in fetuses who were subjected to chronic intrauterine stress [5,6]. However, chronic maternal hypoxia failed to accelerate fetal pulmonary maturation in rats [7].

It has been proposed that delayed pulmonary maturation results from the failure of the placenta to transport to the fetus adequate amounts of certain substrates or to produce adequate amounts of certain hormones [8]. Unfortunately, these same changes could be found in disease states which purportedly accelerate fetal lung maturation. Therefore, at the present time the mechanisms remain unresolved by which some conditions may accelerate and others delay lung maturation.

III. Diabetes Mellitus and Fetal Pulmonary Maturation

A. Introduction

It has been the general feeling among obstetricians for a long time that an infant of a diabetic mother (IDM) is particularly prone to develop RDS. Robert et al. [9] conducted a large retrospective study in which they corrected for factors that influence the incidence of RDS, such as gestational age, route of delivery, Apgar score, and sex. They found that IDMs have a 5.6-fold greater risk of developing RDS than do infants of nondiabetics. Predisposition to RDS in IDMs was evident at gestational ages <38 weeks, with no difference in risk of RDS between IDMs and normal infants at term. Because of the risk of sudden fetal death in diabetic pregnancies obstetricians tend to terminate these pregnancies electively at about 38 weeks. To avoid unnecessary neonatal deaths from RDS, assessment of fetal lung maturity prior to such intervention has become a standard procedure [10,11].

B. Diabetes Mellitus and Surfactant Measurements

In their early investigations, Gluck and Kulovich [12] reported a delayed rise of L/S ratio in White's classes A, B, and C and an acceleration of the rise in classes D, E, and F. Aubry et al. [13] reported delayed maturation in classes A–F. Morrison et al. [8] found delayed maturation in classes B and C but not in class A patients, while Goldkrand et al. [14] reported delayed maturation in classes A, B, and C, and normal maturation in class D patients. On the other hand, other investigators [15,16] could not demonstrate any difference in the rate of pulmonary maturation between the different classes of diabetes and normal pregnancy.

In a later publication, Kulovich and Gluck [17] reported their experience with diabetic pregnancies using the "lung profile." They calculated the regression coefficient of the L/S ratios with gestational age in normal and diabetic pregnancies. Contrary to their earlier studies, they found no significant differences among the different classes and none of the classes differed significantly from normal pregnancy. They found that only seven out of 43 class A patients and only a few patients of classes B and C had delayed maturation of the L/S ratio. They found that L/S ratios in class D did not differ from normal. However, there was a statistically significant delay in the appearance of PG in class A diabetics as compared to normal and to other classes of diabetics. The mean time of appearance of PG in class A patients was 37–39 weeks. In the relatively few classes F and R patients in their study, PG appeared in classes F and R patients before mature L/S ratios were observed. Indeed, in these patients an L/S ratio of 1.8 was never exceeded. Another finding was the delay in the fall of phosphatidylinostitol (PI) levels in class A diabetics. In normal subjects and in other classes of diabetics, the percentage of PI fell no later than 36 weeks. On the other hand, in class A diabetics, a decline was not seen until a mean of 37 or 38 weeks.

Cunningham et al. [18] also reported a significant delay of the appearance of PG in class A diabetics. In nondiabetic patients with L/S ratios of 2.0–2.9, PG was present in 50% of the AF samples; however, PG was present in AF in only 16.7% of diabetic patients with the same L/S ratio.

On the other hand, Bent et al. [19] reported that PG was identified in 35% of overt diabetics between 32 and 34 weeks, a significantly higher percentage than in controls (2.7%). There was no difference between the proportion of patients with classes B and C and those with classes D and R as regards the percentage of patients with identifiable PG. Class A diabetics were not different from controls.

Using fluorescence polarization to measure the microviscosity (MV) of the AF as an index of fetal lung maturity, 16 class A and 62 classes B–R diabetics were studied [20]. The slopes of the regression lines from patients with classes A, B, and C did not differ from normal. The MV values in classes D, F, and R were lower than normal and the difference was statistically significant prior to the thirty-seventh week. They concluded that there was accelerated fetal lung maturation in classes D, F, and R, while there was no change in lung maturation in classes A, B, and C.

It is obvious that no definitive conclusions can be drawn from the many conflicting reports in the literature. One reason for the confusion is the difficulty in obtaining sufficient data from individual classes of diabetes at specific gestational ages to which one could compare statistically control data obtained at the same gestational ages. However, another reason for the conflicting data may be simply the complexity of the disease being studied. Diabetes is really not a single disease entity but rather different syndromes with one common finding, i.e., hyperglycemia with or without ketosis. Some cases are characterized by high insulin levels (insulin-resistant types), while others are insulinopenic. In normal pregnancy, insulin secretion is increased compared to the nonpregnant condition. The insulin response to glucose ingestion is intensified as pregnancy advances. The commonly used White's classification is based on the age of onset and duration of disease. While White's classification emphasizes the presence or absence of vasculopathy, it does not account for different pathophysiological types, i.e., there is no differentiation between insulin-lacking (type I) and insulin-resistant (type II) diabetes. Also, this classification does not take into account the degree of metabolic control achieved. Furthermore, diabetic patients are more prone to develop preeclampsia, and classes D, F, and R are commonly complicated by hypertensive disease. In very few studies was an attempt made to separate the hypertensive from the normotensive diabetic patients in the same class. It may be that the influences on fetal lung maturation of changes in hormonal milieu and carbohydrate metabolism are in the opposite direction to the influences of placental insufficiency thought to be associated with the more advanced stages, especially in the presence of hypertensive disease.

Despite the great variation in the results of different studies, a reasonably consistent finding in at least the more recent reports is the delayed appearance of PG in class A diabetics. The clinical significance of this is as yet undetermined.

C. Possible Mechanisms

Most of the theories of the mechanisms of delayed functional maturation of the fetal lungs in diabetic pregnancies have centered on the role of fetal hyperinsulinemia. Maternal hyperglycemia leads to fetal hyperglycemia which in turn leads to fetal hyperinsulinemia [21]. Insulin is a growth-promoting hormone and anabolic signals provided by continuous insulin exposure may result in lung cell proliferation at the expense of type II pneumocyte maturation. The growth-promoting effects of insulin will increase the substrate demands for fetal growth and lung glycogen deposition, thus limiting the amount of substrate available for surfactant synthesis. In the fetal rat lung there is a progressive increase of glycogen content until the last 2 days of pregnancy when a sharp decline occurs coincident with pulmonary maturation and its attendant increase in phospholipid synthesis. Lung glycogen in the fetal rat may act as a substrate source for pulmonary surfactant. Sustained high levels of insulin will favor continued glycogen synthesis rather than glycogenolysis and surfactant phospholipid synthesis [22]. Along the same lines, hyperinsulinemia favors the incorporation of plasma free fatty acids into adipose tissue and this in turn may lead to a deficiency of palmitic acid in the type II pneumocytes, resulting in decreased phosphatidylcholine (PC) synthesis. In fetal rat lung explants cultured in the presence of insulin, there was an increased level of glycogen and delayed morphological maturation. Electron micrographs revealed a paucity of lamellar bodies in the type II cells of insulin-exposed cultures, as compared to explants cultured in the absence of insulin. Only the latter explants exhibited a normal lamellar body appearance and number after 24 hr of culture [23,24].

Another possible mechanism is that the increased local concentration of insulin may disturb the endocrine milieu which favors maturation of type II cells, particularly by interfering with the actions of glucocorticoids [22]. In rabbit lung tissue culture studies it has been shown that insulin inhibited the cortisol-induced increase in PC synthesis [25]. It was also suggested that insulin may decrease the number of glucocorticoid receptors in rat lungs [26] or perhaps antagonize cortisol binding [27]. Stubbs and Stubbs [28] postulated that hyperinsulinemia activates the pyruvate dehydrogenase pathway of glycolysis; thus glycerol is diverted toward the synthesis of acetyl-CoA, and away from phospholipid synthesis.

However, the central role of hyperinsulinemia has been questioned. The cord blood C-peptide levels (a measure of endogenous insulin production) were not significantly higher in IDMs who developed RDS than in those who did not [29]. Furthermore, decreased biosynthesis of PC and lack of pulmonary morphological differentiation were noted in streptozotocin-treated diabetic rats, where the fetuses are insulinopenic [30]. It has been proposed that fetal blood glucose levels tend to decrease in the third trimester, triggering the observed surge in serum cortisol levels near term. This "steroid surge" may be necessary for the last part of normal lung maturation. Constant fetal hyperglycemia could, therefore, remove the primary stimulus for increased glucocorticoid secretion and thus impede the normal acceleration of lung differentiation in late gestation. The proponents of this theory claim that the lack of pulmonary differentiation is the result of deficient glucocorticoid action rather than antagonism between insulin and cortisol [30].

A decrease in PC biosynthesis has not been observed in some experimental animal models [31,32]. In streptozotocin-treated, glucose-intolerant *Rhesus* monkeys, AF L/S ratio and the rate of incorporation of ^{14}C-choline into PC in fetal lung slices were significantly higher than in control fetuses. However, the PC content of the lungs was significantly greater in the controls [31]. This suggests increased rate of release of surfactant from the type II cells as a result of treatment.

A qualitative rather than quantitative difference in the biosynthesis of surfactant in diabetic pregnancies has been suggested by some experiments. One report was of pregnant rabbits made diabetic by alloxan treatment [32]. The fetal lungs of the diabetic does showed less functional surfactant activity. However, there was no difference in the PC content or L/S ratio in the fetal lung wash, or in the PC content in fetal lung tissue between diabetic and control pregnancies. The observed discordance between surfactant function and the concentration of the major surfactant (PC) may be due to a qualitative difference in the composition of surfactant (possibly the absence of PG or a decreased percentage of dipalmitoyl lecithin with a corresponding increased percentage of lecithin molecules containing other fatty acids).

Whatever the exact mechanisms may be, if such mechanisms exist, the role of the metabolic derangement cannot be underestimated. Actually, it seems reasonable to speculate that the less marked effects of diabetes on fetal lung maturation in recent studies are the result of improved management of diabetic pregnancies with emphasis on strict metabolic control. Hallman and Teramo [33] measured the PG/PI ratio in the AF of diabetics and controls. They found that when the L/S ratio was >2, the PG/PI ratio was significantly lower in the diabetics. They then divided the diabetic patients into three groups: In group 1, the PG/PI ratio was less than 50% of the median; in group 3, the ratio was > 200% of the median; and the remainder constituted group 2. There was a significant increase of the relative birth weight in group 1 as compared to group 3. Half of the newborns in group 1 had hypoglycemia but none in group 3. RDS was more common in group 1. The association of delayed lung maturation (as shown by low PG/PI ratio) with other neonatal complications known to be associated with fetal hyperinsulinemia and indicating poor diabetic control supports the contention that improved management of diabetes in pregnancy with strict metabolic control may result in a more normal maturation of the fetal lungs and in a reduced incidence of RDS in IDM. This view was also expressed by Curet et al. [34], who stated that diabetes may delay normal fetal pulmonary maturation only if it is not properly controlled.

D. Reliability of Surfactant Measurements in Diabetic Pregnancies

Along with the controversy about the effects of different classes of diabetes on the rate of fetal lung maturation, another question of more immediate clinical concern was raised. Do mature and immature L/S ratios have the same significance in diabetic as they have in normal pregnancies? If an infant who is delivered after the L/S ratio was ⩾ 2 develops RDS, the test is falsely positive. Chesley [35] reviewed 13 articles and reported 22 cases of RDS from 1327 deliveries in which the L/S ratio was 2 or greater. This represents an average false positive rate of 1.7%. On the other hand, the false positive rate (using a mature value of 2 or greater) in diabetic pregnancies has been reported to vary between 3 [36] and 30% [37].

In a series involving 210 overt diabetic pregnancies 200 patients were delivered after an L/S ratio of ⩾ 2. Six infants developed RDS, an incidence of 3%. This was not significantly different from the 2.6% incidence observed in 270 nondiabetic patients from the same institution [36]. Tchobroutsky et al. [38] reported two cases of hyaline membrane disease (HMD) out of 67 insulin-dependent diabetics with an L/S ratio ⩾ 2 or a false positive rate of 3%. Tabsh et al. [16] recently reported their experience with 77 insulin-dependent diabetics. The incidence of RDS in newborns delivered after attainment of L/S ratio of ⩾ 2 was 3.9%, which was not significantly different from the 1.5% incidence observed in 130 controls.

Curet et al. [34] measured the L/S ratio by a technique with no acetone precipitation and used an L/S ratio ⩾ 3.5 to indicate fetal lung maturity. They reported on their experience with 108 insulin-dependent diabetics. The incidence of RDS was 1.2% in their diabetic and 1.7% in their nondiabetic population. These workers [34] attributed these excellent results to the strict metabolic control in their patients. Curet et al. [34] postulated that good control of the diabetes results in a normal process of fetal pulmonary maturation with no increased risk of RDS in the presence of a mature L/S ratio. Another reason for the low incidence of RDS in the diabetic patients could be their using an L/S ratio of 3.5 rather than 2.0.

Cruz et al. [39], reporting out of Dr. Spellacy's laboratory, found a 29% (four of 14 cases) incidence of RDS in infants of insulin-dependent diabetics with mature L/S ratios. Dahlenberg et al. [37] reported 14 cases (30%) of RDS from 46 diabetic pregnancies with mature L/S ratios. Likewise, Mueller-Heubach et al. [40] reported that out of the 54 patients delivered after 35 weeks with an L/S ratio of ≥ 2, nine developed RDS (16.7%). They noted that the risk of development of RDS is more the earlier in pregnancy delivery occurs, even with the same numerical value of the L/S ratio. They also reported that the risk of RDS was higher in neonates delivered abdominally, confirming an earlier report [41]. They suggested the use of an L/S ratio of 2.5 as indicative of a mature lung in diabetic pregnancies, and not to deliver before 36 weeks if delivery will be by the vaginal route and not before 37 weeks if delivery is going to be by cesarean section.

O'Brien and Cefalo [42] reviewed the subject in 1980 and found that overall in 495 diabetic pregnancies with an L/S ratio of 2 or greater there were 39 cases of RDS (7.9% false positive rate). They also reported that the incidence of RDS in the presence of a mature L/S ratio decreases with advancing gestational age, 42% at 35-36 weeks, 15% at 37 weeks, and 6.8% at 37-38 weeks. These data are in contrast to an overall false positive rate of 2.2% (56 cases of RDS in 2544 deliveries). This false positive rate of 2.2% is indeed comparable with the 1.7% found in Chesley's review [35]. It would appear then that the L/S ratio does not predict fetal lung maturity as well in diabetic as in nondiabetic pregnancies.

The wide range of the incidence of RDS in diabetic patients with a mature L/S ratio in the different series is difficult to explain. One reason is probably slight differences in method of determining the L/S ratio. Cunningham et al. [18] noted a methodical problem in measuring the L/S ratio. In the commonly used one-dimensional chromatographic method the L/S ratio may be falsely elevated because the PI spot tends to overlap the lecithin spot. They describe a two-dimensional method that avoids this pitfall. However, there is still considerable variation in the ability of different investigators to predict the absence of RDS using the L/S ratio even when similar laboratory procedures are used.

In our hospital we have measured the AF lecithin phosphorus concentration since 1969 [43], and we have used the figure of 0.1 mg/dl to predict fetal lung maturity in all patients [44]. In a recently reported series of 108 pregnant diabetics managed in our institution none of the neonates whose AF lecithin phosphorus concentration was ⩾ 0.1 mg/dl developed RDS, i.e., a false positive rate of 0% [45]. This may be due to the excellent diabetic control achieved in most of these patients, as previously suggested [34]. However, it may also indicate the advantage of measuring absolute lecithin concentrations over L/S ratios. We have previously shown [44] and suggested [46,47] that L/S ratios may be falsely elevated because of low sphingomyelin levels. Some defect in sphingomyelin metabolism (decreased production) may very well be the reason for the reported high false positive rate with the L/S ratio in diabetic pregnancies. Therefore, it is indeed highly possible that the lecithin surge has never occurred in an IDM with a "mature" L/S ratio who develops RDS.

Many other theories have been advanced to explain the apparent increase in RDS in IDM in spite of a mature L/S ratio. Surfactant release and continued production are known to be impaired in the presence of hypoxia and acidosis [15]. Some obstetricians feel that the IDM is more susceptible to asphyxia at birth than normal infants and this may predispose the IDM to a greater risk of developing RDS. Other complications observed in IDM (e.g., hypoglycemia, polycythemia, hypocalcemia) may also increase the predeliction for RDS [48]. The increased incidence of cesarean section delivery in diabetics has also been implicated. In patients delivered before 37 weeks with an L/S ratio ⩾ 2, the incidence of RDS was 0% in the neonates delivered vaginally compared to an incidence of 41% in those delivered by cesarean section [40]. Another theory is that fetal hyperglycemia with resultant hyperosmolality may cause edema of respiratory center and predispose the neonate to RDS [27].

It has also been suggested that fetal hyperglycemia activates fetal breathing [49]. This may result in high transfer of fetal lung lecithin to AF. This could lead to a spuriously high L/S ratio with a lower total lung lecithin content [27]. In support of this concept Epstein et al. [31] reported that pregnant *Rhesus* monkeys rendered glucose-intolerant by streptozotocin treatment had fetuses that demonstrated increased rate of ^{14}C-choline incorporation into lecithin and higher AF L/S ratios *but* decreased lung lecithin content. However, the absence of falsely high AF lecithin in our diabetic patients does not support this hypothesis [45].

Other investigators suggest that the false prediction of absence of RDS in diabetic pregnancies could be due to qualitative changes in the surfactant [29, 30] that cannot be identified by simply measuring the L/S ratio. It has been proposed that the fetal lung near term produces two types of surfactant, one composed of lecithin and PI and the other type composed of lecithin, PI, and PG [50]. Although both types are highly surface active, the second type has lower compressibility on the modified Willrelring balance. Whereas the surfactant containing PI alone is vulnerable to such factors as acidosis, the surfactant containing both PI and PG is more stable. Another possibility is that the fetus of the diabetic mother may make surfactant lecithins which have a smaller percentage of dipalmitoyl lecithin with a correspondingly higher percentage of lecithin containing other fatty acids.

It has been suggested that PG stabilizes the surfactant lipoprotein complex either in its lamellar body storage phase or after secretion into the alveoli [51]. PG has been reported to be absent from the lung effluent more often in newborns with RDS than in healthy controls delivered at similar gestational ages [52]. Some investigators believe that the presence of PG heralds the "final" important step in the biochemical maturation of surfactant. Gluck and his coworkers [53,54] feel that the presence of PG in the amniotic fluid accurately predicts the absence of RDS both in normal and abnormal pregnancies. Cunningham et al. [48] reported on 27 diabetic patients, six of whom delivered neonates with RDS. All six were delivered at or before 38 weeks with mature L/S ratios. PG was present in the amniotic fluid in only one of these cases. In another study, 23 diabetic patients were delivered after the attainment of an L/S ratio between 2 and 3. Four neonates developed RDS and PG was absent in the amniotic fluid in all of them prior to delivery [33]. However, one must remember that PG will be identified in only a proportion of the cases and its absence does not necessarily mean that the neonate will develop RDS. In the latter study, PG was present in only five of the 23 patients. Out of the 18 patients with no detectable PG, only four neonates developed RDS.

E. Conclusions

There seems to be a reasonable consensus in the literature that there is delayed pulmonary maturation in diabetes based on an increased incidence of RDS in IDM compared to matched controls. The L/S ratio data presented in attempts to demonstrate delayed or accelerated lung maturation in various classes of diabetes are inconsistent and inconclusive. However, from a clinical point of view, whether there is a delay or acceleration of lung maturation is not really so important as it is to be able to predict accurately the absence of RDS in the IDM. A mature (≥ 0.1 mg/dl) lecithin phosphorus concentration or the presence of PG in the AF seems to predict reasonably accurately the absence of RDS. There is good evidence suggesting that the L/S ratio will yield a higher percentage of false positive results in diabetic than nondiabetic pregnancies. Therefore, we recommend that obstetricians, utilizing the L/S ratio test, use some number >2 (perhaps 3.0 or 3.5) to predict fetal lung maturity in diabetic pregnancies.

IV. Premature Rupture of the Membranes

A. Introduction

Premature rupture of the membranes (PROM) is defined as rupture of membranes (ROM) at least 1 hr prior to the onset of labor. When PROM occurs after 35 weeks' gestation, labor usually starts shortly afterward, and if it does not, many obstetricians will induce labor and deliver the patient within 24 hr. On the other hand, if PROM occurs prior to 35 weeks, the latent period (interval between ROM and onset of labor) tends to be prolonged. Most patients with preterm PROM will also have prolonged ROM (usually > 24 hr).

B. Effect of Prolonged ROM on Fetal Pulmonary Maturation

Gluck and coworkers [12,17] using L/S ratios reported acceleration of fetal lung maturation with prolonged (> 24 hr) ROM. They reported that the mean L/S ratios were higher, and mature L/S ratios appeared earlier than in normal pregnancy. The slopes of the regression lines describing the relationship of L/S ratio to gestational age were significantly higher in patients with prolonged ROM than in normal pregnant women.

With the introduction of PG measurements more investigators studied the possible relationship. In normal uncomplicated pregnancy PG was reported to appear between 35 and 39 weeks' gestation [54-56]. Stedman et al. [57] performed serial aspirations of vaginally pooled amniotic fluid in 25 patients with preterm PROM between 28 and 34 weeks' gestation. Six fluids (24%) were initially PG positive. Of the 19 patients whose fluids initially lacked PG, three patients received corticosteroids. Of the 16 patients who did not receive corticosteroids, six (38%) converted to PG-positive fluids between 25 and 392 hr (mean 161 hr). They conclude that those who initially lacked PG showed an acceleration of its appearance in the amniotic fluid with time. Surely, from these data this conclusion is highly debatable.

Bent et al. [19] also reported the earlier appearance of PG in AF from patients with prolonged ROM. At 32-34 weeks, PG was present in 2.7% of "normal" pregnant women and in 37.5% of patients with prolonged ROM, a statistically significant difference. These workers [19] reported the presence of PG in two patients < 30 weeks' gestation with prolonged ROM and RDS did not develop in either of their infants. Gluck and his coworkers [17] likewise reported that PG appeared earlier in the amniotic fluid in patients with ROM > 24 hr.

The available data would appear to support a concept that there is an accelerated rise in L/S ratio and an early appearance of PG in the presence of prolonged ROM; however, this assumption is based on very meager evidence and well-designed long-term prospective controlled studies are needed to confirm this supposition.

Richardson et al. [58] reported the incidence of RDS was 64% in 42 infants with an average gestational age of 32.4 weeks born ≤ 24 hours after ROM compared with an incidence of 31% in 22 infants with an average gestational age of 30.4 weeks born > 24 hours after ROM. Yoon and Harper [59] observed a similar decrease in the incidence of RDS with prolonged ROM. In a report by Rajegowda et al. [60] of two sets of twins with PROM, the sib from each set with ROM did not develop RDS, while the other "perfectly matched control" developed RDS and died. However, a large retrospective study from one of the most distinguished perinatal centers in the United States revealed the lack of an association between prolonged ROM and the incidence of RDS [61]. Jones et al. [61] examined the records of 16,458 consecutive live births weighing > 500 g at the University of Colorado Medical Center and found that low 1-min Apgar scores and cesarean section delivery were associated with an increased incidence of RDS compared to matched controls; however, there was no association between prolonged ROM and RDS. They emphasize that the effect of gestational age on the incidence of RDS is so dramatic that an investigator must be extremely careful to ensure that the gestational age distributions within two groups of infants are the same before the incidence of RDS can be tested between the two groups. Jones and coworkers [61] suggest that the apparent relationship between prolonged ROM and RDS which appears in many literature reports may be due to inadequate matching of the control group with the prolonged ROM group with respect to gestational age. Several clinical reports have appeared since then, some claiming a beneficial protective effect of prolonged ROM [62-65], and some denying it [66-70]. Also, Worthington et al. [71] demonstrated a significantly reduced incidence of RDS in association with PROM; however, the duration of rupture did not have an influence on the protection from RDS. They suggested that fetal lung maturity occurs before the membranes rupture.

It is obvious from this review that the final chapter concerning this problem has not yet been written. To quote Roy Pitkin, one of the leading authorities of obstetrics in the United States, as he has said numerous times in his editorial comments in *The Year Book of Obstetrics and Gynecology*, "The relationship between PROM and RDS remains controversial." It may be of interest to our readers that Pitkin's opinion remains the same as of 1984 [72].

C. Possible Mechanisms

If fetal lung maturation is accelerated by prolonged ROM, it does not seem to be caused by the reduction in the volume of AF. In the pregnant ewe removal of large amounts of AF did not accelerate pulmonary maturation as measured by pressure volume curves [73]. It has been postulated that prolonged ROM "stresses" the fetus, resulting in increased endogenuous cortisol production with acceleration of lung maturation. Concentrations of corticosteroids in the peripheral blood of infants delivered following prolonged ROM (> 16 hr) were reported to be higher than in matched controls [74]. This hypothesis was further supported by a study of AF cortisol levels in 12 patients (24-34 weeks' gestation) with ROM for 1-8 days [75]. Samples were obtained from the vaginal pool on one or more subsequent days. In patients with ROM of > 24 hr, AF cortisol levels were higher than in patients in whom ROM was < 3 hr. Moreover, a rise of AF cortisol was found in all six patients studied serially. Since cortisol in AF is considered to originate mainly from fetal adrenal sources, this rise is possibly indicative of enhanced cortisol production by the fetus.

D. Management

The management of preterm PROM is controversial. If labor does not ensue spontaneously within a period of hours, the obstetrician has to decide whether to induce labor and when. Because of possible fetal lung immaturity immediate delivery may result in a high incidence of RDS; whereas delayed delivery with a prolonged ROM may result in an increased incidence of chorioamnionitis and neonatal sepsis.

Kappy et al. [76] reported that in patients with PROM the majority of neonatal deaths are associated with RDS rather than with neonatal sepsis. This suggests that these patients are better managed conservatively to allow further maturation of the fetal lungs rather than by active intervention and immediate delivery. As mentioned previously, some investigators believe that prolonged ROM per se accelerates fetal lung maturity, while others do not. Many obstetricians treat their patients with preterm PROM conservatively and do not induce labor until there is evidence of fetal lung maturity or chorioamnionitis develops.

Although there is as yet no conclusive proof that prolonged ROM accelerates fetal lung development, there is sufficient evidence that this should be considered in formulating a plan of management for patients with preterm PROM. A rational approach would be to balance the risks of infection and the development of RDS in individual patients. In our institution we attempt amniocentesis with real-time ultrasonic guidance, and if we are successful, the AF is analyzed for bacterial counts and maturity studies. If the concentration of lecithin phosphorus is ≥ 0.1 mg/dl or the bacterial counts are > 1000 CFU/ml, labor is induced. If AF culture is negative and the lecithin level is < 0.1, the patient is closely observed for signs of chorioamnionitis or until labor starts spontaneously [77]. This same protocol has been used by others [78].

Because of the high failure rate (50–60%) in obtaining AF transabdominally in PROM, some investigators have obtained it from the vaginal pool. Of course this specimen will be useless for assessment of chorioamnionitis, but it could be used for fetal lung maturity studies. Some authors have suggested the use of the shake test and others utilized the L/S ratio, but the reliability of these tests has not been documented. The potential dilution of amniotic fluid obtained vaginally as well as possible contamination with blood, cervical mucus, semen, or vaginal secretions have provoked skepticism about the value of L/S ratios measured in vaginal pool AF samples. We have measured lecithin concentrations in a few samples collected from the vaginal pool, but because of the many uncontrollable variables involved we have not felt comfortable utilizing the results for clinical management. Because PG is absent from virtually all body secretions (other than lung surfactant) it seems to be the best suited marker for fetal lung maturity in this setting. Dombroski et al. [79] reported that PG was invariably present in the amniotic sac when it was detected in the vaginal pool. Stedman et al. [57] demonstrated the clinical applicability of analyzing the vaginal pool samples from patients with PROM. If PG is present, labor could be induced. If it is absent, the vaginal pool can be aspirated daily and analyzed for PG. If PG becomes positive, labor can be induced. However, it should be remembered that the production of PG represents the endpoint of fetal pulmonary maturity and that an intermediate point exists at which there is sufficient pulmonary maturation to protect the neonate against RDS in the absence of PG. Thus, in some cases, waiting for the appearance of PG might unnecessarily delay active intervention and might cause increased incidence of infectious complications both in the mother and her neonate. We are currently evaluating the usefulness of PG measurements in vaginally obtained AF. Our preliminary results indicate one thing for certain, i.e., a negative PG in fluid collected from the vaginal pool in no way indicates that an infant, if delivered, will develop RDS. The vast majority of infants whom we have delivered with a negative PG have not developed RDS. The few who have were known to be very premature by gestational age estimation and, therefore, were known to be at high risk of developing RDS. At the present time we feel that a positive PG is a useful finding in the management of PROM, but in the face of a negative PG the pregnancy should be managed by clinical parameters and the negative PG should be virtually ignored.

V. Hypertensive Disease

In 1973 Chiswick and Durpard [80] reported that the incidence of neonatal RDS in patients with preeclampsia was significantly less than in their control population despite the fact that the mean gestational age was lower and the cesarean section rate higher in the preeclamptic group. Later, Pardi and Marini [81] reported accelerated fetal lung maturation in preeclampsia both by elevated L/S ratios and lack of RDS in premature gestations. Also, Emara et al. [82] reported an elevated amniotic fluid lipid phosphorus concentration in toxemic pregnancies with living fetuses compared to controls.

Kulovich and Gluck [17] using AF PG measurements reported a dramatic acceleration of fetal lung maturation in the few patients with severe preeclampsia that they studied. PG appeared as early as 29-30 weeks in some cases. However, the time of appearance of PG in AF in the majority of patients with mild preeclampsia was not different from that in normal pregnancies. Yambao et al. [83] also reported the earlier appearance of PG in amniotic fluid of some "stressed" pregnancies, including patients with chronic hypertension and preeclampsia when the L/S ratio was still < 2. Bent et al. [19] measured PG in lamellar bodies from AF samples obtained from normal and hypertensive patients. PG was identified in 2.7% of "normal" pregnancies by the thirty-fourth week but appeared in 12.5% of the hypertensive patients by 32 weeks and in 31.3% of patients by 34 weeks. Fetal lung maturation was evaluated using fluorescence polarization in amniotic fluid from 252 normal and 81 hypertensive pregnancies (27 chronic hypertensive and 54 preeclamptics) [20]. The microviscosity (MV) values were significantly lower than normal in both chronic hypertensive and preeclamptic patients, suggesting acceleration of fetal lung maturation in those conditions. Chronic hypertension had a statistically greater effect, presumably representing the effect of fetal stress of longer duration. However, Freeman et al. [84] did not find evidence of accelerated fetal lung maturation by measuring L/S ratios in stressed pregnancies as defined by low maternal estriol excretion and positive oxytocin challenge tests.

Nevertheless, it would appear that there is reasonable consensus by AF fetal lung maturity studies that there is accelerated fetal pulmonary maturation in hypertensive disorders of pregnancy. Clinical experience also seems to be in accord with these findings. This clinical impression is supported in a recent study of the incidence of RDS in 2105 preterm neonates weighing between 1000 and 2199 g, 250 of whom were delivered from patients with hypertensive disorders of pregnancy. The incidence of RDS in the latter group was significantly less than in the nonhypertensive group. The incidence of RDS was inversely related to the severity of maternal hypertensive disease, suggesting that not only does chronic stress accelerate fetal lung maturation, but also that the more severe the stress is, the more effective is the acceleration of fetal lung maturation [85].

VI. Fetal Growth Retardation

Gunston and Davey [86] reported that the mean L/S ratios in patients with fetal growth retardation (FGR) were lower than matched controls. However, Lindback [87] reported higher AF lecithin concentration levels in pregnancies complicated by hypertensive disease and in which there was FGR than in those in which the fetuses were appropriately grown. When FGR occurred in the absence of hypertensive disease, AF lecithin concentrations were not different from the controls.

Sher et al. [88] measured the foam stability index (FSI) in 27 pregnancies that resulted in low birth weight fetuses: 15 small for gestational age (SGA) and 12 preterm appropriate for gestational age (AGA). Although the mean birth weight of the SGA group was significantly less than that of the AGA group (1254 vs. 1714 g), no cases of RDS occurred in the SGA group; whereas 67% (8) of the preterm AGA neonates developed RDS. The authors [88] report that a FSI of >0.47 predicts the absence of RDS and suggests that a small fetus is SGA as opposed to preterm AGA. Also, in this study, the investigators found that both PG and disaturated PC were increased in AF derived from pregnancies with FGR as compared with those from preterm AGA pregnancies. In four FGR cases, the mean PG concentration was 15.3 mg/liter vs. 1.5 mg/liter in nine AGA cases. The mean values for disaturated PC in the FGR and AGA pregnancies were 83 mg/liter and 15 mg/liter respectively. RDS developed in three of the nine AGA and in none of four SGA neonates. In a similar study [89], 82 low birth weight neonates, 33 SGA and 49 AGA, were investigated. The birth weights were similar in both groups; however, the gestational age was significantly higher in the SGA group. High PG levels (defined as > 7% of total phospholipid) were present in a significantly greater proportion of SGA than in AGA pregnancies (64% vs. 29%). Furthermore, the mean L/S ratios and the mean percentages of PG (expressed as percent of total phospholipid) were found to be significantly higher in the SGA than in the AGA group.

The authors felt that measurements, particularly PG, may be of value in differentiating the SGA fetus from a small preterm AGA fetus. However, these data cannot be construed to indicate acceleration of fetal lung maturation by FGR because in neither study [88,89] were the AF results in the SGA group compared with a normal pregnancy group with corresponding gestational age.

In a more recent study [19], PG was found in the AF of 20% of patients with FGR between 32 and 34 weeks, compared to 2.7% of normal patients at the same gestational age. PG was present in 59% of patients with FGR at 35-36 weeks compared to 46.8% of the normal group.

It is obvious from the above discussion that a clear picture of the effects of FGR on fetal pulmonary maturation has not emerged as yet. However, this is to be expected because FGR may result from a heterogeneous group of conditions with multiple etiologies. It may be that cases that result from "placental insufficiency," whether due to primary placental disease or a maternal disorder such as hypertension, will be associated with accelerated maturation; whereas other cases which are related to an intrinsic defect in the fetus, such as congenital anomaly, chromosomal disorder, or intrauterine infection, etc., will be more commonly associated with delayed pulmonary maturation. At any rate, in future studies involving pregnancies with FGR the study population should be limited to patients with FGR resulting from a single etiology.

VII. Miscellaneous Disorders

A. Incompetent Cervix

There is one report suggesting accelerated fetal lung maturation in patients with incompetent cervix [90]. The incidence of RDS in 19 patients with incompetent cervix with or without cerclage who delivered between 24 and 33 weeks was less than in matched controls. There were no AF studies, but the authors postulated associated changes in maternal or fetal hormonal milieu that could influence fetal lung development [90].

B. Sickle Cell Anemia and Other Hemoglobinopathies

Morrison et al. [8] reported acceleration of fetal lung maturation, defined as L/S ratio of > 2 before 36 weeks, in 26 patients with SS or SC disease, while there was no change noted in another five patients with S-thal and thalassemia. Das and Foster [91] studied AF lipids in four sickle cell patients and four normal pregnant women at 38–40 weeks' gestation. They found the total phospholipid concentration to be 50% lower in the sickle cell patients. Lecithin concentration was markedly reduced; whereas that of other phospholipids was increased. Calculating the mean L/S ratio from their results, it was found to be 8.4 in normal patients and 2.0 in sickle cell patients. There was no attempt to correlate these findings to either the incidence of RDS or to the neonatal outcome. It is obvious that more studies of fetal lung maturation in patients with hemoglobinopathies are needed.

C. Multiple Pregnancy

The L/S ratio in paired twins is usually not significantly different from each other [92,93]. Sims et al. [92] studied nine twin pairs, while Spellacy and associates [93] reported on 14. Picker et al. [94] sampled both sacs in four sets of twins and one set of triplets (one macerated fetus) and found reasonably close L/S ratio measurements in four out of five. In one set of twins the L/S ratio was 9.7 in one sac (infant had mild HMD) and 2.9 in the other (infant had severe HMD). As mentioned previously, if one of the twins has prolonged ROM (> 48–74 hr), this twin may have accelerated fetal lung development [63]. In a recent study Leveno et al. [95] reported on 42 pairs of clear AF samples obtained from twin sacs at cesarean section. The L/S ratio exceeded 2 in both infants in 30 (71%) twins, was < 2 in both infants in seven (17%) pairs and the L/S ratio was > 2 in one twin and < 2 in the other in five (12%). Five infants developed RDS: one pair with L/S ratios of 0.3 and 0.5; twin B with a L/S ratio of 0.5 (unaffected twin A, L/S ratio of 0.6); twin B with a L/S ratio of 0 (unaffected twin A, L/S ratio of 0); twin B with a L/S ratio of 1.4 (unaffected twin A, L/S ratio 2.2). In three twin pairs with birth weight discordancy exceeding

25%, the smaller infant (presumed by some to be malnourished and stressed) did not have a higher L/S ratio as expected. Indeed, in this study the smaller infant had the lower L/S ratio. It is of interest that the means of the L/S ratio were significantly greater at 31-32, 33-34, and 35-36 weeks' gestation compared to those of 137 uncomplicated singleton pregnancies. There was no significant difference between the ratios at 37-38 and 39-40 weeks. These data would suggest that twinning per se accelerates fetal lung maturation. However, this cannot be stated for certainty because complications, such as hypertension, PROM, etc., that led to the early deliveries cannot be ruled out as contributing factors.

D. Nonhypertensive Renal Disease

Although hypertensive renal disease has been reported to enhance fetal lung maturation, nonhypertensive renal disease has been reported to be associated with delayed fetal lung maturation [8,12]. In the first report there were four patients with nonhypertensive chronic glomerulonephritis in whom the L/S ratio was < 2 after 35 weeks' gestation. In the latter study, there were 12 patients with nonhypertensive renal disease in whom the L/S ratio was < 2 after 36 weeks. Obviously, data with so few patients do not establish one way or the other the relationship between nonhypertensive renal disease and fetal lung maturation. However, it is of interest that the tendency in nonhypertensive renal disease is toward a delay rather than an acceleration of fetal lung maturation.

E. Rh Isoimmunization

Aubry et al. [13] reported a delay in the rise of the L/S ratio with the advancement of pregnancy in 69 patients with Rh sensitization. However, they did not report separately on those with hydrops fetalis. A subsequent study also reported a delay of fetal pulmonary maturation (L/S < 2 after 36 weeks) in nine patients with hydrops fetalis, while there was no such delay in 19 isoimmunized pregnancies with no hydrops [8]. Bent et al. [19] as well as Doran et al. [96] found no changes in fetal lung maturation with Rh isoimmunization. The incidence of PG-positive AF samples at 35-36 weeks' gestation was not different from their controls. Likewise, a more recent study did not find any effect of Rh isoimmunization on fetal lung maturation [97]. From the available data no definitive conclusions are apparent concerning Rh sensitization and fetal lung maturity. However, it would appear that in the absence of serious fetal disease Rh sensitization per se has little effect on fetal lung maturation.

VIII. Conclusions

Although there are numerous articles on the subject of the effects of maternal and/or fetal disorders on fetal lung maturation, especially in relation to diabetes mellitus and prolonged ROM, the data are still inconclusive. A major cause for this is that most of the studies do not have sufficient controls matched for gestational age. Obtaining data from adequate numbers of patients with one or more disease entities studied at a certain period of gestation with corresponding matched controls is an extremely difficult thing to do. For instance, suppose you have data from a class B diabetic with twins who develops preeclampsia and has prolonged ROM, what do you compare that data to? Another problem is the number of variations in methodology that have been utilized by different investigators to try to determine acceleration or delay in fetal lung maturation. Also, only a few reports contain any statistical comparisons. Another major concern is that only a few studies have contained data on serial determinations of AF surfactant levels. However, it is not ethically feasible to obtain serial determinations in normal subjects. The only group which could qualify as controls for serial amniocentesis studies would be Rh-sensitized women who subsequently deliver Rh-negative infants. Even they, the pure scientist could argue, are not normal controls. Also, it would be very difficult for an investigator to accumulate a large amount of data on these patients.

Considering the difficulties involved, what is needed most at the present time are reports of prospective studies from a single institution, utilizing the same methodology, encompassing a large number of patients, including an adequate number of matched controls, and subjecting the data to statistical analysis. We would all welcome such information.

References

1. Fencl, M. deM., and D. Tulchinsky, Total cortisol in amniotic fluid and fetal lung maturation, *N. Engl. J. Med.,* **292**:133 (1975).
2. Johnson, B., and P. A. Hensleigh, Surfactant tests and amniotic fluid cortisol, *Am. J. Obstet. Gynecol.,* **129**:105 (1977).
3. Divers, W. A., A. Babaknia, B. R. Hopper, M. M. Wilkes, and S. S. C. Yen, Fetal lung maturation. Amniotic fluid catecholamines, phospholipids, and cortisol, *Am. J. Obstet. Gynecol.,* **142**:440 (1982).
4. Nelson, G. H., K. Eguchi, and J. C. McPherson, Effects of gestational age, dexamethasone, and metopirone on lecithin concentration in fetal lung tissue and amniotic fluid, *Gynec. Invest.,* **7**:337 (1976).
5. Amiel-Tison, C., Neurologic problems in perinatology, *Clin. Perinatal.,* **1**:33 (1974).
6. Gould, J. B., L. Gluck, and M. V. Kulovich, The relationship between accelerated pulmonary maturity and accelerated neurological maturity in certain chronically stressed pregnancies, *Am. J. Obstet. Gynecol.,* **127**:181 (1977).

7. Nelson, G. H., J. C. McPherson, and K. Eguchi, Effect of hypoxia on lecithin concentration in fetal lung tissue and amniotic fluid in rats, *Am. J. Obstet. Gynecol.,* **132**:226 (1978).
8. Morrison, J. C., W. D. Whybrew, E. T. Bucovaz, W. L. Wiser, and S. A. Fish, The lecithin/sphingomyelin ratio in cases associated with feto-maternal disease, *Am. J. Obstet. Gynecol.,* **127**:363 (1977).
9. Robert, M. F., R. K. Neff, J. P. Hubbell, H. W. Taeusch, and M. E. Avery, Association between maternal diabetes and the respiratory distress syndrome in the newborn, *N. Engl. J. Med.,* **294**:357 (1976).
10. Fadel, H. E., Diabetes mellitus and pregnancy. In Diagnosis and Management of Obstetric Emergencies. (Edited by H. E. Fadel.) Menlo Park, California, Addison-Wesley, 1982, p. 264.
11. Fadel, H. E., Management of pregnancy in diabetic women, *Hosp. Form.,* **18**:185 (1983).
12. Gluck, L., and M. V. Kulovich, Lecithin/sphingomyelin ratios in amniotic fluid in normal and abnormal pregnancy, *Am. J. Obstet. Gynecol.,* **115**:539 (1973).
13. Aubry, R. H., J. E. Rourke, R. Almanza, R. M. Cantor, and J. E. Van Doren, The lecithin/sphingomyelin ratio in a high risk obstetric population, *Obstet. Gynecol.,* **47**:21 (1976).
14. Goldkrand, J. W., and D. S. Slattery, Patterns of pulmonary maturation in normal and abnormal pregnancy, *Obstet. Gynecol.,* **53**:348 (1979).
15. Dyson, D., M. Blake, and G. Cassady, Amniotic fluid lecithin/sphingomyelin ratio in complicated pregnancies, *Am. J. Obstet. Gynecol.,* **122**:772 (1975).
16. Tabsh, K. M. A., C. R. Brinkman, III, and R. A. Bashore, Lecithin sphingomyelin ratio in pregnancies complicated by insulin dependent diabetes mellitus, *Obstet. Gynecol.,* **59**:353 (1982).
17. Kulovich, M. V., and L. Gluck, The lung profile. II. Complicated pregnancy, *Am. J. Obstet. Gynecol.,* **135**:64 (1979).
18. Cunningham, M. D., H. E. McKean, D. H. Gillispie, and J. W. Greene, Jr., Improved prediction of fetal lung maturity in diabetic pregnancies. A comparison of chromatographic methods, *Am. J. Obstet. Gynecol.,* **142**:197 (1982).
19. Bent, A. E., J. H. Gray, E. R. Luther, M. Oulton, and L. J. Peddle, Assessment of fetal lung maturity. Relationships of gestational age and pregnancy complications to phosphatidylglycerol levels, *Am. J. Obstet. Gynecol.,* **142**:664 (1982).
20. Simon, N. V., W. A. Hohman, R. C. Elser, J. S. Levisky, M. J. Carp, and S. S. Ashton, Fetal lung maturity in complicated pregnancy, as predicted from microviscosity of amniotic fluid, *Clin. Chem.,* **28**:1754 (1982).
21. Pedersen, J., *The Pregnant Diabetic and Her Newborn,* 2nd ed., Baltimore, Williams & Wilkins, 1977.

22. Warshaw, J. B., Insulin influences on fetal growth. In *The Diabetic Pregnancy and Its Outcome.* Mead Johnson Symposium on Perinatal and Developmental Medicine, No. 13, Vail, Colorado, 1978.
23. Maniscalco, W. M., C. M. Wilson, I. Gross, L. Gobran, S. A. Rooney, and J. B. Warshaw, Development of glycogen and phospholipid metabolism in fetal and newborn rat lung, *Biochem. Biophys. Acta,* **530**:333 (1978).
24. Gross, I., and G. J. W. Smith, Insulin delays the morphologic maturation of fetal rat lung in vitro, *Pediatr. Res.,* **11**:515 (1977).
25. Smith, B. T., C. J. P. Giroud, M. Robert, and M. E. Avery, Insulin antagonism of cortisol action on lecithin synthesis by cultured fetal lung cells, *J. Pediatr.,* **87**:953 (1975).
26. Boutwell, W. C., and A. S. Goldman, Depressed biochemical lung maturation and steroid uptake in animal model of infant of diabetic mother (IDM), *Pediatr. Res.,* **13**:355 (1979).
27. Morrison, J. C., J. M. Schneider, W. D. Whybrew, and E. T. Bucovaz, Lecithin sphingomyelin ratio and RDS in patients with diabetes mellitus; possible mechanisms, *South. Med. J.,* **73**:912 (1980).
28. Stubbs, W. A., and S. M. Stubbs, Hyperinsulinism, diabetes mellitus, and respiratory distress of the newborn. A common link?, *Lancet,* **i**:308 (1978).
29. Sosenko, I. R., J. L. Kitzmiller, S. W. Loo, P. Blix, A. H. Rubinstein, and K. H. Gabby, The infant of the diabetic mother. Correlation of increased cord C-peptide levels with macrosomia and hypoglycemia, *N. Engl. J. Med.,* **301**:859 (1979).
30. Tyden, O., C. Berne, and U. Eriksson, Lung maturation in fetuses of diabetic rats, *Pediatr. Res.,* **14**:1192 (1980).
31. Epstein, M. F., P. M. Farrell, and R. A. Chez, Fetal lung lecithin metabolism in the glucose intolerant Rhesus monkey in pregnancy, *Pediatrics,* **57**:722 (1976).
32. Sosenko, I. R. S., E. E. Lawson, V. Demottoz, and I. D. Frantz, Functional delay in lung maturation in fetuses of diabetic rabbits, *J. Appl. Physiol.,* **48**:643 (1980).
33. Hallman, M., and K. Teramo, Amniotic fluid phospholipid profile as a predictor of fetal maturity in diabetic pregnancies, *Obstet. Gynecol.,* **54**:703 (1979).
34. Curet, L. B., R. W. Olson, J. M. Schneider, and R. D. Zachman, Effect of diabetes mellitus on amniotic fluid lecithin/sphingomyelin ratio and respiratory distress syndrome, *Am. J. Obstet. Gynecol.,* **135**:10 (1979).
35. Chesley, L. C., *Hypertensive Disorders of Pregnancy.* New York, Appleton-Century-Crofts, 1978, pp. 418.
36. Gabbe, S. G., R. I. Lowensohn, J. H. Mestman, R. K. Freeman, and U. Goebelsmann, Lecithin/sphingomyelin ratio in pregnancies complicated by diabetes mellitus, *Am. J. Obstet. Gynecol.,* **128**:757 (1977).

37. Dahlenberg, G. W., F. I. R. Martin, P. E. Jeffrey, and I. Horacek, Amniotic fluid lecithin/sphingomyelin ratio in pregnancy complicated by diabetes, *Br. J. Obstet. Gynaecol.,* **84**:294 (1977).
38. Tchobroutsky, C., C. Amiel-Tison, L. Cedard, E. Eschwege, J. L. Rouvullois, and G. Tchobroutsky, The lecithin/sphingomyelin ratio in 132 insulin dependent diabetic pregnancies, *Am. J. Obstet. Gynecol.,* **130**:754 (1978).
39. Cruz, A. C., W. C. Buhi, S. A. Birk, and W. N. Spellacy, Respiratory distress syndrome with mature lecithin/sphingomyelin ratios. Diabetes mellitus and low Apgar scores, *Am. J. Obstet. Gynecol.,* **126**:78 (1976).
40. Mueller-Heubach, E., S. N. Caritis, D. I. Edelstone, and J. H. Turner, Lecithin/sphingomyelin ratio in amniotic fluid and its value for the prediction of neonatal respiratory distress syndrome in pregnant diabetic women, *Am. J. Obstet. Gynecol.,* **130**:28 (1978).
41. Usher, R. H., A. C. Allen, and F. H. McLean, Risk of respiratory distress syndrome related to gestational age, route of delivery, and maternal diabetes, *Am. J. Obstet. Gynecol.,* **111**:826 (1971).
42. O'Brien, W. F., and R. D. Cefalo, Clinical applicability of amniotic fluid tests for fetal pulmonary maturity, *Am. J. Obstet. Gynecol.,* **136**:135 (1980).
43. Nelson, G. H., Amniotic fluid phospholipid patterns in normal and abnormal pregnancies, *Am. J. Obstet. Gynecol.,* **105**:1072 (1969).
44. Nelson, G. H., Relationship between amniotic fluid lecithin concentration and respiratory distress syndrome, *Am. J. Obstet. Gynecol.,* **112**:827 (1972).
45. Fadel, H. E., and S. Hammond, Diabetes mellitus in pregnancy. Management and results, *J. Reprod. Med.,* **27**:56 (1982).
46. Nelson, G. H., Lecithin/sphingomyelin ratio changes with estrogen or glucocorticoid treatment. Letter to the editor, *Am. J. Obstet. Gynecol.,* **116**:292 (1973).
47. Nelson, G. H., Respiratory distress syndrome with mature lecithin/sphingomyelin ratios. Diabetes mellitus and low Apgar scroes. Letter to the editor, *Am. J. Obstet. Gynecol.,* **129**:231 (1977).
48. Cunningham, M. D., N. S. Desai, S. A. Thompson, and J. M. Greene, Amniotic fluid phosphatidylglycerol in diabetic pregnancies, *Am. J. Obstet. Gynecol.,* **131**:719 (1978).
49. Mintz, D. H., R. A. Chez, and D. L. Hutchinson, Subhuman primate pregnancy complicated by streptozotocin induced diabetes mellitus, *J. Clin. Invest.,* **51**:837 (1972).
50. Hallman, M., and L. Gluck, Phosphatidylglycerol in lung surfactant. III. Possible modifier of surfactant function, *J. Lipid Res.,* **17**:257 (1976).
51. Godinez, R. I., R. L. Sanders, and W. J. Longmore, Phosphatidylglycerol in rat lung. I. Identification as a metabolically active phospholipid in isolated perfused rat lung, *Biochemistry,* **14**:830 (1975).

52. Hallman, M., B. H. Feldman, E. Kirkpatrick, and L. Gluck, Absence of phosphatidylglycerol (PG) in respiratory distress syndrome in the newborn, *Pediatr. Res.,* **11**:714 (1977).
53. Kulovich, M. V., M. Hallman, and L. Gluck, The lung profile. I. Normal pregnancy, *Am. J. Obstet. Gynecol.,* **135**:57 (1979).
54. Bustos, R., M. V. Kulovich, L. Gluck, S. G. Gabbe, L. Evertson, C. Vargos, and E. Lowenberg, Significance of phosphatidylglycerol in amniotic fluid in complicated pregnancies, *Am. J. Obstet. Gynecol.,* **133**:899 (1979).
55. Hallman, M., M. V. Kulovich, E. Kirkpatrick, R. G. Sugarman, and L. Gluck, Phosphatidylinositol and phosphatidylglycerol in amniotic fluid: Indices of lung maturity, *Am. J. Obstet. Gynecol.,* **125**:613 (1976).
56. Skjaeraasen, J., and S. Stray-Pedersen, Amniotic fluid phosphatidylinositol and phosphatidylglycerol. I. Normal pregnancies. *Acta Obstet. Gynecol. Scand.,* **58**:225 (1979).
57. Stedman, C. M., S. Crawford, E. Staten, and W. B. Cherny, Management of preterm premature rupture of membranes. Assessing amniotic fluid in the vagina for phosphatidylglycerol, *Am. J. Obstet. Gynecol.,* **140**:34 (1981).
58. Richardson, C. J., J. J. Pomerance, M. D. Cunningham, and L. Gluck, Acceleration of fetal lung maturation following prolonged rupture of the membranes, *Am. J. Obstet. Gynecol.,* **118**:1115 (1974).
59. Yoon, J. J., and R. G. Harper, Observations on the relationship between the duration of rupture of membranes and the development of idiopathic respiratory distress syndrome, *Pediatrics,* **52**:161 (1973).
60. Rajegowda, B. K., M. D. Freedman, H. Falciglia, M. Exconde, and T. Sukumarar, Absence of respiratory distress syndrome (RDS) following premature rupture of membranes in one sib of a set of twins in 2 cases, *Clin. Res.,* **23**:600A (1975).
61. Jones, M. D., Jr., L. I. Burd, W. A. Bowes, Jr., F. C. Battaglia, and L. O. Lubchenco, Failure of association of premature rupture of membranes with respiratory distress syndrome, *N. Engl. J. Med.,* **292**:1253 (1975).
62. Sell, E. J., and T. R. Harris, Association of premature rupture of membranes with idiopathic respiratory distress syndrome, *Obstet. Gynecol.,* **49**:167 (1977).
63. Berkowitz, R. L., B. W. Bonta, and J. E. Warshaw, The relationship between premature rupture of the membranes and the respiratory distress syndrome, *Am. J. Obstet. Gynecol.,* **124**:712 (1976).
64. Berkowitz, R. L., R. D. Kantor, G. J. Beck, and J. B. Warshaw, The relationship between premature rupture of the membranes and the respiratory distress syndrome, *Am. J. Obstet. Gynecol.,* **131**:503 (1978).
65. Berkowitz, R. L., L. Hoder, R. M. Freedman, D. T. Scott, and M. C. Maltzer, Results of a management protocol for premature rupture of the membranes, *Obstet. Gynecol.,* **60**:271 (1982).

66. Christensen, K. K., P. Christensen, I. Ingemarsson, P. Mardh, E. Nordenfelt, E. Ripa, T. Solum, and N. Svenningsen, A study of complications in preterm deliveries after prolonged premature rupture of the membranes, *Obstet. Gynecol.,* **48**:670 (1976).
67. Barrada, M. I., N. L. Virnig, L. E. Edwards, and E. Y. Hakanson, Maternal intravenous ethanol in the prevention of respiratory distress syndrome, *Am. J. Obstet. Gynecol.,* **129**:25 (1977).
68. Quirk, J. G., Jr., R. K. Raker, R. H. Petrie, and A. M. Williams, The role of glucocorticoids, unstressful labor, and atraumatic delivery in the prevention of respiratory distress syndrome, *Am. J. Obstet. Gynecol.,* **134**:768 (1979).
69. Taeusch, H. W., Jr., F. Frigoletto, J. Kitzmiller, M. E. Avery, A. Hehre, B. Fromm, E. Lawson, and R. Neff, Risk of respiratory distress syndrome after prenatal dexamethasone treatment, *Pediatrics,* **63**:64 (1979).
70. Schreiber, J., and T. Benedetti, Conservative management of preterm premature rupture of the fetal membranes in a low socio-economic population, *Am. J. Obstet. Gynecol.,* **136**:92 (1980).
71. Worthington, D., A. H. Maloney, and B. T. Smith, Fetal lung maturity. I. Mode of onset of premature labor. Influence of premature rupture of the membranes, *Obstet. Gynecol.,* **49**:275 (1977).
72. Pitkin, R. M., Personal communication. March, 1984.
73. Frantz, I. D., III, S. M. Adler, B. T. Thach, I. Wyszogrodski, B. D. Fletcher, H. W. Taeusch, Jr., and M. E. Avery, The effect of amniotic fluid removal on pulmonary maturation in sheep, *Pediatrics,* **56**:474 (1975).
74. Bauer, C. R., L. Stern, and E. Colle, Prolonged rupture of membranes associated with a decreased incidence of respiratory distress syndrome, *Pediatrics,* **53**:7 (1974).
75. Cohen, W., M. deM. Fencl, and D. Tulchinsky, Amniotic fluid cortisol after premature rupture of membranes, *J. Pediatr.,* **88**:1007 (1976).
76. Kappy, K. A., C. L. Cetrulo, R. A. Knuppel, C. J. Ingardia, A. J. Sbarra, J. C. Scerbo, and G. W. Mitchell, Premature rupture of the membranes. A conservative approach, *Am. J. Obstet. Gynecol.,* **134**:655 (1979).
77. Stafford, C. R., and H. E. Fadel, A protocol for the management of preterm premature rupture of the membranes, in preparation.
78. Garite, T. J., R. K. Freeman, E. M. Linzey, and P. S. Braly, The use of amniocentesis in patients with premature rupture of membranes, *Obstet. Gynecol.,* **54**:226 (1979).
79. Dombroski, R. A., J. Mackenna, and R. G. Bramer, Comparison of amniotic fluid lung maturity profiles in paired vaginal and amniocentesis specimens, *Am. J. Obstet. Gynecol.,* **140**:461 (1981).
80. Chiswick, M. L., and E. Durpard, Respiratory distress syndrome, *Lancet,* **i**:1060 (1973).

81. Pardi, G., and A. Marini, Fetal lung maturation in toxemia and estrogen therapy in the management of respiratory distress syndrome, *Lancet,* **ii**:1453 (1974).
82. Emara, S. H., M. F. El-Hawary, H. A. Abdel-Karim, and F. El-Heneidy, Amniotic fluid total lipids, cholesterol, phospholipids, and inorganic phosphorus in toxemia of pregnancy, *Acta Med. Acad. Sci. Hung.,* **33**:179 (1976).
83. Yambao, T. J., D. Clark, C. Smith, and R. H. Aubry, Amniotic fluid phosphatidylglycerol in stressed pregnancies, *Am. J. Obstet. Gynecol.,* **141**:191 (1981).
84. Freeman, R. K., B. G. Bateman, U. Goebelsmann, J. J. Arce, and J. James, Clinical experience with the amniotic fluid lecithin/sphingomyelin ratio, *Am. J. Obstet. Gynecol.,* **119**:239 (1974).
85. Yoon, J. J., S. Kohl, and R. G. Harper, The relationship between maternal hypertensive disease of pregnancy and the incidence of idiopathic respiratory distress syndrome, *Pediatrics,* **65**:735 (1980).
86. Gunston, K. D., and D. A. Davey, Growth retarded fetuses and pulmonary maturity, *S. Afr. Med. J.,* **54**:493 (1978).
87. Lindback, T., Amniotic fluid lecithin concentrations in pregnancies complicated by hypertensive disorders and intrauterine growth retardation, *Acta Obstet. Gynecol. Scand.,* **55**:355 (1976).
88. Sher, G., B. E. Statland, and V. K. Knutzen, Evaluation of the small third-trimester fetuses using the foam stability index test, *Obstet. Gynecol.,* **58**: 314 (1981).
89. Gross, T. L., R. J. Sokol, M. V. Wilson, P. M. Kuhnert, and V. Hirsch, Amniotic fluid phosphatidylglycerol: A potentially useful predictor of intrauterine growth retardation, *Am. J. Obstet. Gynecol.,* **140**:277 (1981).
90. Okada, D. M., and D. W. Thibeault, The incompetent cervix and accelerated fetal lung maturation, *Am. J. Obstet. Gynecol.,* **127**:462 (1977).
91. Das, S. K., and H. W. Foster, Amniotic fluid lipids in sickle cell disease, *Am. J. Obstet. Gynecol.,* **136**:211 (1980).
92. Sims, C. D., D. B. Cowan, and C. E. Parkinson, The lecithin/sphingomyelin (L/S) ratio in twin pregnancies, *Br. J. Obstet. Gynaecol.,* **83**:447 (1976).
93. Spellacy, W. N., A. C. Cruz, W. C. Buhi, and S. A. Birk, Amniotic fluid L/S ratio in twin gestation, *Obstet. Gynecol.,* **50**:68 (1977).
94. Picker, R. H., D. H. Smith, and D. M. Saunders, A new method of amniocentesis using ultrasound in multiple pregnancy to assess the second twin, *Obstet. Gynecol.,* **50**:489 (1977).

95. Leveno, K. J., J. G. Quirk, P. J. Whalley, W. N. P. Herbert, and R. Trubey, Fetal lung maturation in twin gestation, *Am. J. Obstet. Gynecol.,* **148**:405 (1984).
96. Doran, T. A., R. M. Malone, R. J. Benzie, V. J. Owen, D. W. Thompson, and M. L. New, Amniotic fluid tests for fetal maturity in normal and abnormal pregnancies, *Am. J. Obstet. Gynecol.,* **125**:586 (1976).
97. Quinlan, R. W., W. C. Buhi, and A. C. Cruz, Fetal pulmonary maturity in isoimmunized pregnancies, *Am. J. Obstet. Gynecol.,* **148**:787 (1984).

Part Four

PREDELIVERY

11

A Modern Maternal Transport System

DANIEL K. ROBERTS and JOHN F. EVANS

University of Kansas School of Medicine–Wichita
and Wesley Medical Center
Wichita, Kansas

I. Introduction

The May 1983 issue of *Hospital Aviation* [1] lists 46 hospital-based air medical services. Forty of these use only helicopters, one uses fixed-wing only, and five use both fixed-wing aircraft and helicopters. The system described in this chapter is one of the five that use both fixed-wing and helicopters, along with specially equipped vans. This system originated in 1974 as a newborn transport system. Six months later maternal transport began and now it almost equals the number of newborn transports. Recently the transport system has expanded to include nonperinatal transports as well. This chapter will discuss the maternal transport aspect of this system, which is medically justified by improved perinatal outcomes and providing the opportunity for intensive care to everyone.

The expenditure of our health care dollars is becoming increasingly scrutinized. We feel that the care of a mother and her newborn offers the best potential for the highest return. In no other area of medicine can the health care dollar have the longitudinal value extended over the sum of two life expectancies, as represented by the mother and her newborn. If the outcome is good, the mother can continue her contribution to society and her well newborn can likewise have a greater potential for becoming a contributing member of society.

The challenge to identify high-risk pregnancies is not eliminated or changed by maternal transport. We have known for many years that approximately 25-30% of our pregnancies account for 75% of our newborn morbidity and mortality.

Maternal transport has the ability to increase the general awareness of high-risk factors by providing the opportunity for daily dialogue with the receiving facility as well as a mechanism to provide care for the more critically ill pregnancies. In a recent analysis of 2744 consecutively delivered patients, Sokol and Chik [2] noted that the large majority of primary emergency cesarean sections "could not be predicted before the onset of labor." A logical extension of this observation would be that no delivery should take place in a facility that is not equipped to adequately perform an emergency cesarean delivery. The implementation of this philosophy would place severe restrictions on some of our health care facilities. In an attempt to maintain the appropriate intensity of care that may be needed on an infrequent basis, maternal transport systems have been developed. They are designed to provide the appropriate intensity of care by minimizing the problems of distance, time, and lack of appropriate equipment and personnel. Our transport system evolved from the usual "ambulance system." By the mid-1960s, ambulance services were provided by funeral homes (50%), volunteers (24%), fire or police (13%), and hospitals (3%). In this system, only 0.16% of patients received any medical attention while in the "ambulance." In review of cases that required transport of mothers, one-third of the transports required surgery which was not possible under the existing system. Fortunately, ambulance service has improved significantly with the development of the national Emergency Medical System (EMS). We do not feel, however, that this EMS adequately meets the needs of our high-risk mothers.

The EMS is continually raising its standards and upgrading its levels of competency. However, this system differs from the maternal transport in its goals in two major areas. First, it is oriented to on-scene or initial-response care. This is contrasted to maternal care in which the patient is usually already in a controlled hospital environment. Secondly, since the philosophy of the EMS is directed to prehospitalization, even the most intense of paramedic courses spend only a very small fraction of their time dealing with high-risk maternal situations. It is, therefore, necessary to develop a system to meet the unique, peculiar, but highly technical, needs of care for the high-risk mother and her fetus.

We are already seeing administrators of smaller hospitals and low-volume delivery suites discouraging the use of expenditures for sophisticated equipment and specially trained personnel. With the increase in public awareness of modern monitoring devices and with the increasing expectancy of a guaranteed healthy newborn, a heavy financial and medical burden is placed on those providing such care. Balanced against the cost of this equipment and personnel is the devastation that can occur if the outcome of a pregnancy is less than perfect. Physicians and other health care professionals need to respond with an appropriate system. Hopefully, the maternal transport concept can meet the needs for cost containment while providing appropriate intensity of care for those pregnancies that have such needs.

Statistically, the first 24 hr of life carry the highest mortality and certainly the greatest morbidity for the entire life of the individual. Maternal instability due to hypoxia, hypoglycemia, hypertension, anemia, and a host of other factors may further aggravate and compromise the fetus. Transport of a fetus in utero will not reduce the intensity of care needed for maternal conditions, but it would place the newborn in an appropriate intensive care environment should delivery be necessary. With the increased utilization of the maternal transport system our newborn intensive care census has shifted toward a higher percentage of smaller, more immature infants in greater need of neonatal expertise.

It is the goal of this chapter to discuss the organizational units, costs, and perinatal outcome associated with the maternal transport system. In addition, we will present suggestions and guidelines for the establishment of such a system. We base our suggestions on 9 years' experience with our present system in Kansas.

II. Organization

A. General

In the state of Kansas there are two level III perinatal centers to serve the approximately 40,000 annual deliveries. We are fortunate to have the benefit of some appropriated legislative funds allotted to the University of Kansas School of Medicine. The level III center that implements maternal transports is located in Wichita and has a very close working relationship with the community hospital, Wesley Medical Center. The other level III center is at the University of Kansas School of Medicine at Kansas City. These two centers are supported by 11 level II centers, which are distributed throughout the state and are determined not only on the basis of geographical location and delivery volume, but availability of professional personnel, 24-hr registered nurse supervision of nurseries, and administrative commitment. The remaining 121 hospitals are designated as level I centers and vary significantly in their distribution of personnel as well as delivery volume. The maternal transport system serves as one of the links that support the daily dialogue between all providers of obstetrical care throughout the state. Although the major goal of the system is to provide service, additional goals are to provide education and medical treatment updates. Tables 1-3 outline, in brief, the health care providers available and patients eligible for the respective intensity of care levels.

Table 1 Level I Center

Providers:	Ob/Gyn, family physicians
Activities:	High-quality routine prenatal care
	Identification of at risk mothers
	Referral of special laboratory studies
	Phone consultations
	Referral of patients for specific procedures
	Referral of patients in anticipation of NICU needs
	Electronic fetal monitoring in labor
Mothers to be delivered:	Uncomplicated prenatal
	Term gestations
	Stabilization of unexpected problems
	Mild PIH at term
	Newborn without anticipated NICU needs

Table 2 Level II Center

Providers:	Ob/Gyn, pediatricians, family physicians, anesthesiologist, specialty consultants, radiologist with Ob ultrasound training, full-time nursery personnel
Activities:	Level I
	Cerclage
	Amniocentesis for maturity
	Ultrasound for gestational age
	Fetal monitoring, prenatal
	24-hr blood gas availability
	Blood bank with 24-hr technician staffing
	Some special laboratory studies
Mothers to be delivered:	Level I
	Stable gestational diabetics
	Previously complicated pregnancies, controlled
	Mild Rh isoimmunization

Table 2 (Continued)

Mothers to be delivered:	(continued)
	Twins, near term
	Post-term
	Moderate PIH
	Mild IUGR
	Premature but over 32 weeks or 1500 g

Table 3 Level III Center

Providers:	Maternal-fetal medicine, Ob with special high-risk interest and training, neonatologist, subspecialty consultants, Ob/Ped anesthesiologist, ultrasonographer, NICU nursing, full-time medical social service
Activities:	Levels I and II
	Genetic amniocentesis
	Prenatal fetal evaluations for fetal distress
	Diagnostic ultrasound
	Evaluate need for intrauterine transfusion
	All special laboratory studies
Mothers to be delivered:	Levels I and II
	Unstable gestational diabetic
	Insulin-dependent diabetic
	Moderate to severe Rh, other isoimmunization
	Severe PIH
	Moderate to severe IUGR
	Suspected maternal infection, with anticipated neonatal infection
	Congenital anomalies that might require NICU or immediate surgery
	Premature twins, triplets, etc.
	Premature, $<$32 weeks or 1500 g
	Other unstable complicated pregnancies

B. Personnel

The State as a Unit

The organization of the Kansas Regional Perinatal Care Program is outlined in Table 4. The program is governed by the Perinatal Executive Committee, which is organized and directed by the Kansas Department of Health and Environment and the Director of its Bureau of Maternal and Child Health. Its members include the chairmen of the departments of Obstetrics and Gynecology and Pediatrics at the University of Kansas School of Medicine in both Kansas City and Wichita. A representative from the Kansas chapter of the American Academy of Pediatrics and one from the Kansas chapter of the American Academy of Family Physicians attend these meetings along with representatives from the Kansas Obstetrical and Gynecological Society, the Kansas Hospital Association, and the Kansas State Nurses Association. This committee meets on an annual basis and was instrumental in the original organization of the regional system for the state and in providing early support for newborn and maternal transports.

The more functional and operational aspects of the program are accomplished by the Perinatal Medical Council. This council comprises a chairman (currently an obstetrician at a level III center), representatives from obstetrics and neonatology from both level III centers, an obstetrician from a level II center,

Table 4 Kansas Regional Perinatal Care Program

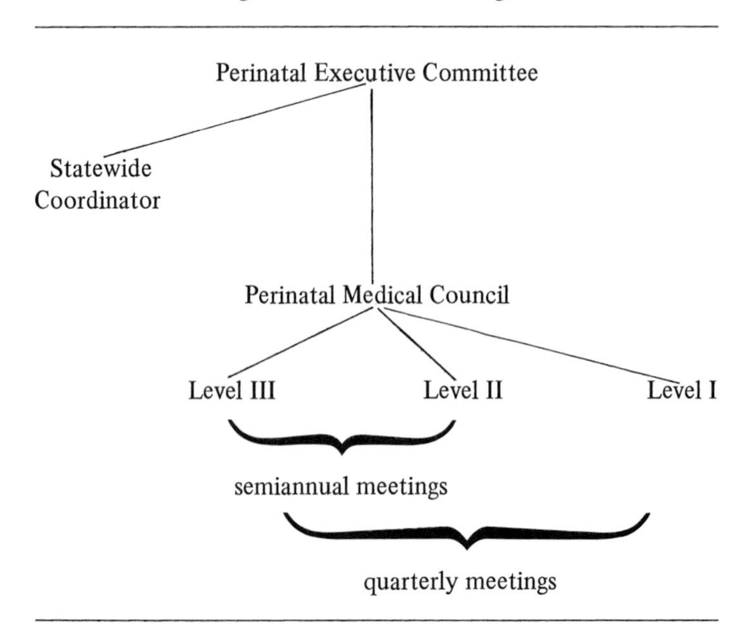

the Director of the Bureau of Maternal and Child Health, a representative from the nursing component of the Bureau of Maternal and Child Health, and various invited health care professionals. The council meets on a monthly basis, and it has been instrumental in the establishment of guidelines for levels II and III centers and has recently recommended guidelines for level I centers. The Council serves as the organizational format for statewide meetings and has also been instrumental in defining areas underserved by newborn and obstetrical health care providers in the state. It has taken steps to assure that medical students desiring to serve in these areas will maintain their eligibility for financial assistance. A statewide administrative coordinator integrates the activities of the Executive Committee and the Medical Council.

The Institute as a Unit

While the Perinatal Transport System in Wichita originated as a newborn system, it was always the goal to have a maternal system that would provide for maternal and fetal stabilization to minimize the need for newborn intensive care services. The need for neonatal transport was more apparent to health care providers and, therefore, this system began approximately 6 months prior to the maternal system. Initially, there was a great deal of resistance to maternal transport within the administrative ranks of the tertiary center hospitals. Their concerns were largely oriented toward the medical-legal implications. Nonetheless, the determination and zeal of the Chairman of the Department of Obstetrics and Gynecology and the Director of Newborn Services prevailed and the maternal transport system was begun. Within several months of operation, the maternal transport system provided the administration with proof of its viability. Subsequently, our hospital administration became a very enthusiastic supporter of the system. An abbreviated organizational scheme is shown in Table 5. As a result of its success, the system has been expanded to include trauma and seriously ill transports. A department has now been formed to coordinate transports of mothers and babies as well as nonperinatal patients.

The maternal transport system represents a unique integration of a private hospital facility and the clinical branch of a university school of medicine. The medical administration of the program is under the direction of the Departments of Obstetrics and Gynecology and Pediatrics at the Medical School as well as the Directors of Ob-Gyn and Pediatric Education at Wesley Medical Center. The Division of Perinatal Medicine represents the cooperative efforts of the education Departments of Obstetrics and Pediatrics at Wesley Medical Center. Continuity of medical personnel is provided by individuals occupying dual offices. The Chairman of the Department of Ob-Gyn at the Medical School is also the Director of Ob-Gyn Education at Wesley Medical Center. The Director of Pediatric Education is also the Associate Head of the Division of Perinatal Medicine.

Table 5 Perinatal Transport Local Organization

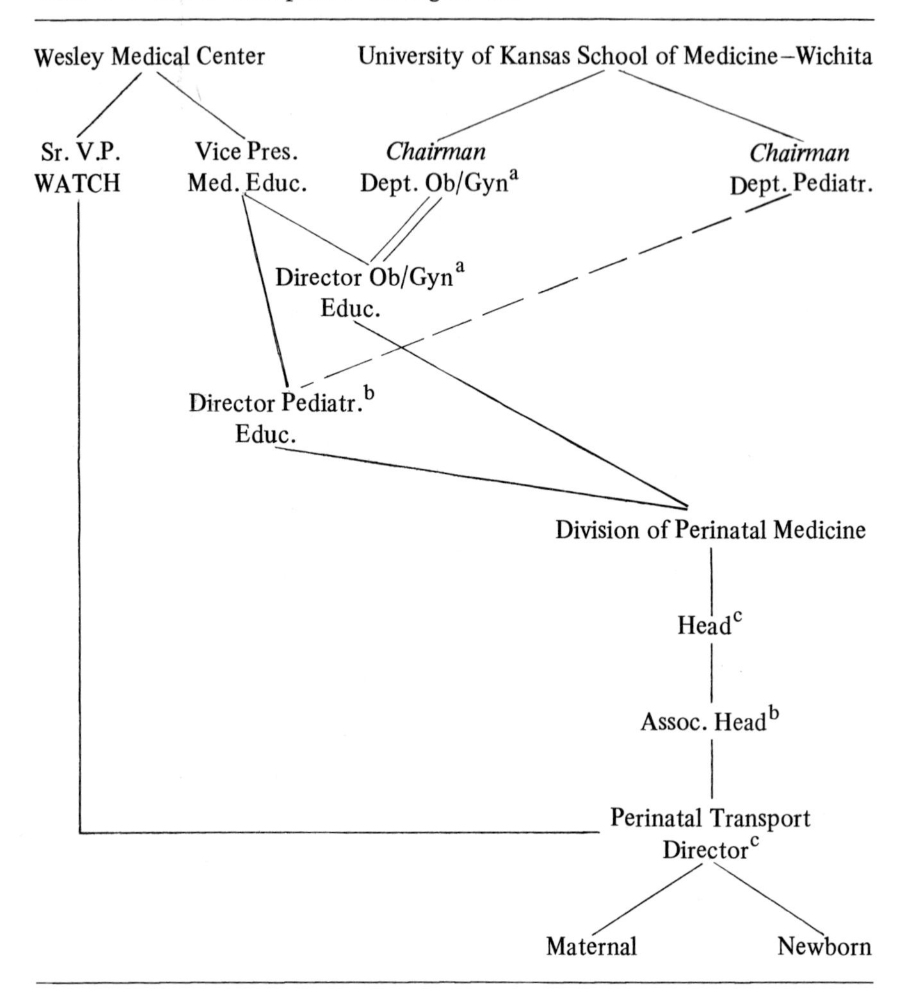

[a]Position occupied by same individual.
[b]Position occupied by same individual.
[c]Position occupied by same individual.
WATCH = *W*esley *A*ir *T*ransport to *C*ommunity *H*ospitals.

The Head of the Division of Perinatal Medicine is the Perinatal Transport Director (PTD) and is a subspecialist in maternal-fetal medicine with special emphasis on maternal transports.

The administrative direction is provided by the Vice President of Medical Education and a Senior Vice President who is presently a registered nurse. It is their responsibility to provide the administrative expertise and budget defense for equipment and personnel.

The Transport Team as a Unit

The members of the maternal transport team are listed in Table 6.

Each member of the maternal transport team has a prescribed role and the success of the transport in large part depends on the presence and abilities of each member. Further descriptions of the roles are as follows:

1. The perinatal transport director should be a board certified obstetrician-gynecologist and preferably should also be board eligible or certified in maternal-fetal medicine. In addition, this individual should be a Federal Aviation Administration Medical Examiner. The responsibilities of the position were developed by the American Society of Hospital-Based Emergency Air Medical Services. These include but are not limited to establishing medical guidelines and serving as overall supervisor for the medical transport team. The PTD also provides liaison between the obstetrical resident staff and the referring physician and staff from the referring hospital; assists in the provision of continuing education for the transport team, including members at referring facilities; supervises the quality control aspects of the program and certifies the competency of the medical personnel to perform skills required for the stabilization and delivery of high-risk mothers; communicates closely with the hospital administration to assure compliance with hospital policies; serves as coordinator between the referring physicans and neonatologists and assures that appropriate follow-up

Table 6 Maternal Transport Team

Medical	Support
Perinatal transport director	Dispatchers
Upper level Ob residents	Drivers
Transport nurses	Pilots
NICU respiratory therapists	Security officers
Referring physicians	Local EMS
Staff from referring hospital	

care is received by each transport patient; participates in the marketing of the program, particularly to physician and nursing groups; and meets the recommended Federal Aviation guidelines as an aeromedical consultant as both a military trained flight surgeon and as an FAA aviation medical examiner.

2. The upper level obstetrical residents for the high-risk maternal service work closely with the PTD. Patient status for both undelivered and delivered patients and their newborns are evaluated and reviewed each day. The obstetrical resident serves as liaison between the PTD and the neonatologist on call and must be knowledgeable concerning maternal and neonatal bed availability as this may affect the routing of a maternal transport. Each resident receives clear instructions not only in the procedures and policies of the transport system, including patient management, but he must also have a clear understanding of how each transfer is to be handled. The resident's performance is closely scrutinized by the PTD and follow-up concerning the resident's performance is obtained from the referring physician. We feel that this responsibility provides a very unique opportunity for obstetricians-in-training to exercise their judgment and abilities as consultants, to function in different surroundings, and to receive exposure to communities and medical personnel within the referral area. Each maternal transport is attended by either an upper level obstetrical resident or the PTD. Often, the PTD accompanies the resident on his initial transport in order to familiarize him with the routine and supervise his performance. The resident or PTD coordinates call-backs to the referring physician so that he is notified if delivery occurs, or at least within the first 24 hr should stabilization and evaluation still be in progress. The referring physician is updated after delivery on a weekly basis and notified shortly before the patient's discharge.

3. The transport nurses fill very critical roles in the medical team. They have received extensive training in the labor-delivery unit and they participate in a surgical scrub course. In conjunction with perinatal flights, transport nurses rotate on a regular basis through labor and delivery and the newborn intensive care unit for maintenance of maternal and newborn skills. They follow the transported patients and assist in delivery and/or the stabilization of the newborn.

Orientation to the perinatal transport team includes an intensive 9-month program, if they have not had any previous obstetrical or newborn exposure. For the maternal transport component, they function in the labor and delivery suite initially with low-risk patients. Here they learn the nursing charting procedures and techniques regarding hospital patients. From there, they spend a period of time with high-risk mothers in both antepartum and postpartum monitoring. During their rotation they participate in a surgical scrub class that is oriented toward obstetrical needs. Their work schedules are flexible and adjustable to meet patient care needs to provide maximum continuity. During their last month in labor and delivery, they are assigned to the obstetrical resident on labor and delivery for 24-hr periods. This allows them to function more in a physician-extender role. Their clinical exposure and training are supported by 2 weeks (approximately 60 hr) of intensive didactic instruction, approximately two-thirds of which is provided by obstetrical physicians.

In order to comply with the standards of the American Society of Hospital-Based Air Medical Services (ASHBEAMS) and recommendations by the Nurses Association of the American College of Obstetrics and Gynecology (NAACOG), transport nurses receive didactic training regarding the physiological effects of flight taught by the PTD. This is augmented by a physiological training course in Oklahoma City, Oklahoma, during which an altitude chamber "ride" is included. During aeromedical orientation, the procedures and processes regarding air medical transports are presented. Transport nurses receive an aviation flight physical to the standards of a private pilot. They also receive basic orientation to aviation communication systems and flight procedures. They are required to maintain their cardiopulmonary resuscitation (CPR) and ACLS certifications up to date.

Evaluations of transport nurses are done on the basis of case reviews held at weekly transport meetings and are supplemented with laboratory procedures for intubation and chest tube placement on animals. Evaluators consist of the PTD, staff physicians, referring physicians, and the chief flight nurse, who is the most senior member of the transport nurse team.

4. A newborn intensive care unit respiratory therapist may be invited to participate in a maternal transport if there is any possibility of delivery at the referral center or en route. This is determined by the referring physician and the consulting transport physician. The intensive care respiratory therapists are registered and have had at least 1 year's experience in the newborn intensive care unit. They are represented at all transport meetings for both mothers and newborns. They receive instruction in aeromedical physiology. They have a primary responsibility for intubation, airway management, stabilization, and respirator monitoring. During a maternal transport, they are responsible for maintaining adequate oxygenation of the mother during transport and assisting the transport nurse as needed.

5. Referring physicians are also an integral part of the maternal transport team. They provide the history and medical evaluation of the patient. They are also an excellent source of additional professional help should delivery be necessary prior to transport and are very helpful in assisting in the coordination of hospital staff and in complying with hospital policies.

6. The staff from the referring hospital assist the patient in preparation for transport as well as initial stabilization. Almost all transports are received at the referring hospital under hospital conditions. This allows for a more controlled transfer of charts, monitor leads, and labor evaluations. If procedures such as bladder catheterization, vaginal examination, or changing from glass to

plastic bottles are necessary, these can be more easily done in the referring hospital.

In addition to the medical component of the transport team, the support team members are equally important for the safety and efficiency of a smooth maternal transport.

7. Coordination for each transport is a very complicated and important task. This is managed by the WATCH dispatchers (see Table 7). They are certified emergency medical technicians with experience in medical dispatching. They maintain a 24-hr a day, 7 days a week schedule. Through a unique ground-to-air frequency supplied by the FAA and emergency medical channels they have the capability to be in contact with all transport vehicles, the sheriff, and highway patrols. They are responsible for logging times of calls, departures, arrivals, and coordinating transport assistance at the referral site, if necessary. They also maintain the communication logs as well as the logs of each transport and the tapes of all recorded communications to and from the dispatch center. They have been approved to meet federal aviation requirements for handling flight plans under visual flight rules. They are also responsible for relaying communications regarding restocking of equipment and supplies with security division and drivers.

8. Whether by land or by air, the transport drivers usually are involved in maternal transport. Even when the helicopter comes from the airport to the hospital roof, the drivers assist in the preparation of necessary medical equipment and assist with the loading and unloading of the patient. When fixed-wing aircraft are used, they transport the team to the airport and assist in loading of the aircraft. Upon the transport arrival, they again return to the airport to transfer the patient and equipment back to the hospital. These drivers are hospital employees and are licensed ambulance drivers.

9. Flight personnel are provided by the air-taxi operator from whom the aircraft and maintenance services are leased. The pilots are required to comply with all FAA regulations and maintain the proficiency standards required by commercial air-taxi operators. These standards are usually exceeded and the average pilot-in-command often has greater than 5000 hr flight time. Helicopter operations take place both day and night, but they are limited to visual flight rules so that flying through clouds is not permitted. Fixed-wing flights require a crew of two pilots, and proficiencies are maintained to allow instrument flight conditions.

10. The security officers at Wesley Medical Center play an integral role in assisting patient handling as well as standing as firewatch for helicopter landings on the rooftop helipad. They have also been used as parttime standby mobile intensive care van drivers and they assist in the movement of transport personnel to areas of need within the hospital campus and to and from the airport facility.

Table 7 Maternal Transport Call Sequence

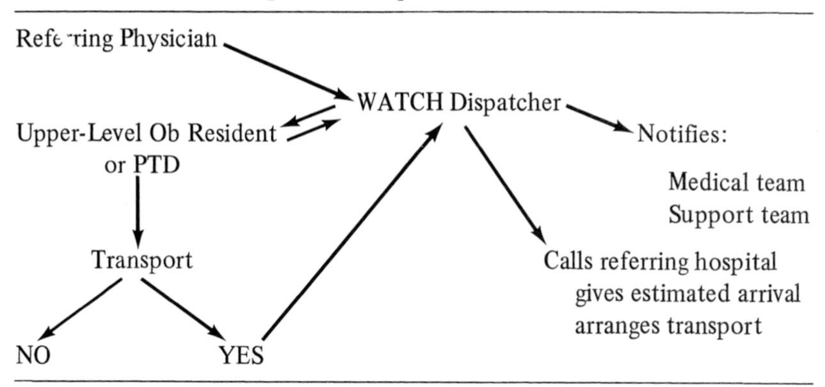

11. The local emergency medical service corps at the referring centers also provides a very important role in the management of maternal transports. When fixed-wing aircraft are used, transport to and from the referring hospital is done with the assistance of local EMS services. Even with some helicopter flights, the landing site may be one or two blocks from the hospital entrance, requiring the use of local emergency medical personnel.

Meetings

Monthly task force meetings are composed of the chairman of the Critical Care Committee at Wesley Medical Center, the PTD, the senior vice president WATCH, nonperinatal transport director, interested staff physicians, chief flight nurse, and representatives of the leasing company for aircraft and pilots. The establishment of policies and philosophy is largely determined at these meetings. Plans for major equipment purchase or leasing are established as well. The development of outreach education programs and public relations are frequent topics of discussion.

The monthly crew meetings are held with the PTD, chief flight nurse, transport nurses, representative from the county emergency medical service, representative respiratory therapist from the Newborn Intensive Care Unit, and chief dispatcher. These meetings provide a forum for discussing matters that affect the transport system as a whole. A significant portion of the time is devoted to a review of the previous month's transports and problems that may have developed on a nonmedical basis. Such situations and problems would include delays due to equipment malfunction, weather factors, locating standby personnel, etc. Aspects regarding medical problems will be discussed later. The monthly crew meetings represent the more "grass roots" application and implementation of policies established at task force meetings.

C. Equipment

Mobile Intensive Care Vans

The earliest maternal transports were done with the use of ground vehicles. A major donation was provided for the purchase of a motor home that was converted to meet the needs of a mobile intensive care van. Conversions consisted of rearrangement of interior components with the exclusion of tables and sitting areas. The capacity of the auxiliary power unit was increased. A significant modification was needed for mounting brackets for instrument platforms, countertops, medical kits, and approved cot security mechanisms. Extensive electrical modification was done, permitting contact with citizens' band frequencies, sheriff, highway patrol, and emergency medical channels. Despite the increased utilization of the maternal transport system, the time required to get to the referring hospital by ground in the rural setting of Kansas frequently resulted in a return transport with the newborn only. This meant that the standard procedure was to initiate each maternal transport as a double team transfer in anticipation of returning with either mother or newborn. This time factor and the distances required were the major incentives for use of air transport. The transport program now has three mobile intensive care vans, one of which is used primarily for maternal transports in town and to and from the airport following fixed-wing flights. One other unit is used for out-of-town transports when conditions do not permit the use of the helicopter in areas inaccessible to the fixed-wing aircraft.

Fixed-Wing Aircraft

In Kansas, the terrain is fairly flat and the population density is low. Consequently, transport distances of several hundred miles are not unusual. During World War II many military aircraft were assembled in the Wichita area. Extensive pilot training took place within the state. To accomodate the larger aircraft, many large runways were built and are still used by the local communities for general aviation and commuter traffic. Before the addition of fixed-wing aircraft, it was not unusual to spend up to 12 hr on a transport, particularly if it involved a newborn that required stabilization. Patient care needs as well as personnel time required more efficient transport. Our first aircraft was a Beech Queen Air that provided us with a very rugged aircraft and adequate cabin size. However, the engines were frequently prone to problems and the desire for cabin pressurization strongly influenced consideration of a turbine-powered aircraft. Our second aircraft selection was a Beech King Air, which has served us well. The all-weather, turbine-powered, pressurized aircraft has been very satisfactory and enables us to cover distances rapidly that are outside helicopter range and to provide transport in weather conditions not conducive to helicopter transfers.

Our fixed-wing aircraft have been equipped with special ambulance modifications and are certified by the FAA. These ambulance modules provide us with ample oxygen and alternating and direct current to power monitoring equipment, respirators, pumps, etc. The transport stretcher is securely attached to the module, and the EKG monitor rests in its own mounting tray. For long-distance flights or when the King Air is not available, a Cessna Citation jet can be used.

Helicopters

Helicopter transfer was the third means of transport added to our system. It has found a unique place for patient transport when time is very important, road conditions are bad, and/or transport range is outside the city but within approximately 110 miles of the hospital. The helicopter has the advantage of landing much closer to the hospital and it often eliminates the need for local emergency medical service transfers. The helicopter has a limitation of noninstrument flight conditions and of small cabin size. While the Beech King Air fixed-wing aircraft provides flexibility for additional crew members and options for maternal and/or newborn transfer, helicopter transfers commit the team to either one or the other. The transport team for the helicopters consists of the physician and transport nurse. Oxygen is carried in either a separate small tank or internally mounted tanks. On several occasions the helicopter has been launched with the maternal transport crew, only to find on arrival that the maternal condition has significantly changed, requiring delivery at the local facility. In those cases an intensive care van is dispatched with a neonatal transport crew and newborn equipment. However, the helicopter has enabled us to fly to a nearby referring hospital, pick up a mother with premature twins and delivery imminent, return and deliver the twins by cesarean section, and have them in the Neonatal Intensive Care Unit, all within an hour.

Medical Supplies

The evolution of equipment over the years has been most interesting. Initially, we carried enough surgical instruments to be the envy of a cardiac surgeon. The mobile intensive care vans were indeed equipped with stretcher mounts, oxygen and suction outlets, as well as lighting to facilitate emergency cesarean delivery in the van. With decrease in transport time facilitated by fixed-wing and helicopter transfer, the extent of our medical supplies has significantly diminished. With the advent of the helicopter, weight considerations became significant and the supply roster was again reduced. Our experience and interaction with referring hospitals has also enabled us to develop and use more of their equipment should operative deliveries be necessary. Since the helicopter is equipped for trauma flights as well, many of the "code blue" medications and equipment remain on the helicopter. The maternal medications are now contained in a small box approximately 4 by 6 by 2 in. All the additional equipment is carried in a knapsack mounted to the helicopter bulkhead. On fixed-wing or ground transports, the obstetrical kits number 1 and number 2 are taken (Appendix A). A life pack 4 (ECG monitor) is carried on all maternal transports and mothers are monitored as needed, especially those on tocolytic agents. They are transported in the lateral supine position, all have IVs running, and 90% have indwelling Foley catheters. Fetal heart tones are obtained with a Doptone prior to leaving the hospital, prior to take off, and just after landing at the home-based airport.

Several sources are available for equipment lists. Some of these include the Federal Aviation Air Ambulance Guidelines Manual, ASHBEAMS literature, and the bulletin from the Nurses Association of the American College of Obstetricians and Gynecologists, number 8, June 1983.

We have found that the equipment necessary is greatly influenced by the extent of the facilities referring the patient and the anticipated duration of transfer. Contingencies always have to be available for providing extended patient care due to landings outside the home base during inclement weather conditions, or for extended travel time due to weather diversions or road detours, traffic mishaps, and/or mechanical malfunctions. The goal of each maternal transport is to continue to provide the most appropriate intensity of care for the mother and her fetus during transfer. If either the mother or her fetus is placed in undue jeopardy because of the weather, we feel it is not justified to leave the security of the referring hospital with its staff and controlled environment, even though the intensity is not that afforded at a tertiary level center.

W. Wingert, in his introduction to *Air Ambulance Guidelines*, 1981 [3], made a very appropriate statement: "A physician who would never dream of releasing a patient from the hospital to the care of a cab driver for an unsupervised drive across town to another hospital may inadvertently do the same when ordering an air-taxi vehicle which happens to have removable seats and is free of passengers at the moment." The mad dash by the well meaning to transport the abnormal pregnancy by the undertrained, who are not prepared for the unknown, and in an ill-equipped vehicle, has no place in modern medical care.

D. Communications

As previously mentioned, the WATCH dispatcher is the central link in the system. To facilitate calls and consultations, an 800 number is used. The consultation call is received by the dispatcher, and the appropriate physician is connected with the referring physician. If transport is not necessary, the system has filled another one of the vital roles of a level III center, i.e., consultation. Should a transport be deemed advisable, the dispatcher is notified at the conclusion of the call and the maternal transport system is activated. The obstetrician receiving the call is expected to complete the transfer unless other arrangements are made and the dispatcher is appropriately notified. On the basis of the information provided, if the obstetrician feels delivery may be a possibility, he requests the dispatcher to notify any additional crew such as respiratory therapist and neonatologist. The choice of vehicle is made by consideration of distance, existing weather, and availability of vehicles. That decision is either immediately known or, if consultation with the flight crew is necessary, the obstetrician is notified as soon as possible so that he knows when and where to report to meet the remainder of the crew. The dispatcher notifies the driver if a ground transport is indicated or the driver and fixed-wing or helicopter pilots should fixed- or rotory-wing transport be selected. The transport nurse is likewise notified plus any necessary additional crew. The dispatcher notifies the referring facility as to estimated time of arrival and any transfer needs that might be required at the receiving site. Each crew member is equipped with a two-way walkie-talkie and a pager. A network has been established to allow communication contact anywhere in Kansas or its surrounding areas. Thus, it is possible for the PTD to monitor any changes in the patient's status and make suggestions for enroute treatment.

E. Regulations

Operation of a ground or air transport service that merits credibility by the medical community requires the compliance with specific federal and state guidelines. The term "ambulance" is defined in Kansas legislation, KSA 65-4301 (B), as "Any privately or publicly owned motor vehicle, airplane, or helicopter, designed, constructed, repaired and equipped for use in transporting and providing emergency care for individuals who are ill, injured, or otherwise disabled, including any specially constructed or equipped motor vehicle, airplane, or helicopter which is capable of providing life support services for extended periods of time." Most states have similar definitions.

We found our purposes were better served by equipping and staffing our ground vehicles as mobile intensive care vans rather than as standard ambulances. While standard ambulances could be used, the vans have equipment specially designed for the care of high-risk mothers and possibly their newborns.

Federal Aviation Regulations are very specific regarding commercial aircraft. Operators of air-taxi and commercial air services are governed under Federal Aviation Regulations found in Part 135 Air Taxi Operators and Commercial Operators. Any air-taxi operator being considered for use in a maternal transport system should be licensed under Part 135 and have a certificate which is dated and current. This regulation is very extensive, and depending on the size of the operation the operator may or may not need to comply with all of its components. The equipment that is necessary for maternal transports must be available, i.e., pressurization, multiengine, turbo-prop, etc. The operator will need to comply with the regulations governing the operations of these aircraft. Such an operator needs to be willing to make such adjustments, and it would be to the sponsoring institution's advantage to have someone knowledgeable in this area to make sure that all parties agree and that misunderstandings are avoided. Copies of Part 135 of the Federal Aviation Association Regulations are available at federal bookstores, through government printing offices, and general aviation facilities that sell various aircraft information booklets. This regulation also specifies a minimum number of flight hours' experience for pilots and the requirements for continued flight experience and proficiency evaluations.

ASHBEAMS has also recommended a minimum experience level which is slightly above that of the Federal Aviation Association requirement. We are currently requiring that a pilot has 3000 hr of fixed-wing experience with 1000 hr of multiengine experience, and a commercial license with both multiengine and instrumental ratings. Helicopter pilots have similar requirements, with the exception of multiengine and instrument rating requirements.

Only officially approved airports are used for landing sites, and a minimum field requirement of 2600-ft runways is required for the Beech King Air aircraft. No helicopter landing site is used until the chief pilot has been able to evaluate the landing site and be assured that it can be used by all helicopter pilots. Hospitals are encouraged to develop landing sites and helipads complying with FAA guidelines and regulations. Hospital liability insurance requires that no pilot land on a rooftop helipad without its thorough evaluation and check-out by an approved federal aviation flight examiner or the company's designated chief pilot.

III. Cost

A. Introduction

To the disgruntled hospital employee having just been told that he will not receive the anticipated cost-of-living increase and to the recently hospitalized patient reviewing his hospital charges, the air transport overhead may represent an unnecessary extravagance. However, to the disgruntled hospital employee, those transport flights may mean increased bed utilization and his continued employment. To the recently discharged hospital patient, those transport flights may represent a potential for reduced tax burden because of less economically dependent newborns.

Each time a maternal transport patient arrives, it represents at least two patients if she is delivered. It also represents a potential for stabilizing that pregnancy under a maternal admission and minimizing or eliminating the need for the more intense care of a newborn nursery. In our hospital, a mother can be hospitalized with intensive antepartum evaluation for approximately 5 days for the cost of each day of a newborn in the Intensive Care Unit. Not only do we have the potential for realizing an overall savings in hospitalization, but we are also dealing with "front-end" beginning of life treatment that hopefully provides a better chance for a productive citizen than a near "end-stage" condition associated with many other adult transports. Reimbursement for maternal transport is often determined by third-party payors. A cursory review of the last several years of maternal transports reveals a payment pattern similar to general hospitalized patients. Two-thirds of our patients have some insurance coverage which provides for approximately 85-90% of the charges. The remaining third are equally divided between Medicaid and self-pay.

B. Personnel

As with any personnel intense program, the medical and support crews represent a significant portion of the operating cost. For those familiar with the problem of staffing a labor and delivery unit, the problems of unanticipated patient load can be appreciated in terms of staffing a transport system. Over the years, our transport nurse call system has changed from having a few nurses available and subject to call to a more defined duty schedule. We have found that the defined schedule has been much more conducive to personal life and staff morale. Efforts were made to have 12- or 18-hr shifts, but it was found that transports frequently overlapped a shift and overtime charges placed an increased financial obligation on administrative budgets. Our current 24-hr shift schedule also allows for updating and evaluation rotations in the Newborn Intensive Care Unit or the labor and delivery suites. These shifts are rotated on a 6- to 8-week basis for each transport nurse. The hospital is also responsible for the salaries of the full-time intensive care van drivers, fill-in security officers, and dispatchers. It is essential that these positions be filled on a 24-hr, 7 days a week basis. The duration of their shifts is somewhat more flexible, but it is usually 8-12 hr. The salary scale for dispatchers and drivers would be comparable to the security officers in our hospital.

In addition, the salary of the statewide administrative coordinator, as well as a small portion of the two neonatologists and maternal-fetal medicine specialists, is provided by state funds. State funds also help underwrite outreach education expenses, long distance telephone calls, and a portion of secretarial expenses for the level III centers. The remainder of the funds required for outreach and personnel support are dependent on professional charges generated by patient care. For the maternal transport system at Wesley Medical Center in Wichita, Kansas, state funds account for less than 10% of the perinatal division's operational expenses and significantly less than 10% of the actual transport costs.

Since the financial burden of the day-to-day operation rests largely on patient care revenue, operational policies and transport system development have rested largely with the governing bodies of Wesley Medical Center and the University of Kansas School of Medicine at Wichita.

C. Equipment

Mobile Intensive Care Vans

We currently maintain and operate two mobile intensive care vans for maternal transports. One of them is a converted GMC motor home, which now has approximately 80,000 miles. Our newest van was manufactured by Horton and is one of their new Perinatal vans. This new unit represents over $70,000, with much of the equipment having been donated by local organizations and manufacturers. We were also fortunate to have a major local contributor underwrite the basic cost of the van itself. The maintenance costs for these vehicles are significantly higher than the average motor coach. Even though the frequency of red light and siren trips has diminished over the years, these vehicles are expected to run on demand in all kinds of environmental conditions. The increase in power requirements with auxiliary power units as well as converters, pumps, and related equipment add to the maintenance costs.

Capital Aircraft

Aircraft expenses vary with different hospitals and transport programs. Some hospitals purchase their own aircraft, while others have a lease arrangement with an air-taxi operator. Some share a cooperative lease arrangement.

The relationship of the hospital to the flight crew usually parallels the relationship of vehicle acquisition, i.e., leasing arrangements usually include the flight crew, and hospital ownership usually means that the flight crew are hospital employees. The pros and cons of these approaches, in large part, are related to the philosophy of the hospital and its administration as well as to the real or implied liability of ownership vs. exclusive leasing.

A cost comparison of seven maternal transport programs is depicted in Table 8. This information was tabulated in March 1982. As can be seen, the charges vary considerably as well as the factors that are chosen to be itemized. Some of the systems receive direct governmental support, and others have grants that help underwrite expenses. The charges that are developed for any particular service represent a reflection of philosophy for which the service was implemented. Hospital-owned services rely heavily on hospital charges to defray the transport costs and, therefore, will transport patients only to their facility. Independently owned services have a more liberal concept of patient transport and are willing to serve other community hospitals without transport systems. However, they need to recover more of the transport expenses directly.

Table 8 Selected Air Ambulance Programs and Charges

Program	Helicopter				Fixed-wing			
	$ Start-up	$/pt. mi.	Med. crew	Miscellaneous	$ Start-up	$/pt. mi.	Med. crew	Miscellaneous
1.	150	9.50	MD, RN	$20 Supplies	125	7.50	MD, RN	$75 equipment and van
2.	150	10.00	RN	$40/hr				
3.	150	4.00	RN	None				
4.	None	9.50	RN ± MD	$35/hr	195 295	8.20 11.20	RN ± MD RN ± MD	$35/hr King Air $35/hr Lear Jet
5.	100	6.00	RN ± MD	None				
6.	110	5.00	MD, RN	$60/hr $15–30 Equip.	None	4.80	MD, RN	$60/hr $15–30 Equip.

Whatever arrangement is used, someone attending the task force meetings must have an understanding of maintenance requirements and aircraft expenses to help interpret the financial complexities of the system. Such a person would also facilitate communication between the hospital and the air-taxi operators. For example, most air-taxi operators relate their expenses to flight hours or the number of hours the aircraft engines are actually running. However, insurance companies and hospital administrators can more easily account for expenses in terms of number of transports or distance of transport in miles. Factors that affect these differences are much greater than just taking the average air speed of an aircraft and dividing by the distance. Even though a tail wind may help in one direction, it never quite equalizes or makes up for the time lost in the other direction. Trips to certain locations may require a route of flight other than a straight line for deviation around weather. The flight plan may require flight under instrument conditions along prescribed airways. Also, initiation of transports without the transfer of a patient will generate nonrevenue miles. Some of these variations may seem like a small difference, but in the over 240,000 miles flown by our transport team last year, a few cents variation on the estimated cost per mile may make a significant difference in the overall accounting of the program.

Medical Equipment

One of the major advantages of maternal transport vs. newborn transport is the decreased need for neonatal medical equipment. In our experience, it has been very rare to need respirator equipment for maternal transports. Through 1983 we have transported over 900 mothers and have not had a delivery enroute on any of our transport vehicles. Intravenous fluids can be administered by conventional means or, if medication is necessary, insulin pumps have been utilized. Most adult equipment can be adapted for use in maternal transports. However, whatever equipment is used on transport will experience increased breakdown and a shorter life span. This equipment needs to be replaced on a regular basis as even infrequent failures cannot be tolerated on transport equipment. We do not expect to use monitoring equipment longer than 5 years for maternal transports. This expense of replacement and repair also needs to be considered in the overall cost evaluation. There is a very distinct financial and physiological advantage to transporting a fetus in utero rather than transporting an unstable newborn in a very expensive transport incubator.

D. Summary

Given a list of lease contracts, hourly wages for members of the transport team, and a rather liberal equipment cost maintenance and replacement schedule, a good accountant can arrive at a total maternal transport system cost. This cost can then be weighed against the increased bed occupancy resulting from an increased delivery rate from maternal transports. Then dividing the number of maternal transports into the previously established cost for the transport system will result in a cost per transport. To many, this average cost per transport may seem unrealistically high and beyond a reasonable expectation for recovery. There are, however, other significant advantages to a maternal transport system which include:

1. Maternal transport equals two patients, so that cost recovery needs to consider newborn care as well.
2. We may be able to significantly reduce hospital costs by stabilizing the mother before delivery of a premature infant.
3. We are initiating intensive medical care at the beginning of life when it will have the maximum effect on long-term quality of life.
4. If the maternal transport concept for newborn care is perceived by the referring physician and family in a very positive manner, they may also consider the tertiary facility for other major medical problems.
5. There will be decreased capital costs for the referral hospital for specialized newborn equipment and trained personnel.

Other intangible advantages include:

1. Increased intensity of care at referral hospital should delivery be necessary
2. Decreased referral center liability when team comes to receive patient
3. Improved public trust in all health care providers

Consequently, there are often many advantages to maternal transport, not realized in the short term, but which have very positive overall social, economic, and medical implications.

IV. Impact on Perinatal Outcome

A. Maternal

The improved outcome of high-risk pregnancies delivering at tertiary centers is becoming more apparent [4,9–11]. The mechanism that will make the availability of tertiary center births for those pregnancies requiring that intensity of care will be the maternal transport system.

Besides the potential for better newborn outcome, there should also be a decrease in maternal morbidity and mortality. Of our over 900 maternal transports, none has resulted in a maternal death. Most of the transports were made because of prematurity and the need for better newborn care. However, some of these transports were made because of severe maternal complications requiring intensive stabilization and treatment. A review of the last 350 maternal transports reveals that approximately 8% of the mothers remained undelivered to return to their primary care area which provided the appropriate intensity of care following stabilization and further fetal development.

B. Neonatal

Despite the fact that Anderson et al. [4] did not find a significant difference in neonatal survival in comparing 100 neonatal transports with 85 maternal transports, the neonatal transports had a significantly longer hospitalization and a significantly greater hospital cost. Subsequent studies have shown a more direct relationship regarding survival with maternal transports. Specifically, Boehm and Haire [5] felt that over 50% of their stillbirths could have been prevented with consultation and/or maternal transport prior to fetal death. Harris et al. [6] found that the overall neonatal mortality of maternal transport patients was 9.6%, contrasted with newborn transport patients of 12.5%. Although these numbers are not significantly different, the lower mortality was achieved in maternal transports in the face of significantly lower birth weights (2215 g vs. 2563 g, $p < 0.001$) and earlier gestational ages (34.7 vs. 36.8 weeks, $p < 0.001$). We obtained similar results when analyzing our maternal transports. Our study was also consistent with Modanlow et al. [7] who compared 50 neonatal with 50 maternal transports. These workers compared the type of delivery, 5-min Apgar score, length of hospital stay, admitting diagnosis, need for assisted ventilation, and length of time on assisted ventilation [7]. They found two factors to be of significance. One was an increase in cesarean section rate of 50% in maternal transports vs. 24% in neonatal transports ($p < 0.025$) and a lower morbidity among the premature neonates born to maternal transports ($p < 0.05$). A more recent report by Paneth et al. [8] describes a study of 13,560 singleton, low birth weight infants from the New York area. They concluded that delivery in a level III center results in a lower neonatal mortality in low birth weight infants. Approximately 10% of our last 350 maternal transports resulted in stillbirths or neonatal deaths. However, most of these were for extreme prematurity and/or stillbirth when transfer was politically motivated or at the patient's request. Eighty-two percent of the transports resulted in delivery and a favorable neonatal outcome. Sixty-five percent of this group required neonatal intensive care.

C. Indirect

In addition to the increased data supporting the improved outcome of maternal transports, we feel that there are some significant indirect benefits as well. First, it assures that the mother and newborn will be together, at least during her hospital stay. This time together, even though the maternal visits may be infrequent to the intensive care nursery, seems to be very important in the development of parental bonding [12]. We have also noted, but not quantified, an increased tendency for maternal transports to have their newborns followed in our high-risk follow-up clinic with greater regularity. Since the follow-up clinic serves a vital function for our ongoing evaluation of treatment protocols for our intensive care patients, we feel maternal transport has been a very significant contributing factor to the overall goals for improved maternal and neonatal care.

V. Suggestions and Guidelines

A. General Considerations

If the hospital is already serving as a tertiary center, unless it is in a very densely populated area, one of the strong recommendations for all level III centers is the provision of a transport system. Most often these systems are oriented toward newborn transports. However, acceptance of the maternal transport concept is continually increasing. The major goal of the maternal transport system is to improve the outcome of mother *and* newborn. High-risk pregnancy identification and conditions that lead to newborn distress need to be emphasized in the regional area. Once this process has been implanted, the implementation of a maternal transport system seems to be easier and its successful utilization much more assured.

Any system that is developed needs a sound, philosophical approach as to its mission. It also needs to consider strongly the feeling of third-party payors and maintain an active liaison and communication with them to: (1) establish the need for such a service, and (2) educate them in terms of the difference between a maternal transport system and a conventional ambulance service. It is obvious that the operation of an ambulance service is less costly compared to a maternal transport system.

In explaining the higher cost we have found it helpful to emphasize the level of professional attendance to each patient during transport. Maternal transport patients are considered critical patients on the basis of their referring physician's evaluation and the potential of delivery of a high-risk newborn. These factors help establish the distinction between an ambulance service which provides transportation in an environment staffed by paramedics with training oriented to prehospital admission problems. Optimal care cannot be provided to high-risk mothers by the conventional ambulance system.

B. Medical Profession

The existence of a maternal transport system is vitally dependent upon the availability of qualified and interested medical professionals. These include: (1) obstreticians with interests and preferably special training in high-risk obstetrics, (2) neonatologists, (3) intensive care nurses in both obstetrical and neonatal areas, (4) respiratory therapists oriented toward newborn care, (5) medical social workers, (6) nutritionists with special interests in maternal and infant needs, and (7) last but not least, dedicated referring physicians.

The attending obstetricians must have a close working relationship with the neonatologists. It is very easy for the neonatologist to feel he is not included in patient care decision making. Without appropriate professional communication, resentment can easily be fostered by the increased burden of the high-risk newborn resulting from maternal transports.

Before implementing a maternal transport system there needs to be a clear understanding of the priority for maternal transports. The system must have the support of the neonatology service because the potential for neonatal and maternal transports vying for the same newborn intensive care bed is an untenable situation.

It is ideal for the neonatologist to meet with the mother and father prior to delivery if possible. This fosters a good relationship between the neonatologist and the parents before they are confronted with the technology of the intensive care unit. It also provides the format and the concept of a team approach toward maximizing maternal and newborn care.

A forum for discussions relating to maternal treatment protocols must be developed. This provides an excellent opportunity for an interchange of professionals from their perspectives of patient management. It again provides another mechanism to minimize misunderstandings regarding the use of medications prior to delivery and the use or misuse of diagnostic procedures. For example, the use of antibiotics antepartum for prolonged rupture of membranes may be a topic for which the neonatologist may have some valuable information to contribute to overall patient care. A mechanism for providing follow-up information for both the mother and newborn is a valuable adjunct to future patient care.

The success of a program is related to the enthusiasm of those participating. The system works best if it is not assigned as an additional task to an already overburdened staff member.

C. Administrative Considerations

It has already been mentioned that administrative support is essential for the implementation of a maternal transport system.

Before embarking on an aggressive campaign for the purchase or lease of very expensive equipment, initiate a market survey to evaluate the need for a maternal transport system as well as the activity generated from such a system.

Encourage or cultivate those in administration with a particular interest in this area who have the concept of long-term planning rather than short-term gains. If a transport system already exists, the administrative mechanism may already be in place to implement the maternal transport aspect. If a transport system does not exist, then the selection of consultants for a marketing survey is of utmost importance.

D. Organizational Considerations

If given the opportunity of initiating a program of maternal transport, select equipment that seems most appropriate for the area served. Be willing to work with existing equipment if at all possible or to suggest less than optimal equipment to test the principle of maternal transport.

Use knowledgeable people in the appropriate areas of administration, emergency medical systems, communication systems, aircraft selection, etc.

Make liberal use of experience gained from other systems. This can be done relatively easily by using long-distance phone calls. Publications are available through the *Journal of Hospital Aviation* and through the association of ASHBEAMS for the appropriate names and phone numbers for personnel to contact. If possible, make site visits to maternal transport systems. Join interest groups related to this area of medical care.

Do not start a program unless the hospital is willing to stay with it for several years because it often takes this long to establish the confidence of referring physicians.

Do not assign the day-to-day management to someone not vitally interested in the project.

Do not oversell the system's abilities. An area that is often exaggerated is the promise of arriving at the referral site in much less time than it is possible to do. The personnel at the referring hospital measure time in minutes and are not at all aware of the problems incurred in locating a crew, assembling equipment, and other time spent prior to departure.

Be prepared to spend time in outreach education. One of the ways to improve the receptivity of referral hospitals is to offer continuing education programs. The face-to-face contact with referring physicians also improves the probability of future referrals.

Always keep the referring physician informed of the patient's status. News always seems to travel back home very fast. In very small communities, your patient's transfer from the small community hospital in a bright shiny, noisy helicopter may merit front page headlines. Consequently, it is important that the referring physician receive information from the receiving physician as soon as possible and definitely before the information is published in the local paper.

Have a simple and effective means for contacting responsible personnel at the tertiary center. This can be provided by an 800 number, and it serves a vital function for feedback, professional communication, and consultation.

VI. Conclusions

Maternal transport has a definite place in our overall health care system. It maximizes the use of the health care dollar by minimizing developmental problems at the front end of the life span spectrum. Even though the initial costs are great, it has been very rewarding to see our hospital administration become supportive of our efforts with personnel, equipment, and time. While for some the bottom line is the challenge of organization, and for others the challenge of minimizing costs, for us it has been the improved outcome of the low birth weight and distressed newborn and the decreased morbidity of the high-risk mother. Where a maternal transport service is available, it is to the best interest of the patient, her fetus, and her physician to utilize the service. Hopefully, time will also support the preliminary data that show an improved quality of life through maternal transport in terms of bonding, frequent pediatric follow-up, and a lifetime of productivity. It is our sincerest belief that society will ultimately reap enormous benefits from maternal transport systems.

Appendix

Obstetric Kit No. 1

Top Shelf

Narcotic box:

2 Diazepaon (Valium) 10 mg/2cc
2 Morphine sulfate 10 mg/cc
2 Phenobarbital 130 mg/cc

Laerdol ET tube adaptor

1 $NaHCO_3$
2 $CaCl_2$ 1 gr
2 Atropine 1 mg
1 Lidocaine (Xylocaine) 2 gm
3 Epinephrine 1 mg 1:10,000
1 Normal saline
2 Sterile H_2O
Medication labels

Band-Aids
1 Lidocaine (Xylocaine) 1%
Tongue blade
5 Amylnitrite inhalants
5 Dimenhydrinate (Dramamine) tablets

Second Shelf

Back row:

3 Hydralazine (Apresoline) 20 mg/cc
1 Epinephrine 1:1000
2 Ampicillin 500 mg
1 Phytonadione (Aquamephyton) 10 mg/cc
1 Diphenhydramine (Benadryl) 50 mg/cc
2 Phenytoin (Dilantin) 250 mg/5cc
2 Ephedrine 50 mg/cc
1 Gentamicin (Garamycin) 80 mg/2cc
1 Mepivacaine (Carbocaine) 1% Red label
2 Cord clamps
2 Heparin 1000 U/cc
2 Inderal 1 mg/cc
1 Isoproterenol (Isuprel) 1:5000
2 Digoxin (Lanoxin) 0.5 mg/2cc
2 Furosemide (Lasix) 20 mg/2cc
2 Methergine 0.2 mg/cc
1 Naloxone (Narcan) 0.4 mg/cc
1 Nitrazine paper

Front row:

4 Oxytocin (Pitocin) 10 U/cc
3 Ritodrine 10 mg/cc
1 Clinistix bottle
KY jelly
Assorted needles

Third Shelf

Top:

1 $MgSO_4$ 50% 5 g
2 $MgSO_4$ 10% 2 g
Gel for Doppler
1 35-cc syringe
Suture:
4 3-0 Vicryl # J-316
4 0 Vicryl # J-518
2 Culturettes

2 Blood culture tubes
1 Metal tubex syringe
1 1-in Adhesive tape
Benzoin applicators
Needles
  22 X 3 1/2
  20 X 3 1/2
  18 X 3 1/2
2 16-gauge Jelco
2 18-gauge Jelco
2 20-gauge Jelco
1 Tape measure
1 1-in Transpore tape
1 Tourniquet
1 Thermometer
2 Scapels # 1
Assorted syringes
  TB, 3 cc, 6 cc, 12 cc

Bottom:
Clipboard with
  1 Mother chart
  1 Infant chart
3 Betadine solution
1 Holter pump 'C' Ext. tubing
Sterile gloves
  1 – 7
  1 – 7 1/2
  1 – 8
1 Solution set
1 Minidrip
1 Buretrol
1 Blood tubing
1 Mylanta
4 4 X 4s
1 Solu-Cortef 250 mg
2 Terbutaline 1 mg/cc
Alcohol and Betadine swabs
1 Afrin nasal spray
1 Tourniquet
1 Short armboard
1 Amniohook
1 3-mm ET tube

1 6-mm ET tube
2 7-mm ET tube
1 Adult Laerdol mask
1 Laerdol bag with connecting tubing
1 Adult O_2 mask
1 Nasal cannula
1 35-cc syringe
Doppler
Stethoscope
Adupt BP cuff
Black bag
  1 Laryngoscope handle with batteries
  Blades
    Miller 2
    Miller 0
    MacIntosh 2
  2 extra 'C' batteries
Extra laryngoscope bulbs (2 sizes)
3 Airways
1 Sims connector

Obstetric Kit No. 2

1 C-Section set up
1 Needleholder
1 K-67
2 14 Fr suction catheter
1 8 Fr suction catheter
Infant NRPR with mask
Plasma 250 cc
1 Dextrose 50%
3 $NaHCO_3$
1 Transport precip. pack
1 Pressure bag
1 Bulb syringe
1 Disposable skin stapler
1 DeLee trap 10 Fr
1 Surgipad
4 Exam gloves (sterile)
1 1000-cc D_5 LR
1 1000-cc $D_{5\ 1/2}$ NS
1 500-cc D_5

References

1. Hospital-based aeromedical services directory, *Hospital Aviation*, May 1982, p. 9ff.
2. Sokol, R., and L. Chik, A perinatal database system for research and clinical care, *Acta Obstet. Gynecol. Scand.* (*Suppl.*), **109**:57–59 (1982).
3. Wingert, W., *Air Ambulance Guidelines*. U.S. Department of Transportation, U.S. Government Printing Office, 26–798/1444, p. viii (1981).
4. Anderson, C., S. Aladjem, O. Ayuste, C. Caldwell, and M. Ismail, An analysis of maternal transport within a suburban metropolitan region, *Am. J. Obstet. Gynecol.*, **140**:499 (1981).
5. Boehm, F., and M. Haire, One-way maternal transport: An evolving concept, *Am. J. Obstet. Gynecol.*, **134**:484 (1979).
6. Harris, T., J. Isman, and H. Giles, Improved neonatal survival through maternal transport, *Obstet. Gynecol.*, **52**(3):298 (1978).
7. Modanlow, H., W. Dorchester, A. Thorosian, and F. Freeman, Antenatal versus neonatal transport to a regional perinatal center: A comparison between matched pairs, *Obstet. Gynecol.*, **53**(6):725 (1979).
8. Paneth, N., J. Kiely, S. Wallenstein, M. Marcus, J. Pakler, and M. Susser, Newborn intensive care and neonatal mortality in low-birth-weight infants, *N. Engl. J. Med.*, **307**:149–155 (1982).
9. Miller, T. C., M. Densberger, and J. Krogman, Maternal transport and the perinatal denominator, *Am. J. Obstet. Gynecol.*, **147**:19–24 (1983).
10. Crenshaw, C., P. Payne, L. Blackman, et al., Prematurity and the obstetrician, *Am. J. Obstet. Gynecol.*, **147**:125–132 (1983).
11. Pomerance, J. J., C. T. Ukrainski, T. Ukra, D. H. Henderson, A. H. Nost, and J. Meredith, Cost of living for infants weighing 1000 gm. or less at birth, *Pediatrics*, **61**:908–910 (1978).
12. Klaus, M., K. Jerauld, N. Kreger, W. McAlpine, M. Steffa, and J. W. Kennell, Maternal attachment: Importance of the first postpartum days, *N. Engl. J. Med.*, **286**:460–463 (1972).

General References

1. *Maternal-Neonatal Transport*, NAACOG Bulletin No. 8, June 1983.
2. Committee on Perinatal Health, *Toward Improving the Outcome of Pregnancy*, National Foundation – March of Dimes, 1977.
3. *Guidelines for Perinatal Care*, American Academy of Pediatrics, American College of Obstetrics and Gynecology, 600 Maryland Avenue SW, Suite 300, East, Washington, D.C., 20024, 1983.
4. ASHBEAMS quality standards, *Hospital Aviation*, Jan. 1983, p. 12.

12

Preterm Labor and Delivery

FRITZ FUCHS

Cornell University Medical College
New York, New York

I. Introduction

The most challenging problem in regard to preterm birth is prevention, since prematurity accounts for >75% of the perinatal mortality. But preventive measures, including treatment of preterm labor with tocolytic agents, can only hope to prevent 30-40% of the present incidence of prematurity. Proper obstetrical management and above all intensive care of the premature neonate, therefore, are of paramount importance, not only to reduce the perinatal mortality but also to prevent the development of permanent handicaps. In the present chapter, management of preterm birth will be discussed before prevention, which has been the subject of a large number of recent publications. After all, the transition from intrauterine to extrauterine life is much more perilous for the preterm fetus than for the mature fetus which has gone through a maturation process designed specifically to facilitate this transition, but the perils can be reduced by proper management and care.

II. Terminology

A widely accepted definition of premature or preterm birth is delivery before the completion of 36 weeks of gestation, calculated from the first day of the last menstrual period. Infants born between 20 and 28 weeks of gestation are considered immature rather than premature, and the best term to describe labor between 20 and 36 weeks is therefore preterm labor. Threatened premature labor is an ambiguous term which should not be used.

Premature rupture of the membranes (PROM) is a term that will be difficult to eradicate, although "prelabor" rupture of the membranes is more logical. The abbreviations AROM and SROM are often used for artificial rupture of the membranes and spontaneous rupture during labor, respectively.

III. Preterm Labor

A. Risk Factors

Epidemiological studies have identified a number of conditions which are associated with an increased incidence of preterm delivery. Although the cause-relationship is far from clear in all instances, such conditions may be considered as predisposing factors. As shown in Table 1, it is practical to divide these factors into maternal, placental, fetal, and iatrogenic. In some cases, more than a single such risk factor may be present, but in about half the cases, no predisposing factor can be identified. In such instances, one has to assume that the timing mechanism, which normally prevents the initiation of labor before fetal maturity, is either not functioning or overruled by a strong, though unidentifiable, stimulus.

Many studies have documented the association of premature birth with maternal age below 20 or above 35 years at the time of the first birth, with primiparity, small stature of the mother, and socioeconomic deprivation. The association of low birth weight with maternal cigarette smoking is also well documented. While the causal relationship to the demographic and constitutional factors is unclear, the relationship between maternal smoking and low birth weight is thought to be due to the increased uptake of carbon monoxide in smokers.

The increased incidence of premature birth in mothers with congenital heart diseases and other severe cardiovascular disorders is probably due to a relative insufficiency of the transport of nutrients to the fetus. The same explanation must pertain to the relationship between small heart volume relative to body size and increased incidence of prematurity, which was first reported by Finnish workers [1,2].

The relationship of urinary tract infection and prematurity is well documented, and it has been shown that even asymptomatic bacteriuria is a predisposing factor. The relationship between febrile conditions and prematurity is

Table 1 Risk Factors in Preterm Labor

- Maternal factors
  - Age < 20 or >35 years at first delivery
  - Primiparity
  - Small stature
  - Low socioeconomic status
  - Cigarette smoking
  - Small heart volume
  - Congenital cardiac disease
  - Chronic debilitating diseases
  - Anatomical defects of the uterus
    - Congenital uterine malformations
    - Uterine synechiae
    - Fibromyomas
    - Incompetent cervix
  - Pregnancy complications
    - Urinary tract infection
    - Intercurrent febrile infections
    - Accidental traumas
    - Mental and physical stress
- Placental factors
  - Abruptio placentae
  - Placenta previa
  - Placental insufficiency
- Fetal factors
  - Multiple gestation
  - Anencephaly
  - Adrenal hyperplasia
  - Anomalies associated with poly- and oligohydramnios
- Iatrogenic factors
  - Induction of labor for pregnancy complications
    - Preeclampsia
    - *Rhesus* isoimmunization
    - Diabetes mellitus
  - Elective induction of labor
  - Intrauterine contraceptive device in utero

presumably due to the increased motility of the myometrium at high body temperatures.

Anatomical defects of the uterus as causes of preterm labor are not very common, but easily understood. Malformations due to incomplete fusion of the Müllerian ducts may prevent the normal growth of the uterus or interfere with placental development. The same mechanism applies to excessive scarring of the uterus, including the formation of synechiae, and to submucous fibromyomas. The incompetent cervix, resulting in mid-trimester abortion or premature birth, may be due to a congenital defect or to a traumatic lesion inflicted in connection with induction of abortion. Thus, it may occasionally belong in the category of iatrogenic factors.

The placental factors are obvious. Placental insufficiency may be due to malformations or infarcts, or it may be purely functional without any anatomical defects.

The association of fetal factors and prematurity is easy to understand. In multiple gestation the nutritional transport system may become insufficient for the adequate supply of the fetuses. This occurs frequently in twin gestation, and if there are three or more fetuses, the pregnancy is practically never carried to term. However, this does not preclude the pharmacological treatment of preterm labor, which is often successful. The high incidence of prematurity in association with anencephaly [3] and other severe malformations of the fetal central nervous system supports the assumption that the center controlling the length of gestation is located in the fetal brain. The anomalies associated with hydramnios probably cause premature labor indirectly by rapid distention of the uterus. Potter's syndrome, with oligohydramnios, is also associated with an increased incidence of prematurity for unknown reasons.

Induction of labor before term is indicated in a number of pregnancy complications, and the risk of the fetus remaining in utero must be balanced against the risk of prematurity in each individual case. Induction merely for the convenience of the patient or the obstetrician should not be done at all, and where geographical or similar factors justify induction, it should not be done without ascertaining fetal maturity by amniocentesis or sonographic evaluation of placental maturity.

The increased risk of prematurity in pregnancies with an intrauterine contraceptive device (IUD) has recently been documented. Because of this and the increased risk of abortion, occasionally septic, the general opinion is that when pregnancy occurs with an IUD in situ the IUD should be removed.

B. Preventive Measures

From the list of predisposing factors (Table 1) it is evident that in some instances premature birth may be prevented by proper management of the pregnancy.

Thus, mothers should be warned against the harmful effects of heavy smoking. If they have congenital heart disease, or for that matter any heart disease, they should be advised to rest as much as possible and to avoid all sources of infection. Urinary tract infection should be treated vigorously in pregnancy, and febrile conditions should be treated with antipyretics to avoid activation of the myometrium.

Anatomical defects of the uterus may require operative correction. Cervical incompetence, which is the most common reason for operative prevention of preterm birth, should be diagnosed before the beginning of pregnancy as part of the work-up for previous pregnancy failures. The Shirodkar or McDonald cerclage operations to reinforce the cervix are best performed at 12–16 weeks of gestation, when the presence of the living fetus can be confirmed by ultrasound. Bleeding, contractions, or rupture of the membranes are contraindications to the operation. In over 80% of the cases, patients with cerclage operations for proper indications deliver healthy infants.

Multiple gestation should be diagnosed as early as possible, and the increased use of ultrasonography is very helpful in this regard. Most obstetricians advocate increased bedrest to mothers with twin pregnancies, although the opinions are divided as to whether this will improve the outcome. If there are three or more fetuses, discontinuation of work and increased bedrest become mandatory.

It has been clearly demonstrated that programs to identify patients at risk for preterm birth and to reduce the impact of the risk factors can be successful [3–6]. Such programs deserve to be applied on a broad scale, and it is probable that they might have a greater effect than treatment of preterm labor with tocolytic agents.

C. Diagnosis

The diagnosis of preterm labor requires observation of one or more uterine contractions in a 10-min period, leading to some effacement and/or dilatation of the cervix in a patient before the completion of 36 weeks of gestation. Examination of the patient suspected to be in preterm labor should include palpation of the uterus to determine the presence of myometrial contractions, and external cardiotocography to document these contractions and to observe the fetal heart rate. Unless there are signs of rupture of the membranes or vaginal bleeding, a sterile vaginal examination should be done to determine the degree of cervical effacement and dilatation and also to verify the fetal presentation found by external palpation. In order to rule out false labor, which will stop by itself after a period of bedrest, a second sterile vaginal examination may have to be performed half an hour or an hour later to determine changes in cervical effacement and/or dilatation.

If, after careful examination, the patient is judged to be in true labor, one has to determine whether or not it is preterm labor. In order to answer this question, it is essential to know the length of gestation. As obvious as this may seem, it is often a cause of confusion. The history must include not only the date of the last menstrual period but also the length of previous cycles as well as the occurrence of a spontaneous or induced abortion or delivery with or without lactation shortly before conception. Discontinuation of oral or intrauterine contraception is also relevant. The history should include signs and symptoms from the early part of the current pregnancy, growth of the uterus, time of quickening, and the results of pregnancy tests or ultrasonography early in gestation. In some cases, the true gestational age still remains unclear. Of all methods described to help the obstetrician in this particular situation, ultrasonographic determination of the biparietal diameter and other fetal measures seems to be best suited and therefore should be performed if available. Even if gestational age cannot be determined accurately because intrauterine growth retardation may confuse the picture, ultrasound can at least help estimate the fetal weight, which is known to be a major prognostic factor.

IV. Mechanism of Preterm and Term Labor

To remain essentially at rest during pregnancy and to contract when the fetus is mature, the uterine muscle must possess a control system which inhibits its response to activating stimuli during gestation and facilitates its response at term. The myometrium contains the contractile proteins and the enzymes involved in the contraction-relaxation process throughout gestation and is thus capable of contracting at any time, as evidenced by its behavior in elective abortion.

Uterine activity is suppressed when myometrial sensitivity to oxytocic stimuli is low, and when circulating or locally produced oxytocic agents are not present in sufficient concentrations. The most powerful oxytocic substance in pregnancy is oxytocin; the second most powerful is vasopressin, which is even more oxytocic than oxytocin during the menstrual cycle [7]. The third most powerful endogenous oxytocic agent is prostaglandin E_2 (PGE_2), followed by prostaglandin $F_{2\alpha}$; however, the threshold dose of prostaglandins at term is some 500 times greater than the oxytocin threshold dose [8]. Oxytocin can be demonstrated in the blood throughout pregnancy in more than 80% of random samples [9], but the sensitivity of the uterus, which rises steadily during pregnancy, remains too low until term. Vasopressin is also present throughout pregnancy because of its role in regulation of diuresis, but the concentration stays far below the threshold level.

In contrast, the sensitivity of the myometrium to prostaglandins is already high during pregnancy and does not show the marked increase which is characteristic of the oxytocin sensitivity. The circulating prostaglandin levels remain very low during pregnancy and it is not until labor is well under way that a marked rise in the levels of prostaglandins (as measured by their stable metabolites) is observed [10]. Thus, both mechanisms for the prevention of uterine stimulation, namely, low sensitivity to oxytocin and low concentration of prostaglandins, operate in the human.

The increasing uterine sensitivity to oxytocin at term is due to a great increase of the concentration of myometrial receptors [11] which reach a maximum in early labor. The response of a target tissue to a hormone depends both on the concentration of hormone in the blood reaching the tissue and on the ability of the tissue to bind the hormone to cellular receptors. Therefore, the absence of a dramatic rise in plasma oxytocin concentration at the onset of labor does not preclude a role for oxytocin in the initiation of labor, since the ability of the myometrium to bind oxytocin goes up dramatically.

The decidua contains the same concentration of oxytocin receptors as the myometrium [11]. Far from being an active buffer tissue between the myometrium and the fetal membranes, the decidua is one of the sites of prostaglandin synthesis during labor, and perhaps the most important site in quantitative terms. We have recently shown that oxytocin stimulates the synthesis of prostaglandins E_2 and $F_{2\alpha}$ in the decidua, of PGE_2 but not $PGF_{2\alpha}$ in the amnion, and of neither in the myometrium [12]. We, therefore, have formulated the hypothesis of a dual function of oxytocin: (1) stimulation of the contractile process in the myometrium; and (2) stimulation of prostaglandin synthesis in the decidua, which in turn acts on the adjoining myometrium in synergy with oxytocin [11].

In infants born after spontaneous onset of labor, whether vaginally or abdominally, the umbilical arterial blood contains a much higher concentration of oxytocin than the umbilical venous blood or the maternal venous blood which have about equal levels [13]. In infants born after cesarean section at the very beginning of labor, the oxytocin level in the umbilical artery was considerably higher than in infants born at the same gestational age without labor [14]. The high umbilical arterial level, the large arteriovenous difference, and the fact that oxytocin can pass between fetus and mother [13] indicate that a considerable amount of oxytocin from the fetal side is added to the level in the maternal blood. It, therefore, is reasonable to assume that initiation of labor is achieved by a moderate rise in maternal oxytocin secretion, supplemented by a considerable amount of fetal oxytocin which stimulates the myometrium; the myometrium has by then reached a high level of sensitivity because of the sharp increase in the concentration of oxytocin receptors. Subsequently, the prostaglandins produced in the decidua and amnion in response to the large amounts of oxytocin reaching these tissues from the fetus as well as the mother will stimulate the uterine activity further.

If we accept this hypothesis for labor at term, what happens then in preterm labor? We have shown that blood taken in the early phases of preterm labor contains higher levels of both oxytocin and prostaglandins than blood from pregnant patients at the same gestational age but not in labor [14]. The myometrium also contains a considerably higher concentration of oxytocin receptors in preterm labor than at the same stage without labor [11]. Thus, the mechanism of preterm labor seems to depend on the same factors as at term; in addition, we have indirect evidence that both oxytocin and prostaglandins are involved, since inhibition of oxytocin secretion with ethanol [15,16] and inhibition of prostaglandin synthesis with indomethacin [17,18] can arrest premature labor.

It appears possible that the second most potent oxytocic agent, vasopressin, may also play a role in preterm labor. The fetus appears to secrete large amounts of vasopressin in response to stress [19-21], and there is a large arteriovenous difference in cord blood, suggesting a transfer to the mother.

Many of the predisposing factors in preterm birth subject the fetus to some degree of stress. Is it unreasonable to assume that by adding the oxytocic activity of a vasopressin concentration in the umbilical artery, which can be as high as 15-20 times the concentration of oxytocin, the fetus can trigger preterm labor? The fact that ethanol can inhibit preterm labor does not exclude this possibility, since ethanol also inhibits secretion of vasopressin from the neurohypophysis [22].

It probably is not justified to count out a role for the sex steroids in the mechanism of labor, although scores of studies have failed to demonstrate any consistent changes in the levels of estrogen and progesterone at the onset of labor. These steroids probably have subtle but vital functions, such as controlling the enzymes involved in prostaglandin synthesis, controlling the formation of oxytocin receptors, and influencing the biochemical changes of the collagen and glycosaminoglycans in the cervix during the process of ripening [23]. Only a few investigators have studied the levels of estrogen and progesterone in preterm labor, but the results are as divergent as at term [24-27].

So far, there is no evidence to suggest that the mechanism of preterm labor is different in principle from that of term labor, apart from the timing. More basic research on the mechanism of human parturition is therefore urgently needed. In the meanwhile, we must utilize the current knowledge, particularly about the oxytocic agents in the body, as best we can.

V. Choice of Appropriate Mode of Treatment

One of the most difficult aspects of preterm labor is the decision whether to try to stop it or to let it continue to preterm birth. In evaluating this problem, one must analyze the benefits and risks of the different modalities as well as the chances of success with each of them. The assessment on which to base the decision must include the degree of fetal maturation (estimated fetal weight, index of lung maturation, etc.), the fetal condition, the stage of labor (cervical dilatation and effacement, strength of contractions), the risk for the mother and the fetus if labor is arrested, and the risks of the tocolytic treatment itself if attempted. There are essentially three options: (1) to let labor continue on the assumption that it is not in the best interest of the fetus or the mother to continue the pregnancy, or that tocolytic treatment is futile because labor is already too advanced; (2) to arrest labor for a period of 48-72 hr in order to try to accelerate fetal lung maturation; and (3) to arrest labor in order to prolong pregnancy and postpone delivery until term or as close to term as possible. In the following, the criteria upon which the decision is based and the optimal management with each of the three modalities will be discussed.

A. Management of Preterm Labor and Delivery

Many patients arrive at the hospital in such an advanced stage of preterm labor that any attempt to arrest labor is futile and, therefore, contraindicated. In other instances, complications in the mother and/or the fetus contraindicate tocolytic treatment. When preterm delivery is anticipated, the first concern should be whether the mother is in a hospital which can provide the optimal care for her and her preterm infant, or whether transfer to a better equipped facility is desirable and, in regard to time, possible. This is not an easy decision. There is no doubt that it is better to have the delivery take place in the best-equipped place, so that the infant can get expert care from the moment of birth. However, delivery in an ambulance, even with qualified staff, is not desirable, and preterm labor, once in progress, can be of short duration even in primiparas.

Once the decision as to where the delivery will take place has been made, it is the obligation of the obstetrician to conduct labor and delivery in such a way that the neonate is turned over to the pediatrician in the optimal condition. Since the preterm fetus does not have the same tolerance of uterine contractions as the mature fetus, careful monitoring of the fetal heart rate and the uterine activity is mandatory. If external monitoring is unsatisfactory, internal electrodes and pressure catheters must be applied. Definite signs of fetal distress require early intervention and it is essential that the staff is well trained in the detection of the early signs of distress. Analgesics should be used sparingly. Mothers will usually accept pain if it is explained to them that analgesics could be harmful to a very small baby. It is, as always, essential to ascertain the fetal presentation. In addition, when dealing with a very small fetus it may be important for the decision how to deliver it to have a better estimate of the fetal weight than that provided by external examination. Sonography is of great value in such cases, if it is available.

There is no doubt that delivery by cesarean section is less traumatic to a preterm fetus than vaginal delivery, and section should be used, therefore, whenever there is a suspicion that other modes of delivery will stress the fetus beyond endurance. It has even been proposed that all fetuses with an estimated weight < 1500 g should be delivered by section. While this has not gained wide support, there is general agreement in the United States today that a preterm fetus in breech position should invariably be delivered by cesarean section if it is deemed to be viable.

If vaginal delivery is decided upon, the second stage should not be allowed to extend beyond one hour. A low forceps delivery is often less traumatic than a spontaneous delivery, and episiotomy may also be used to facilitate delivery.

It is very important to have a pediatrician trained in neonatology present in the delivery room in order to resuscitate the preterm infant and to transfer it to the Neonatal Intensive Care Unit if necessary and if one is available. In hospitals where no special facilities for the care of sick and small neonates are available, the question of transfer of the baby to a hospital with adequate facilities must be considered. However, before transport is undertaken, the infant must be resuscitated and stabilized. Occasionally, special procedures may have to be carried out in the delivery room, such as laparocentesis in an infant with hydrops and marked ascites preventing lung expansion.

It is essential for the pediatrician responsible for the neonatal care to be fully informed of all medication, including tocolytics, given to the mother during labor and delivery, and that he be familiar with the possible effects of such medication on the newborn. Thus, he must look out for hypotension, hypoglycemia, hypocalcemia, and ileus if β-mimetics have been used, and for persistent fetal circulation if prostaglandin synthetase inhibitors have been used.

B. Short-Term Tocolytic Treatment

The demonstration by Liggins and Howie [28] that administration of corticosteroids to the mother can accelerate the formation of surfactant in the fetal lungs at certain stages of pregnancy gave us a new modality for the treatment of preterm labor. The principle of short-term tocolytic treatment is to arrest labor for 36-72 hr and to give the mother corticosteroids for 2 days, and then to deliver the infant if labor recurs or if delivery is otherwise indicated. This principle is particularly useful in cases of premature rupture of the membranes, and in multiple pregnancies with triplets or quadruplets, which rarely can be brought to term with tocolytic treatment. In such and other cases, where complications preclude extension of the pregnancy to term but do not require immediate delivery, the respite gained by short-term tocolysis can be used not only for corticosteroid therapy but also for transfer, if necessary, of the mother to a hospital with adequate facilities for management of preterm newborn infants.

The principles of short-term tocolytic treatment do not differ from those of long-term tocolysis which will be discussed in detail next. The same agents are used, and the same principles of monitoring apply. It is of importance to realize, however, that the use of corticosteroids in combination with β-mimetics accentuates the metabolic effects of the latter, and greatly increases the risk of pulmonary edema in the mother [29]. The combined effect of corticosteroids and β-mimetics on blood sugar levels is marked hyperglycemia, and the combination is therefore contraindicated in pregnancies complicated by diabetes mellitus. It should be mentioned that maternal pulmonary edema has also been observed after treatment with magnesium sulfate and corticosteroids [30].

Because of the indications for short-term treatment the risk of failure is even greater than in the long-term treatment group. The same considerations apply to both groups in regard to the risk of the tocolytic agent affecting the premature neonate.

A particular point to bear in mind when patients with premature rupture of the membranes are given corticosteroids is that the steroids can mask the symptoms of chorioamnionitis, the dominant risk in such cases. Before short-term tocolysis is even considered, infection must be ruled out.

C. Long-Term Tocolytic Treatment

Whenever possible, and provided it is not contraindicated due to a maternal or fetal complication, the best treatment of preterm labor is to inhibit the uterine activity and prolong the pregnancy. The best incubator for a preterm fetus is a resting uterus in a healthy mother. For long-term tocolysis to be the treatment of choice, the following criteria should be fulfilled: (1) the gestational age should be between 18 and 34 completed weeks; (2) the fetal weight should not exceed 2500 g (about 5.5 lb) by clinical estimation or 2000 g by the much more accurate sonographic estimation; (3) the membranes should be intact and not bulging through the cervix; (4) the cervix should be < 5 cm dilated; (5) the fetus is alive and well; and (6) a diagnosis of true labor has been established.

As already mentioned in previous sections of this chapter, there are a number of contraindications to long-term tocolysis, including: (1) intrauterine fetal death; (2) persistent fetal distress; (3) gross fetal malformations verified by sonography; (4) abruptio placentae; (5) ruptured membranes; and (6) medical or surgical diseases of the mother requiring termination of pregnancy.

In addition to these relatively strict criteria, there are some relative indications and contraindications. Thus, placenta previa is a contraindication if the bleeding is severe and persistent; on the other hand, many pregnancies with placenta previa have been brought closer to term by tocolytic treatment.

Ruptured membranes has been listed as a contraindication because tocolytic treatment is often unsuccessful in such cases. However, this is an area of dispute, and under the most favorable conditions patients with ruptured membranes may be considered for long-term tocolytic treatment.

Based upon our present experience in the United States, β-mimetic drugs are the tocolytic agents of choice in most instances. But if there are contraindications to the use of β-mimetics, one of the other tocolytics may be chosen, such as magnesium sulfate or ethanol. Swedish workers have recommended the use of nonsteroidal anti-inflammatory agents before the twenty-eighth week on the consideration that if birth should occur this early in spite of treatment, the chances of survival of the newborn are so slim and the incidence of persistent fetal circulation so great that the agent in itself does not increase the neonatal mortality [31]. In a review published in 1981, Niebyl concludes that limiting the use to under 34 weeks and discontinuing the drug as soon as failure becomes apparent will minimize the risks [32].

Combinations of tocolytics would seem to offer an advantage which needs to be explored further. Because of the fact that different groups of tocolytics have different mechanisms of action and different types of side effects, it is conceivable that they may have additive or perhaps even synergistic effects upon the uterus with much less pronounced side effects. Thus, Suranyi and coworkers in Hungary [33] have reported that the use of a combination of 20% of the standard dose of ethanol and 25% of the usual dose of ritodrine has the same efficacy as either of those tocolytics in the standard dose. Likewise, Gamissans and coworkers in Spain [34,35] have used a combination of ritodrine and indomethacin with excellent results.

VI. Tocolytic Agents

A. β-Mimetics

According to the concept of Ahlquist [36], one can differentiate between two types of adrenergic receptors, the so-called α- and β-receptors. The β-receptors may be divided into β_1- and β_2-receptors. A variety of effects may be obtained by stimulating or blocking these receptors. In most organs, including the uterus, stimulation of α-receptors causes excitation; stimulation of the β-receptors causes relaxation except in the heart. This concept was elaborated by subdivision into β_1- and β_2-receptors; β_1-receptors are in the heart, and β_2-receptors are present in the uterus, vascular smooth muscle, bronchial smooth muscle, etc. The first β-stimulant to be introduced in obstetrics was isoxsuprine [37]. After more than a decade in clinical use, its value in premature labor remains unproven in large controlled studies, and its cardiovascular effects make its use difficult. Therefore, the introduction of newer agents such as ritodrine, fenoterol, hexoprenaline, salbutamol, and terbutaline, all of which appear to have a stronger affinity to the β_2-receptors, is a major breakthrough in the treatment of premature labor. The relative merits of the different agents are difficult to evaluate, since there are very few comparative studies. A large body of information is available for ritodrine hydrochloride (Yutopar), which was approved for use in preterm labor by the FDA in 1980 [38]. The first prospective, double-blind placebo-controlled study of ritodrine in the treatment of preterm labor was reported in 1971 by investigators at seven hospitals in four European countries [39]. Another study was carried out in three medical centers in the United States where ritodrine was compared to ethanol [40]. An excellent review of the pharmacology and clinical use of β-mimetic compounds was published by Lipshitz in 1981 [41].

The currently available β-mimetic agents are closely related in regard to chemical structure. All β-mimetic agents presently available also stimulate the β-receptors in the heart, and any form of cardiac disease or even a suspicion of heart disease is therefore a contraindication. Thus, an evaluation of the cardiac status with an ECG before initiating treatment is essential. Another contraindication is uncontrolled hyperthyroidism. Because of their metabolic effects, β-mimetics should not be used in diabetes mellitus, unless the patient is well controlled. Careful monitoring of the blood sugar during treatment is necessary.

For the initial treatment, where it is important to find the proper therapeutic level as early as possible, intravenous infusion is preferable, but β-mimetics are also active when given intramuscularly, orally, or by nasal spray. The infusion fluid should be made fresh according to the recommendation of the manufacturer. Since some of the side effects seem to be related to the volume of fluid infused, recording of fluid intake and output is mandatory, and if attempts have been made to hydrate the patient before deciding to use a β-mimetic, this should be taken into account (doubling the concentration of β-mimetic in the infusion fluid may be appropriate in such instances, but such deviations from routine must be made clear to the personnel responsible for patient management to avoid unintentional overdosage).

In order to establish the therapeutic level, it is generally recommended to begin with a low dose and increase it every 10 min. For ritodrine, the recommended schedule is 0.50 μg/min up to 3.50 μg/min. However, it is often difficult to ascertain the clinical effect on the uterus in a single 10-min period, and unless the uterine activity is very strong, it may be prudent to extend the period before going to the next level of infusion.

The tolerance to β-mimetics is better in the lateral than in the supine position, but in positioning the patients, it is important to ascertain that the uterine activity is accurately recorded by the tocograph.

When the uterine activity has been arrested it is often possible to reduce the infusion rate by one or two steps. In the absence of contractions, this level is then maintained for about 11 hr. Oral treatment is begun 30 min before discontinuation of the IV treatment, and is then maintained according to the manufacturer's recommendations. Since the half-life of β-mimetics in the maternal circulation is relatively short, some patients will do better on oral medication every 2 hr than on the double dose every 4 hr. Thus, there is a need to individualize the oral treatment to achieve the best effect. Oral treatment can be maintained after discharge from the hospital, but the patient should be able to reach the obstetrician easily, and she should be checked frequently.

The ultimate aim of long-term tocolytic treatment is to bring the pregnancy to term. Whereas treatment usually is not initiated after 34 completed weeks, oral treatment begun earlier may be extended to 36 or 37 weeks, if tolerated well.

Although it is often claimed that the newer β-mimetics are predominantly β_2-stimulators, there is currently no agent devoid of cardiovascular side effects. β-mimetics have a distinct chronotropic effect as well as a weaker inotropic effect on the maternal heart and, as they cross the placenta, on the fetal heart as well. Hypotension may occur, but the usual effect is a widening of the difference between the systolic and the diastolic blood pressures. Through an increase of the maternal cardiac output and a lowering of the peripheral resistance, β-mimetics lead to an increase in placental perfusion which in combination with the relaxation of the myometrium lead to improved oxygenation of the fetus. However, the cardiac effects and the possibility, widely discussed in Europe, that β-mimetics can cause permanent damage to the heart remain concerns which have led to the use of calcium antagonists or β-blockers to counteract this effect of β-mimetics [42]. The value of such treatment remains to be proven, however.

In general, β-mimetics have distinct metabolic side effects [43,44]. Their lipolytic action is evidenced by an increase in serum fatty acid concentrations and their glycogenolytic action by rises in maternal and fetal serum glucose levels. This rise is further increased if glucocorticoids are given to accelerate fetal lung maturation. There is an increase in serum lactate and a fall in serum potassium. The potassium levels will sometimes drop below the normal limits, requiring a substitution. It is not clear whether there is a true potassium loss in the body. These metabolic changes do not seem to affect the mother to any large extent, but if the treatment fails to arrest labor, they may cause metabolic derangements in the newborn which can increase the management problems of the preterm infant. There have been cases reported of infants with sustained hypoglycemia, hypocalcemia, hypotension, and ileus due to the effect of the β-mimetic on intestinal motility, and these changes can lead to neonatal death if not discovered and corrected.

In animal experiments, β-mimetics cause fluid retention in the maternal lungs. This effect may be increased by corticosteroids if given concomitantly for the induction of fetal lung maturity. Several cases of pulmonary edema have been observed after such combined treatment, but pulmonary edema can also occur after β-mimetics alone.

B. Ethanol

Since the first publications on the use of ethanol in threatened preterm birth in 1965 [45] and 1967 [46] this treatment has been widely accepted. The fact that ethanol inhibits the secretion of oxytocin had been demonstrated in the human both during lactation [47] and labor [48]; more recently, we have found the same effect in preterm labor [14]. There is some evidence to suggest that ethanol may also have some direct action on the myometrium, the mechanism possibly being a reversible interaction of ethanol with calcium ions in the myometrial cells [49]. However, there is no doubt that the primary effect of ethanol is suppression of oxytocin secretion, and that the myometrium, even at high ethanol levels, remains sensitive to exogenous oxytocin stimulation. Recently developed radioimmunoassays for the detection of oxytocin in blood [50-53] have provided an unequivocal demonstration of oxytocin both in maternal and fetal blood at delivery.

Ethanol is effective by both oral and intravenous administration in threatened premature birth. The intravenous route is preferable because gastrointestinal absorption of ethanol depends on the amount of food present, whereas intravenous administration gives a constant rate of uptake and permits calculation of blood concentrations on the basis of body weight. However, oral administration can be used at home or under circumstances where transport to a hospital takes a long time.

Contraindications to the use of ethanol in preterm labor include the following: altered mental status, history of current drug abuse, liver disease, poorly controlled diabetes mellitus, peptic ulcer, epilepsy (ethanol shortens the half-life of diphenylhydantoin), and current use of anticoagulants (ethanol shortens the half-life of warfarin). A history of alcohol abuse is not considered a contraindication by us, unless there are signs of liver cirrhosis, and it does seem to work in such cases.

The recommended dosage of ethanol is the following. Initial dose: 7.5 ml of a 10% (v/v) solution of ethanol (preferably ready-made) per kilogram of body weight per hour for 2 hr. Maintenance dose: 1.5 ml of 10% ethanol per kilogram of body weight per hour for 10 hr. The maintenance dose has been calculated to maintain the blood level at the end of the initial dose, usually between 0.12 and 0.18% (120-180 mg/dl). The initial dose in a woman weighing 60 kg would be 900 ml over a period of 2 hr, corresponding to the oral intake of about 200 ml or 7 oz, of an 86-proof liquor.

During treatment, the patient's vital signs and uterine activity are monitored closely. If there are side effects, the rate of infusion may have to be adjusted. It is helpful to determine the blood alcohol levels, but if the dosage schedule is followed, and the patient is closely observed, this may not be needed.

The most frequent side effect is urinary incontinence, although nausea, vomiting, and headache may also occur. Antiemetics and antacids should be used routinely to avoid such symptoms.

It is advisable not to discontinue the infusion of ethanol as soon as contractions stop, but to continue it for several hours. The total course should be at least 6 hr and preferably longer. After the infusion is discontinued, it takes about 10 hr to eliminate the ethanol from the body. If a second course has to be given within 10 hr after discontinuation of the first course, the initial dose must be reduced, or the blood alcohol will reach dangerous levels. The repeat initial dose should be 10% of the original dose times the number of hours from the time of discontinuation. The maintenance dose should not be changed in repeat courses [16]. There is no consensus about the number of repeat courses which is safe, but it would appear prudent to change to another tocolytic agent after three or four courses of ethanol, or to interpret the recurrence of preterm labor as a signal that the fetus is better off outside the uterus.

Although ethanol is readily transferred to the fetus, no harmful effect has been observed, except when the baby is born while the mother still has a high blood level of alcohol. Such infants seem to be at increased risk for the development of respiratory distress syndrome [54]. It is therefore suggested that treatment with ethanol be interrupted as soon as it becomes evident that labor cannot be arrested. On the other hand, once the ethanol has been eliminated by mother and fetus, treatment seems to reduce the risk of occurrence of respiratory distress syndrome in the newborn infant [55].

We do not advocate continuous oral treatment with ethanol after arrest of labor by intravenous administration, but a number of patients have described how they have been able to stop mild contractions at home with a drink.

The result obtained in about 400 patients with intact membranes has been a delay of at least 72 hr in two-thirds of the cases [56]. We have defined success as delay of birth by at least 72 hr [46], and in the comparative study with ritodrine, the success rate for ethanol was 73% and for ritodrine 90% [40]. The average gain for the ethanol group (including failures) was 28 days and for the ritodrine group 44 days. At the stage of gestation where ethanol has been used to control preterm labor, the fetus is fully formed and the fetal alcohol syndrome is probably not a risk. However, it is difficult to tell pregnant women to abstain from alcohol and then to use alcohol to prevent preterm birth. We therefore have to reserve ethanol treatment for cases where other tocolytic agents are contraindicated or not effective.

C. Prostaglandin Synthetase Inhibitors

Prostaglandins E_2 and $F_{2\alpha}$ are powerful oxytocic agents, although on a molar basis they are 100–1000-fold less oxytocic on the pregnant human uterus than oxytocin [8]. Uterine tissues, including myometrium, decidua, and amnion, have a high capacity for prostaglandin synthesis, and during labor the concentrations of the two prostaglandins and their more stable metabolites increase rapidly in the maternal blood [10,57] and the amniotic fluid [58,59]. These prostaglandins interact with oxytocin in the mechanism of labor as indicated above, and if their synthesis is inhibited in early labor, the uterine contractions will stop [17,32,60].

Unfortunately, prostaglandins have many physiological functions in the mother and the fetus, including control of the blood flow through the fetal ductus arteriosus. This makes use of prostaglandin synthetase inhibitors, the so-called nonsteroidal anti-inflammatory drugs, less than ideal in premature labor [31].

However, the careful study by Niebyl et al. in Baltimore [61] and studies by Zuckerman et al. in Israel [17] have shown promising results. It is therefore important that further clinical studies be carried out. It would appear that prostaglandin synthetase inhibitors could be particularly useful in premature rupture of the membranes, since this complication is often associated with an increased level of circulating prostaglandins [62,63]. At the present time, none of the many nonsteroidal anti-inflammatory drugs, which inhibit prostaglandin synthesis, has been approved for use in preterm labor. Practicing obstetricians should avoid these compounds until more experience has been gathered in well-controlled studies in tertiary centers.

D. Magnesium Sulfate and Calcium Antagonists

The so-called calcium antagonists are agents which interfere with the function of the calcium ions in the contraction mechanism of smooth muscles. As such, they have definite tocolytic properties. They have been used in Europe both as single tocolytic agents and in combination with β-mimetics to protect the heart against the potentially dangerous effects of the latter [64]. One such drug, nifedipine, has been found efficacious in a small group of patients in preterm labor [65]. Magnesium sulfate is not, strictly speaking, a calcium antagonist, but it does interfere with the function of calcium, and this is supposedly the basis for its tocolytic effect [66]. Both magnesium sulfate and the specific calcium antagonists need further studies of their efficacy in preterm labor.

Many consider magnesium sulfate the drug of choice in severe preeclampsia, at least in the United States. Strangely enough, when used for this purpose, the tocolytic effect of magnesium sulfate is only slight. Nevertheless, magnesium sulfate has been advocated for premature labor on the basis of a study by Steer and Petrie [67].

Contraindications for the use of magnesium sulfate include reduced renal function, myocardial damage or heart block, and mental disease. Before its use, the serum levels of calcium and magnesium should be measured.

Usually, the treatment is begun with a dose of 4 g (equal to 40 ml) injected intravenously over a 10-min period. The maintenance dose is 2 g/hr in the form of a slow intravenous infusion of a 4% solution. During treatment the reflexes should be examined every hour, and the urine output must be monitored to ascertain a urine flow of at least 25 ml/hr. Use of magnesium sulfate must be discontinued if maternal side effects do not respond to reduction of the infusion, or if the serum level of magnesium exceeds 8 mg/dl.

VII. The Role of Nursing in Tocolytic Treatment

The outcome of tocolytic treatment for preterm labor depends not only on the right choice of agent and dosage but to a large extent upon the nursing care during the treatment. The nursing staff must be thoroughly familiar with the agents and their effects and side effects. They must be able to assure that the monitoring devices function continuously, and that appropriate blood samples are drawn at the right intervals for monitoring of electrolytes, glucose, etc. Because of the cardiovascular effects of tocolytics pulse rate and blood pressure must be recorded accurately and frequently; likewise, fluid intake and output must be measured and recorded.

Of paramount importance for the successful outcome is the ability of the obstetrical nurses to reassure and comfort the patients, and to explain the side effects; in other words, to provide tender loving care. Whenever possible, the patient should be kept on the labor floor until the uterus is completely at rest. Once the patient has been sent to the obstetrical floor, recurrence of uterine activity may not be detected as readily and valuable time may be lost.

VIII. Failure of Tocolytic Treatment

Failure of tocolytic treatment not only results in preterm birth, but it may even compound the problems of the premature neonate due to the metabolic effects of tocolytics on the fetus. This applies to all categories of clinically useful tocolytics. As a consequence, it is important to make the decision whether to discontinue treatment as early as possible, so that as much tocolytic agent as possible is eliminated from the fetus before birth. In addition, it is absolutely essential that the neonatologist be informed about the tocolytic treatment given and that he also be familiar with the metabolic and other effects of the tocolytic agent on the newborn.

Recurrence of preterm labor after successful treatment with a tocolytic agent is not infrequent. If it happens after a brief interval, treatment should be repeated, or a different tocolytic agent should be considered. Swedish investigators have noted that the sensitivity of the uterus to β-mimetics decreases with time, possibly through a down regulation of the β-receptors [68]. If the interval between treatment and recurrence is longer, many days or even weeks, the fetus may have come close enough to maturity to justify a decision not to repeat the treatment.

IX. Conclusions

To solve the problem of preterm birth, the most challenging one in obstetrics and neonatology, it is necessary to increase our endeavors to identify the risk factors in order to eliminate them where possible, or to reduce their impact by proper precautions. It is equally necessary to improve the tocolytic agents which are used when preterm labor begins, to increase the number of patients carried to term, and to reduce the side effects on mother and fetus. When both prevention and tocolytic treatment fail, expert management of labor and delivery, immediate resuscitation of the newborn, and high-quality intensive neonatal care are essential in order to obtain the best results. While the most efficient care can be provided in tertiary centers, it is very important that the expertise and skills not be limited to these places. Every obstetrician and pediatrician must be sufficiently trained to deal with the problems of preterm birth at all levels of care.

References

1. Räihä, C. E., Relation of maternal heart volume in pregnancy to prematurity and perinatal mortality, *Bull. WHO,* **26**:296 (1962).
2. Kauppinen, M. A., The correlation of maternal heart volume with the birth weight of the infant and prematurity, *Acta Obstet. Gynecol. Scand.,* **46** (Suppl. 6):1 (1967).
3. Creasy, R. K., B. A. Gummer, and G. C. Liggins, System for predicting spontaneous preterm birth, *Obstet. Gynecol.,* **55**:692 (1980).
4. Fredrik, J., Antenatal identification of women at high risk of spontaneous preterm birth, *Br. J. Obstet. Gynaecol.,* **93**:351 (1976).
5. Papiernik, E., and M. Kaminski, Multifactorial study of the risk of prematurity of 32 weeks of gestation, *J. Perinat. Med.,* **2**:30 (1974).
6. Herron, M. A., M. Katz, and R. K. Creasy, Evaluation of a preterm birth prevention program: Preliminary report, *Obstet. Gynecol.,* **59**:452 (1982).
7. Coutinho, E. M., and A. C. V. Lopes, Response of the nonpregnant uterus to vasopressin as an index of ovarian function, *Am. J. Obstet. Gynecol.,* **102**: 479–489 (1968).

8. Fuchs, A.-R., The role of oxytocin in human parturition. In *Current Topics in Experimental Endocrinology*, vol. 5, *Endocrinology of Pregnancy*. Edited by L. Martini and V. H. James. New York, Academic Press, 1983.
9. Dawood, M. Y., O. Ylikorkala, D. Trivedi, and F. Fuchs, Oxytocin in maternal circulation and amniotic fluid during pregnancy, *J. Clin. Endocrinol. Metab.*, **49**:429-434 (1979).
10. Fuchs, A.-R., K. Goeschen, P. Husslein, A. B. Rasmussen, and F. Fuchs, Oxytocin and the initiation of human parturition. III. Plasma concentrations of oxytocin and 13,14-dihydro-15-keto-prostaglandin $F_{2\alpha}$ in spontaneous and oxytocin-induced labor at term, *Am. J. Obstet. Gynecol.*, **147**: 497-502 (1983).
11. Fuchs, A.-R., F. Fuchs, P. Husslein, M. S. Soloff, and M. J. Fernström, Oxytocin receptors and human parturition: A dual role for oxytocin in the initiation of labor, *Science*, **215**:1396-1398 (1982).
12. Fuchs, A.-R., P. Husslein, and F. Fuchs, Oxytocin and the initiation of human parturition. II. Stimulation of prostaglandin production in human decidua by oxytocin, *Am. J. Obstet. Gynecol.*, **141**:694-697 (1981).
13. Dawood, M. Y., C. F. Wang, R. Gupta, and F. Fuchs, Fetal contribution of oxytocin in human parturition, *Obstet. Gynecol,*, **52**:205-209 (1978).
14. Fuchs, A.-R., P. Husslein, L. Sumulong, J. P. Micha, M. Y. Dawood, and F. Fuchs, Plasma levels of oxytocin and 13,14-dihydro-15-keto-prostaglandin $F_{2\alpha}$ in preterm labor and the effect of ethanol and ritodrine, *Am. J. Obstet. Gynecol.*, **144**:753-759 (1982).
15. Fuchs, F., A.-R. Fuchs, V. F. Poblete, Jr., and A. Risk, Prevention of premature labor by ethanol infusions, *Am. J. Obstet. Gynecol.*, **99**:627-636 (1967).
16. Fuchs, F., Prevention of prematurity, *Am. J. Obstet. Gynecol.*, **126**:809-817 (1976).
17. Zuckerman, H., U. Reiss, and I. Rubinstein, Inhibition of human premature labor by indomethacin, *Obstet. Gynecol.*, **44**:787-792 (1974).
18. Wiqvist, N., V. Lundström, and K. Gréen, Premature labor and indomethacin, *Prostaglandins*, **10**:515-526 (1975).
19. Pohjavuori, M., and F. Fyhrquist, Hemodynamic significance of vasopressin in the newborn infant, *J. Pediatr.*, **97**:462-465 (1980).
20. Rurak, D. W., Plasma vasopressin levels during hypoxaemia and the cardiovascular effects of exogenous vasopressin in foetal and adult sheep, *J. Physiol. (Lond.)*, **277**:341-357 (1978).
21. Stark, R. I., S. L. Wardlaw, R. S. Goland, M. K. Husain, R. L. Vande Wiele, and L. S. James, β-Endorphin, adrenocorticotropin, and vasopressin in the human at birth. *Pediatr. Res.*, **14**:473 (1980).

22. Van Dyke, H. B., and R. Ames, Alcohol diuresis, *Acta Endocrinol.,* **7**:110-121 (1951).
23. Fuchs, F., Endocrinology of parturition. In *Endocrinology of Pregnancy,* 3d ed. Edited by F. Fuchs and A. Klopper. New York, Lippincott-Harper, 1983.
24. Csapo, A. I., O. Pohanka, and H. L. Kaihola, Steroid profile of threatened premature labour, *Lancet,* **ii**:1097 (1973).
25. Csapo, A. I., O. Pohanka, and H. L. Kaihola, Progesterone deficiency and premature labour, *Br. Med. J.,* **1**:137-140 (1974).
26. TambyRaja, R. L., A. B. M. Anderson, and A. C. Turnbull, Endocrine changes in premature labour, *Br. Med. J.,* **4**:67-71 (1974).
27. TambyRaja, R. L., and K. C. Lun, Plasma estriol as a predictor of preterm labor, *Int. J. Gynaecol. Obstet.,* **15**:535-538 (1978).
28. Liggins, G. C., and R. N. Howie, A controlled trial of antepartum glucocorticoid treatment for prevention of the respiratory distress syndrome in premature infants, *Pediatrics,* **50**:515-525 (1972).
29. Abramovici, H., A. Lewin, A. Lissak, and A. Palant, Maternal pulmonary edema occurring after therapy with ritodrine for premature uterine contractions, *Acta Obstet. Gynecol. Scand.,* **59**:555-561 (1980).
30. Elliott, J. P., D. F. O'Keeffe, P. Greenberg, and R. K. Freeman, Pulmonary edema associated with magnesium sulfate and betamethasone administration, *Am. J. Obstet. Gynecol.,* **134**:717-719 (1979).
31. Wiqvist, N., Preterm labour: Other drug possibilities including drugs not to use. In *Preterm Labour.* Edited by M. G. Elder and C. H. Hendricks. London, Butterworths, 1981, pp. 148-175.
32. Niebyl, J. R., Prostaglandin synthetase inhibitors, *Semin. Perinatol.,* **5**:275-287 (1981).
33. Suranyi, S., I. Endrödi, I. Ban, J. Nagy, and K. Zsigmond, Uterine relaxation with betamimetics and alcohol. In *Labour Inhibition: Betamimetic Drugs in Obstetrics.* Edited by H. Weidinger, G. Fischer. Stuttgart, Thieme, 1977, pp. 153-157.
34. Gamissans, O., E. Cañas, V. Caracach, J. Ribas, B. Puerto, and A. Edo, A study of indomethacin combined with ritodrine in threatened preterm labor, *Europ. J. Obstet. Gynec. Reprod. Biol.,* **3**:123-128 (1978).
35. Gamissans, O., V. Caracach, and J. Serra, The role of prostaglandin-inhibitors, beta-adrenergic drugs, and glucocorticoids in the management of threatened preterm labor. In *Beta-mimetic Drugs in Obstetrics and Perinatology.* Edited by H. Jung and G. Lamberti. Stuttgart, Thieme, 1982, pp. 71-84.
36. Ahlquist, R. P., A study of the adrenotropic receptors, *Am. J. Physiol.,* **153**:586-595 (1948).

37. Hendricks, C. H., The use of isoxsuprine for the arrest of premature labor, *Clin. Obstet. Gynecol.,* **7**:687–696 (1964).
38. Barden, T. P., J. B. Peter, and I. R. Merkatz, Ritodrine hydrochloride: A betamimetic agent for use in preterm labor, *Obstet. Gynecol.,* **56**:1–6 (1980).
39. Wesselius-de Casparis, A., M. Thiery, A. Yo Le Sian, K. Baumgarten, I. Brosens, O. Gamissans, J. G. Stolk, and W. Vivier, Results of double-blind, multicentre study with ritodrine in premature labour, *Br. Med. J.,* **3**:144–147 (1971).
40. Lauersen, N. H., I. R. Merkatz, N. Tejani, K. H. Wilson, A. Roberson, L. I. Mann, and F. Fuchs, Inhibition of premature labor: A multicenter comparison of ritodrine and ethanol, *Am. J. Obstet. Gynecol.,* **127**:837–845 (1977).
41. Lipshitz, J., Beta-adrenergic agonists, *Semin. Perinatol.,* **5**:252–265 (1981).
42. Jung, H., and G. Lamberti, (Eds.), *Beta-mimetic Drugs in Obstetrics and Perinatology.* Stuttgart, Thieme, 1982.
43. Borberg, C., M. D. G. Gilmer, R. W. Beard, and N. W. Oakely, Metabolic effects of beta-sympathomimetic drugs and dexamethasone in normal and diabetic pregnancy, *Br. J. Obstet. Gynaecol.,* **85**:184–189 (1978).
44. Kirkpatrick, C., M. Quenon, and D. Desir, Blood anions and electrolytes during ritodrine infusion in preterm labor, *Am. J. Obstet. Gynecol.,* **138**:523–527 (1980).
45. Fuchs, F., Treatment of threatened premature labour with alcohol, *J. Obstet. Gynaecol. Br. Commwlth.,* **72**:1011–1013 (1965).
46. Fuchs, F., A.-R., Fuchs, V. F. Poblete, Jr., and A. Risk, Prevention of premature labor by ethanol infusions, *Am. J. Obstet. Gynecol.,* **99**:627–637 (1967).
47. Fuchs, A.-R., and G. Wagner, Effect of alcohol on the release of oxytocin, *Nature,* **198**:92–93 (1963).
48. Gibbens, D., and T. Chard, Observations on maternal oxytocin release during human labour and the effect of intravenous alcohol administration, *Am. J. Obstet. Gynecol.,* **126**:243–246 (1976).
49. Fuchs, A.-R., and F. Fuchs, Ethanol for prevention of preterm birth, *Semin. Perinatol.,* **5**:236–251 (1981).
50. Chard, T., N. R. Boyd, M. L. Forsling, and A. S. McNeilly, The development of a radioimmunoassay for oxytocin. The extraction of oxytocin from plasma, and its measurement during parturition in human and goat blood. *J. Endocrinol.,* **48**:223–234 (1970).
51. Chard, T., C. M. Hudson, C. R. W. Edwards, and N. R. H. Boyd, Release of oxytocin and vasopressin by the human foetus during labour, *Nature,* **234**:352–353 (1971).

52. Dawood, M. Y., K. S. Raghavan, and C. Pociask, A radioimmunoassay for oxytocin, *J. Endocrinol.,* **76**:261–270 (1978).
53. Kumaresan, P., P. B. Anandarangam, W. Dianzon, and A. Vasicka, Plasma oxytocin levels during human pregnancy and labor as determined by radioimmunoassay, *Am. J. Obstet. Gynecol.,* **119**:215–223 (1974).
54. Zervoudakis, I. A., A. Krauss, F. Fuchs, and K. H. Wilson, Infants of mothers treated with ethanol for premature labor, *Am. J. Obstet. Gynecol.,* **138**: 20–25 (1980).
55. Barrada, M. I., M. L. Virnin, and L. E. Edwards, Maternal intravenous ethanol in the prevention of respiratory distress syndrome, *Am. J. Obstet. Gynecol.,* **129**:25–29 (1977).
56. Fuchs, F., A.-R. Fuchs, N. H. Lauersen, and I. A. Zervoudakis, Treatment of preterm labour with ethanol, *Danish Med. Bull.,* **26**:123–124 (1979).
57. Dubin, N. H., J. W. C. Johnson, S. Calhoun, R. B. Ghodgaonkar, and J. C. Beak, Plasma prostaglandin in pregnant women with term and preterm deliveries, *Obstet. Gynecol.,* **57**:203–208 (1980).
58. Keirse, M. J. N. C., M. D. Mitchell, and A. C. Turnbull, Changes in prostaglandin F and 13,14-dihydro,15-keto-prostaglandin F in amniotic fluid at the onset of and during labour, *Br. J. Obstet. Gynaecol.,* **94**:743–748 (1977).
59. Dray, F., and R. Frydman, Primary prostaglandins in amniotic fluid in pregnancy and spontaneous labor, *Am. J. Obstet. Gynecol.,* **126**:13–19 (1976).
60. Schwartz, A., I. Brook, V. Insler, F. Kohen, U. Zor, and H. R. Lindner, Effect of flufenamic acid on uterine contractions and plasma levels of 15-keto-13,14-dihydro-prostaglandin $F_{2\alpha}$ in preterm labor, *Gynecol. Obstet. Invest.,* **9**:139–149 (1978).
61. Niebyl, J. R., D. A. Blake, R. D. White, K. M. Kumos, N. H. Dubin, J. C. Robinson, and P. G. Egner, The inhibition of premature labor with indomethacin, *Am. J. Obstet. Gynecol.,* **136**:1014–1019 (1980).
62. Mitchell, M. D., A. P. F. Flint, J. Bibby, J. Brunt, J. M. Arnold, A. B. M. Anderson, and A. C. Turnbull, Rapid increases in plasma prostaglandin concentrations after vaginal examination and amniotomy, *Br. Med. J.,* **2**:1183–1185 (1977).
63. Husslein, P., E. Kofler, A. B. Rasmussen, L. Sumulong, A.-R. Fuchs, and F. Fuchs, Oxytocin and the initiation of human parturition. IV. Plasma oxytocin and 13,14-dihydro-15-keto-prostaglandin $F_{2\alpha}$ concentrations during labor induced by artificial rupture of membranes, *Am. J. Obstet. Gynecol.,* **147**:503–507 (1983).
64. Forman, A., K.-E. Andersson, and U. Ulmsten, Inhibition of myometrial activity by calcium antagonists. *Semin. Perinatol.,* **5**:288–294 (1981).

65. Ulmsten, U., K.-E. Andersson, and L. Wingerup, Treatment of premature labor with the calcium antagonist nifedipine, *Arch. Gynecol.,* **229**:1–5 (1980).
66. Petrie, R. H., Tocolysis using magnesium sulfate, *Semin. Perinatol.,* **5**:266–273 (1981).
67. Steer, C. M., and R. H. Petrie, A comparison of magnesium sulfate and alcohol for the prevention of premature labor, *Am. J. Obstet. Gynecol.,* **129**:1–4 (1977).
68. Rydén, G., R. G. G. Andersson, and G. Berg, Is the relaxing effect of β-adrenergic agonists on the human myometrium only transitory?, *Acta Obstet. Gynecol. Scand.,* **61**(Suppl. 108):47–51 (1982).

Part Five

THE DELIVERY ROOM

13

Attempts at Prevention of Hyaline Membrane Disease in the Delivery Room

GORAN ENHORNING

University of Toronto
Toronto, Ontario, Canada

I. Introduction

A smooth transfer from intra- to extrauterine life requires the ability on the part of the neonate to switch immediately the site of gas exchange from placenta to lungs. It is clear from previous chapters that the principal cause of the inability to make such a switch, and to maintain adequate pulmonary function, is immaturity, particularly regarding the synthesis and/or release of pulmonary surfactant. Birth at too low a gestational age is the main reason for pulmonary immaturity, leading to the respiratory distress syndrome (RDS). Correct dating of the pregnancy and analysis of amniotic fluid for accurate assessment of pulmonary maturity aid the obstetrician in preventing preterm delivery and, therefore, RDS. Socially favorable circumstances, including good prenatal care, are essential in the avoidance of premature delivery, but tocolytic agents also may be of some value. When it is feared that the infant might be born prematurely, or when the intrauterine milieu is less than favorable and preterm delivery is contemplated, glucocorticoids could be used to accelerate the lungs' maturation process [1,2].

In spite of all the measures alluded to above, and fully covered in previous chapters, the situation often arises where preterm delivery is imminent, and the infant in all likelihood will be born with a surfactant deficiency. It is then of utmost importance that delivery be atraumatic, that drugs be avoided which when transferred to the fetus might inhibit normal function of the respiratory center, and that delivery take place in a hospital where optimal neonatal care can be provided.

II. Surfactant Supplementation

A. The Concept

With the milestone paper of Avery and Mead [3], the pathogenesis of RDS became better understood. Their findings gave evidence that infants developing RDS had a surfactant deficiency, more than likely causing the breathing problem. Such being the case, one would expect it to be possible to prevent, or at least alleviate, the condition by supplying the neonate with the surfactant so desperately needed. A deposition into the upper airways prior to the first breath is a relatively simple procedure. The moment immediately following birth, and preceding the first breath, offers a unique opportunity for effective administration of the missing surfactant. When instilled into the pharynx or upper trachea, the concentrated surfactant will be where it is urgently needed, i.e., at the air-liquid interface. There it will lower surface tension, thus facilitating initial aeration. As the surfactant is distributed to various sections of the lungs, it remains in the menisci, where its activity is exerted, leaving behind perhaps only a monomolecular layer of the surface-active phospholipids outlining the airways. Also, in the alveoli a stabilizing monomolecular layer will be formed at the air-liquid interface, below which there will be more or less of a surfactant reserve in the hypophase. Figure 1 illustrates how surfactant deposited into the upper airways can be expected to be distributed with the first breath.

B. Early Experiences

With some hesitance, administration of surfactant directly into the airways is becoming an accepted principle for treating a clearly established, severe RDS. Yet, when first put to the test in Canada 20 years ago the method did not seem particularly promising [4]. Even more discouraging was an article by Chu et al. [5]. After extensive studies, these investigators were unable to report that the treatment was beneficial. Their lack of success made them doubt that RDS was caused mainly by a surfactant deficiency. Instead, they concluded that the problem was primarily one of pulmonary ischemia. In the two pioneering studies just referred to [4,5], only the main component of surfactant, dipalmitoyl

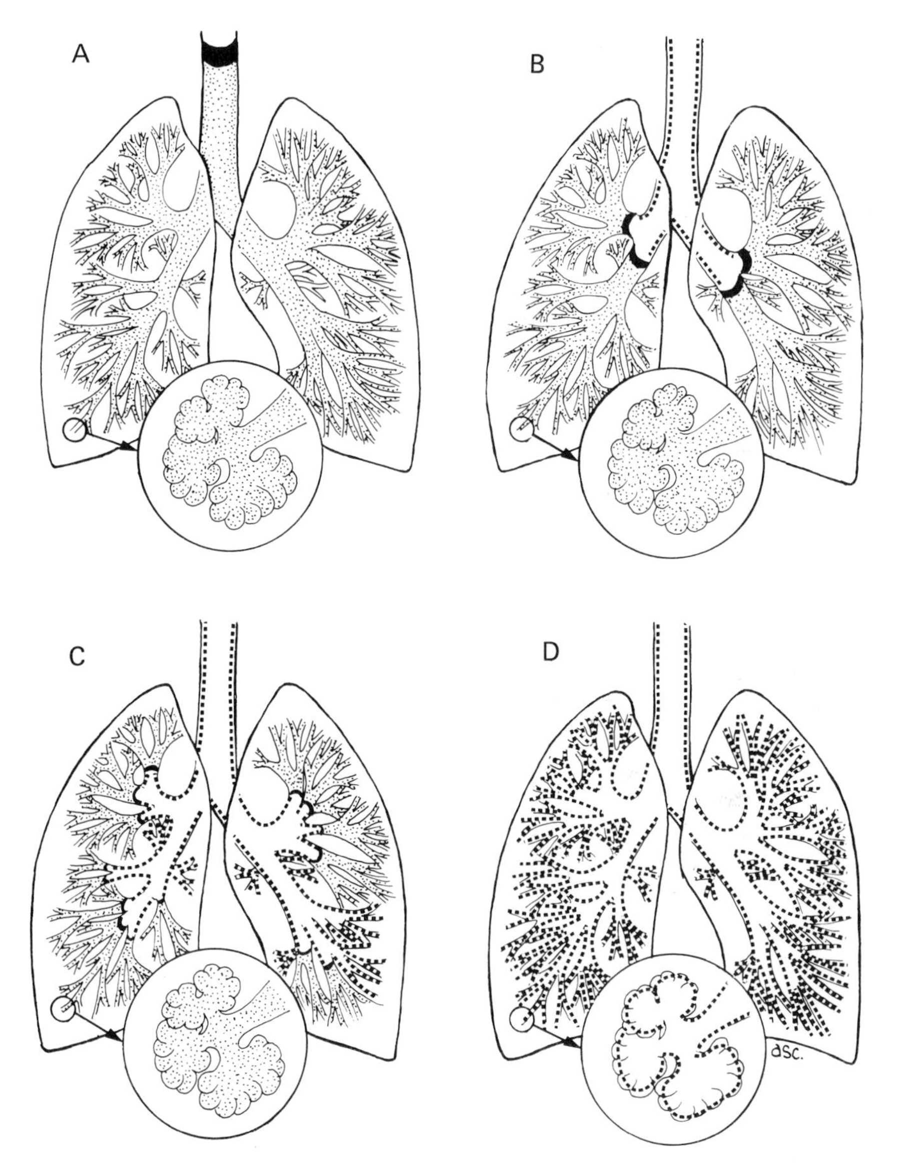

Figure 1 Principle of depositing a concentrated surfactant into the upper airway prior to the first breath. In the various stages of the initial aeration (A–D), the surfactant moves down the airways, always remaining in highest concentration at the air-liquid interface. Finally (D), the surfactant is outlining the terminal airways, offering stability.

phosphatidylcholine (DPPC), was supplied as an aerosol. As will be discussed later, DPPC without at least the initial aid of other phospholipids is unlikely to be able to express the surface properties of natural surfactant, and an aerosol probably would be distributed only to airways already open. The closed bronchioli and alveoli, perhaps in the greatest need of surfactant, are not likely to receive the DPPC dispersed as an aerosol. For those reasons, it seems clear today that mixing the inhaled air with a DPPC aerosol is not apt to result in a substantially improved compliance or gas exchange, even though there are more recent reports [6,7] indicating that this mode of therapy may be of some value.

C. The Key to Success

If the concept that RDS is an expression of surfactant deficiency is correct, then it certainly should be possible to improve the situation for a preterm neonate and prevent, or at least inhibit, the development of RDS by replacing the liquid in the upper airways with a surfactant concentrate. This instantaneous upgrading of the neonate's lung maturity prior to the first breath was put to the test in a series of animal experiments carried out by Enhorning et al. [8–14]. Natural surfactant, obtained from young adult rabbits, was used. The lungs were lavaged with saline solution and the surfactant was concentrated, with a simple centrifugation procedure, so that there were approximately 20 mg phospholipids/ml in the final product. The surfactant suspension thus obtained was tested on rabbit neonates delivered on the twenty-seventh or twenty-eighth day of gestation, a few days prior to term. They were then clearly surfactant deficient and, for this reason, were almost completely unable to aerate their lungs and seldom survived. A tracheal deposition of the crude natural surfactant prior to lung aeration resulted in increased compliance, as previously reported by Rüfer [15], improved histological [8–11] as well as radiological expansion [12], and an increased survival rate [9,10,12,13]. Figure 2 shows chest radiograms of preterm rabbit neonates, surfactant treated and controls, during the first 2 hr of extrauterine life. For details, including lower tracings, see Ref. 12.

When the same surfactant preparation was tested on preterm primates (*Rhesus* monkeys delivered at a gestational age of 130–132 days, i.e., about 35 days prior to term), there was, in comparison with untreated controls, an improved gas exchange and survival [13], and the surfactant also seemed to prevent hyaline membranes from developing [14]. Nilsson et al. [16] presented further data in support of the observation that the presence of surfactant will inhibit the development of cellular necrosis and other morphological derangements otherwise seen following respirator use. These and other aspects of surfactant replacement were covered in reviews by Robertson [17] and Notter and Shapiro [18].

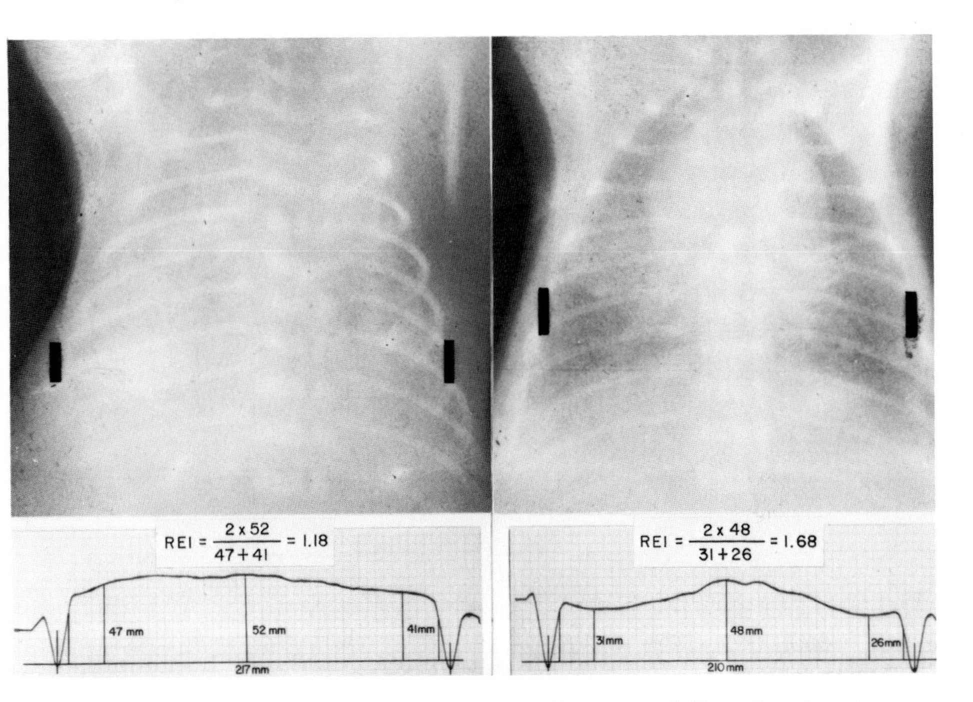

Figure 2 Chest radiograms of two rabbit pups, littermates delivered on twenty-seventh day of gestation. Control on the left, surfactant-treated pup on the right. (From Ref. 12.)

The lamb delivered by cesarean section at a gestational age of 120–130 days (term 150 days) has proven to be an ideal, large animal model for neonatal RDS. The surfactant deficiency at 120 days is so severe that without supplementation early respiratory failure is certain. Adams et al. [19] found that treating 120-day lambs with tracheal instillation of natural surfactant in a dose of 50–170 mg total lipids per kilogram of body weight protected against the early features of RDS. Jobe et al. [20] gave the treatment at birth, or shortly thereafter, when respiratory failure was established. Either way, the treatment initially was extremely effective, when six lambs treated at birth were compared with their twins receiving no surfactant. The results were very convincing. At birth, the conditions of the two groups were almost identical but, whereas the treated lambs immediately reached a very high PO_2 (270 + 35 mmHg), the untreated twins deteriorated quickly and within an hour had developed severe acidosis (Fig. 3). Although the treated lambs were supported on infant ventilators with 100% oxygen, or possibly because of this unnecessarily high oxygen

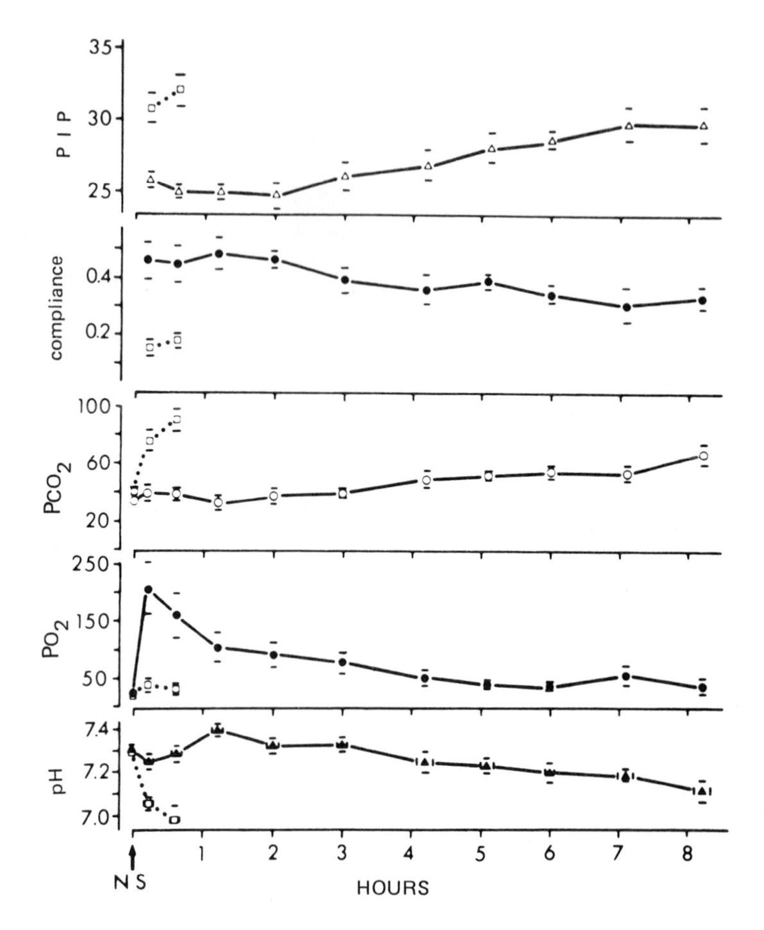

Figure 3 Sequential measurements for six lambs treated with natural surfactant (NS) at birth (solid lines) and for six untreated lambs (interrupted lines). Peak inspiratory pressure (PIP) is in centimeters of water. Initial PCO_2, PO_2, and pH values were from cord blood. The conspicuous effect was not as dramatic when the surfactant treatment was withheld until respiratory failure had been documented. (From Ref. 20. Copyright 1981 by the American Society for Clinical Investigation.)

supplementation, they deteriorated and were in severe respiratory distress at the end of the 8-hr study period. The lambs treated when respiratory failure had already occurred were older and weighed more than those treated at birth. Even so, they required a higher maximal ventilatory pressure and their response to treatment was of shorter duration. Jobe et al. [20] concluded that the intercurrent episode of severe hypoxia, hypercarbia, and acidosis had adversely affected the response to treatment. They also considered though that the reason the treatment was less effective once respiratory failure had become established might have been due to uneven distribution of the surfactant. The nonuniform aeration observed on chest radiograms was compatible with this latter interpretation.

In experiments on surfactant-depleted adult rats [21], and later on premature lambs [22], the efficacy of natural surfactant was compared with that of an artificial preparation consisting of a 9:1 mixture of DPPC and phosphatidylglycerol (PG). The natural product was superior to the artificial, in vitro as well as in vivo, but those treated with the artificial surfactant had a higher PO_2 than the untreated controls.

Based on the aforementioned experiences, it seems safe to say that the key to success was the tracheal instillation of a natural surfactant suspension rather than an administration of aerosolized DPPC as in the very early clinical trials [4,5]. Furthermore, the animal experiments offer evidence that for even distribution of the surfactant and an optimal effect administration should be at birth prior to the first breath. Only then can one expect the surfactant to be evenly dispersed to all airways as illustrated in Figure 1. Animal experiments demonstrating that surfactant supplementation will prevent development of neonatal RDS strongly support the concept that surfactant deficiency is the cause of RDS and will give rise to the morphological consequences of the breathing difficulty—atelectasis and, eventually, hyaline membranes.

D. Problems with Clinical Application

Instillation of a natural surfactant concentrate into the upper airway prior to the first breath (Figs. 1 and 2) results in instantaneous upgrading of the preterm neonate's lung maturity. However, there are obvious reservations to the application of this treatment in human subjects. A major concern is that crude natural surfactant prepared from lung lavage would not be sterile and could be antigenic. Sterilization by autoclaving inactivates the natural surfactant, probably because of its high protein content. The latter makes the surfactant potentially antigenic, and although the risk of immunization is minimal in view of the low immune response of the preterm infant, and because the surfactant most likely would be used only once, it would certainly be preferable if the surfactant administered to the human neonate contained little or no protein.

The mode of administration may also have its drawbacks, even though instillation of a concentrated suspension prior to the first breath is likely to be very effective. It probably can be accomplished rather easily if delivery is vaginal in cephalic presentation and epidural anesthesia is used. Once the head has been delivered, the shoulders can be rotated, turning the face upward. Vaginal pressure on the thorax would render breathing efforts ineffective while the upper airways are sucked clean and the surfactant deposited. However, breech presentation will be relatively frequent when labor starts prior to term. It would then be necessary to restrain the chest manually until the airways were sucked clean and the surfactant administered. The same procedure would have to be used when delivery is by cesarean section. Once the lungs are aerated, administering the surfactant as a suspension is not so appealing, since tracheal instillation of a liquid would seriously interfere with gas exchange, at least momentarily. It would be preferable if the surfactant were carried to the alveoli by air rather than by liquid.

Efforts to make surfactant treatment clinically more acceptable for the most part have taken two directions: (1) production of a sterile, nonantigenic preparation, and (2) development of methods for surfactant administration. The following sections will deal with some of the problems encountered in these endeavors.

Preparing an Artificial Surfactant

Composition of Natural Surfactant

Producing an artificial surfactant may seem easy enough—simply a matter of putting together the components of natural surfactant, preferably with the exclusion of proteins. The first question requiring an answer then would be, what are these components, i.e., what is natural surfactant? Is it the material present in the airway fluid of a fetus at term? Is it the material obtainable with a lung lavage? These two types of fluid obviously may contain not only pulmonary surfactant but various contaminants as well, such as cell debris and mucus from goblet cells in the larger airways. In an effort to overcome this problem, efforts have been made to purify the fluid. There is no absolute evidence, however, that selective material resulting from fractionating procedures, such as density gradient centrifugation, can be said to be true pulmonary surfactant. One might suppose that if it were possible to harvest the lipids in the monolayer outlining the alveolar spaces, this would truly be surfactant. By the time a monolayer is formed, however, it is conceivable that there has been a concentration of certain phospholipids at the expense of others [23]. The excluded phospholipids might have been important initially for rapid creation of a monolayer, i.e., for a fast adsorption. Furthermore, an alveolar monolayer probably undergoes cyclical changes in its composition [24]. When the film is compressed during expiration,

Table 1 Composition of Canine Surfactant

		Study 1[a] (%)	Study 2[b] (%)
Saturated phosphatidylcholines		45	40
Unsaturated phosphatidylcholines		25	21
Phosphatidylglycerol		5	8
Phosphatidylethanolamine		3	5
Other phospholipids		2	9
	Total phospholipids	80	83
Neutral lipids		10	10
	Total lipids	90	93
Protein		8	7
Carbohydrate		2	0

[a]Data from Ref. 26.
[b]Data from Ref. 27.

certain molecules are squeezed out, but they reenter more or less completely during inspiration to become again part of the monolayer.

For the above reasons, it is impossible to give an exact definition of pulmonary surfactant. It would seem reasonable, though, to consider a material to be surfactant if it is obtained from the airways and has certain physical properties deemed necessary for initial lung aeration and airway stability, hence normal pulmonary function. Perhaps the most important of these properties are: (1) fast adsorption, (2) very low surface tension with compression, and (3) moderate elastance (change in surface tension with change in surface area). Materials fulfilling these criteria have been carefully analyzed [25-27]. Table 1 gives data from two studies of canine surfactant. The composition is not species-specific [28], but there are changes occurring with increasing fetal maturity, and the appearance of PG is relatively late in ontogenesis [29].

Phospholipid Characteristics

Pulmonary surfactant consists primarily of phospholipids, i.e., amphipathic lipids characterized by a glycerol nucleus to which are bound two hydrophobic fatty acids, turned toward the air phase in the monolayer, and the hydrophilic polar

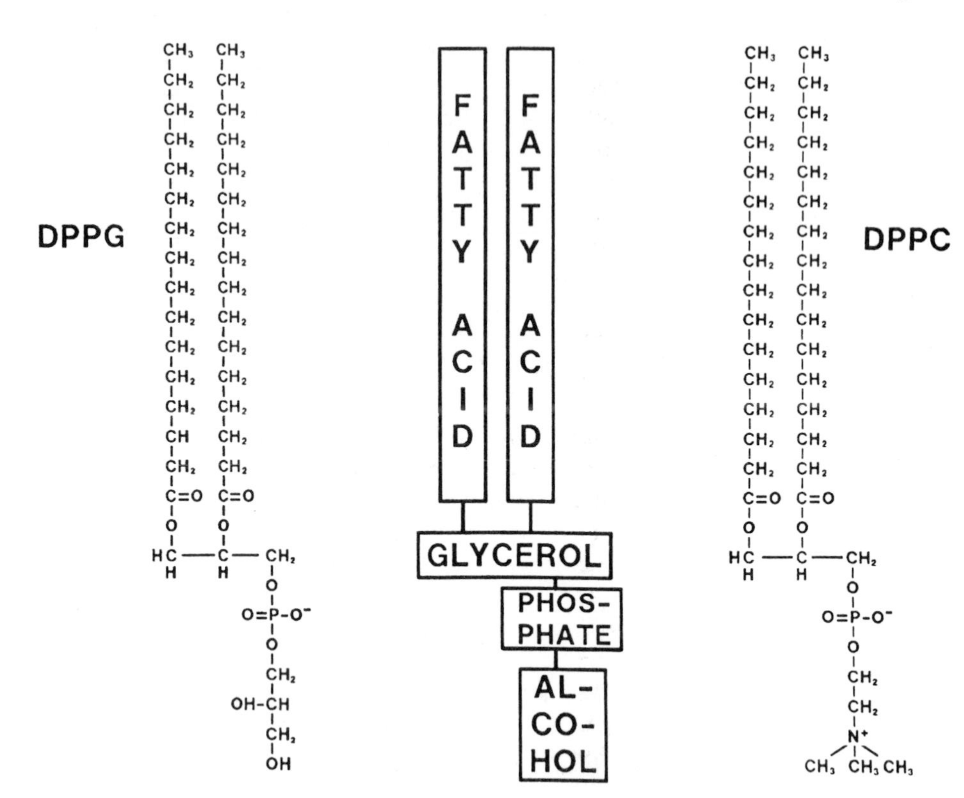

Figure 4 Principle of the molecular architecture of amphipathic phospholipids and two important surfactant components, dipalmitoyl phosphatidylglycerol (DPPG) and dipalmitoyl phosphatidylcholine (DPPC).

head group, surrounded by water (Fig. 4). The polar head in turn consists of a phosphate group and an alcohol. The latter most often is choline and the phospholipid is then known as phosphatidylcholine or lecithin. In the membranes of various kinds of cells, lecithin is an important building block, but the type found in pulmonary surfactant is characterized to a large extent by being disaturated, i.e., the fatty acids have no double bonds; they are both saturated. There are an even number of carbon atoms in the fatty acid chain, 14, 16, 18, 20, or 22. Palmitic acid is saturated and has 16 carbon atoms. Two such chains are found in DPPC, the most abundant phospholipid in pulmonary surfactant. Like any amphipathic lipid, DPPC has the ability to form a monomolecular film at an air-water interface. When forced to occupy a compressed surface area, as will be the case in the lung at end-expiration, such a film exerts a high surface pressure, i.e., it will reduce surface tension to an extremely low value (close to zero). In this respect, DPPC fulfills the requirements of pulmonary surfactant as well as or better than any other phospholipid. However, DPPC differs from pulmonary surfactant in two important ways. Its surface elastance is too great, and without the aid of other phospholipids, or possibly proteins, DPPC is almost totally unable to move from a water-suspended form, e.g., a liposome, to an air-water interface. In other words, its adsorption rate is extremely low, which may be especially detrimental to the neonate, quickly creating a large air-liquid interface with the first breath.

Knowing that the principal ingredient of pulmonary surfactant does not work on its own, it was necessary to find out what other components would have to be included to give the mixture the desired surface properties of natural surfactant. Because the cell membrane has the basic structure of a phospholipid bilayer, a broad knowledge of phospholipid characteristics and physical behavior has been acquired by membrane investigators. See review articles by Bangham [30], Chapman [31], and Phillips [32]. Using differential scanning calorimetry, the gel-to-liquid crystalline transition temperature has been determined for the various phospholipids. Only above that temperature are the fatty acids sufficiently motile to allow interface adsorption at a reasonable rate. For DPPC the transition temperature is 41°C, and to bring it below body temperature another lipid must be added [33]. Cholesterol could be considered, or another phospholipid with one or both fatty acids being shorter and/or having double bonds. Replacing the choline of DPPC with another alcohol, e.g., glycerol, will have a similar effect [32]. Notter et al. [34,35] and Hawco et al. [36] have systematically investigated the effect of various additions to DPPC. It certainly is possible to prepare a mixture with appropriate transition temperature. This has been found to increase the adsorption rate, but often at the expense of a lost high surface pressure during film compression.

Because the surface-active phospholipids are poorly soluble in water, or even insoluble, they must be suspended by shaking or with the aid of ultrasound. Sonication is effective in dispersing the lipids into liposomes, but these may have high stability and will not break up to form a monolayer at the air-water interface. Duration and intensity of sonication and the temperature at which it is performed will affect the size and shape of the lipid aggregates formed, influencing adsorption rate [37].

The search for an artificial pulmonary surfactant necessitates the testing of a very large number of samples. The pulsating bubble technique [38], first described by Adams and Enhorning [39], makes such screening feasible. The principle is simple. A bubble, communicating with ambient air, is like a model of an alveolus made to expand and pulsate in the sample (20 μl) to be studied. Since the radius (r) of the bubble is known, and the pressure (P) around it is recorded, surface tension (γ) can be calculated with the law of Laplace, $\Delta P = 2\gamma/r$.

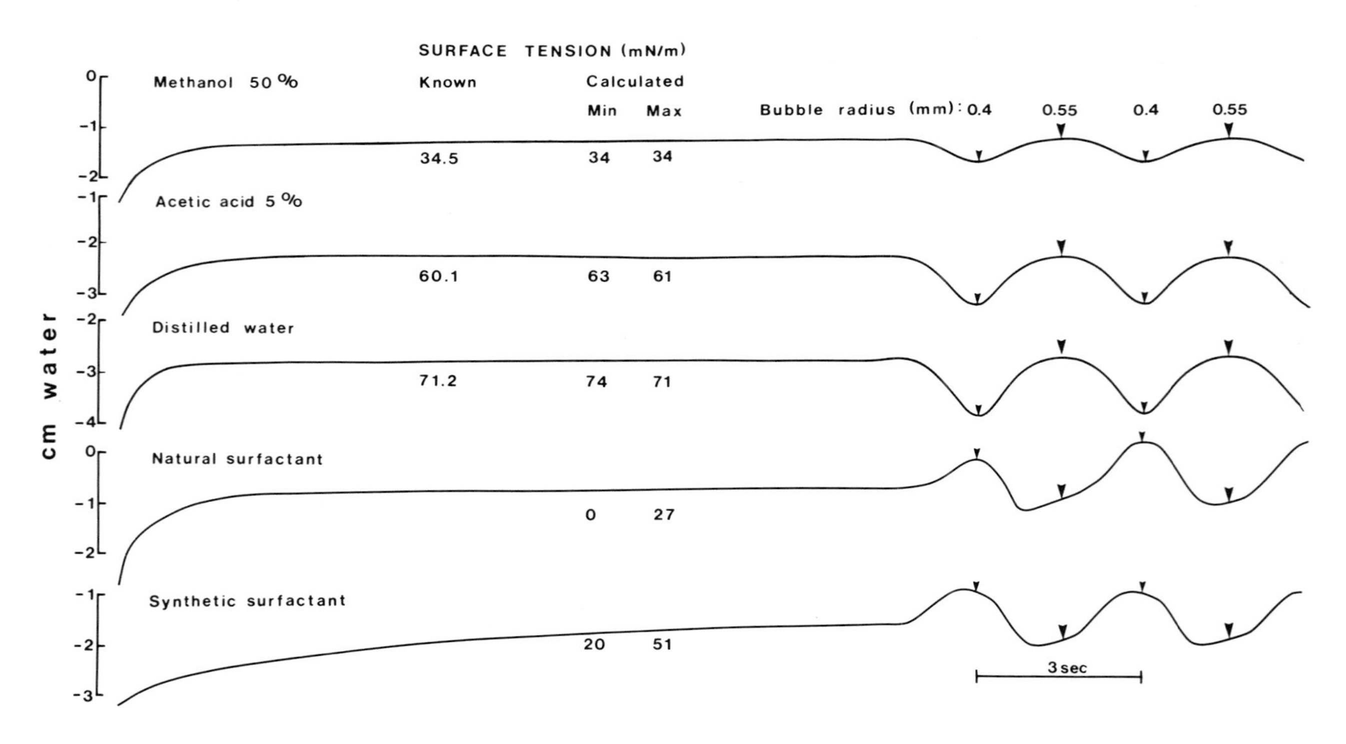
SURFACE TENSION (mN/m)
Known
Calculated
Min
Max
Bubble radius (mm): 0.4
0.55
0.4
0.55
Methanol 50 %
34.5
34
34
Acetic acid 5 %
60.1
63
61
Distilled water
71.2
74
71
Natural surfactant
0
27
Synthetic surfactant
20
51
3 sec
cm water

Figure 5 shows tracings obtained with this technique. The rate of change in pressure when the bubble has just been expanded reflects the speed with which a monolayer is formed (= adsorption rate). The tracing obtained when the expanded bubble is oscillating in crude natural surfactant expresses the monolayer's ability to exert high surface pressure at minimal bubble size, i.e., at end-expiration. The tracing also demonstrates moderate surface elastance, in that surface pressure is also relatively high at maximal bubble size, i.e., end-inspiration.

The surfactometer based on the pulsating bubble technique made it feasible to screen thousands of phospholipid combinations. It has not been possible so far to find a mixture of only synthetic lipids with the desirable surface properties of natural surfactant. The reason for persisting in a search for an artificial surfactant consisting of lipids only has been a desire to exclude proteins that might be antigenic. Could it be though that the proteins are necessary ingredients?

In highly purified canine surfactant, King [26] found 8% protein. In fact, further analysis revealed the presence of two proteins, one with a molecular weight of 35,000-40,000 daltons; the other even smaller, 12,000 daltons. That these apoproteins serve a useful purpose cannot be ruled out, but as yet there is no clear evidence of this. Observations by Metcalfe et al. [27] infer that if proteins are needed, their concentration can be $<0.5\%$. An extract of canine lung lavage was very surface active, although its protein content was extremely low. Strong support for the concept that proteins are not needed was offered by Bangham et al. [40], who observed that a dry, protein-free powder consisting of DPPC and PG in a molar ratio of 3:1 would spread quickly at an air-liquid

---

Figure 5 Tracings obtained with the pulsating bubble surfactometer. The abrupt pressure increase at the far left of the tracing corresponds to the expansion of a bubble, or model "alveolus," with a radius of 0.55 mm. That bubble size is maintained for 10 sec before pulsation is started, forcing the radius to oscillate from 0.55 to 0.4 mm. Liquids with known surface tension at 37°C are studied with the upper three tracings. At maximal bubble size, measured most accurately, the value obtained with the bubble surfactometer is in good agreement with the known value for surface tension. The upper three tracings are principally different from the lower two. In the latter, pressure is increased as the bubble is forced to become smaller. This reflects the presence of a monomolecular phospholipid film in the bubble surface. Natural surfactant is characterized by a fast adsorption (pressure quickly reaches a stable value in the first 10 sec) and a surface tension of zero at minimal bubble size. The synthetic surfactant is inadequate in that it has low adsorption rate and high surface tension at minimal bubble size (= end-expiration).

interface, forming a monolayer exerting high surface pressure. The PG was thought to be squeezed from the film during compression, leaving DPPC in high concentration. It was essential, though, for rapid film formation that the phospholipids be supplied at the air-liquid interface in a dehydrated form. The possibility remains that when suspended in water an apoprotein is needed for fast adsorption.

Preparations Used as of Today

Dipalmitoyl phosphatidylcholine alone was used in the early clinical trials of Robillard et al. [4], Chu et al. [5], and more recently Shannon and Bunnell [7]. Due to the limited success of these trials, Ivey et al. [41] decided to include PG. They felt that an artificial surfactant ought to contain this anionic phospholipid because its presence enhances cell fusion [42]. They gave a nebulized suspension of DPPC and dipalmitoyl phosphatidylglycerol (DPPG) (9:1) to 21 severely ill infants. The dose given to each neonate was estimated at 3 mg phospholipids per kilogram.

The preparation developed by Fujiwara et al. [43] was carefully tested before use in a clinical trial [44]. It was prepared from extracts of lyophilized bovine lung minces. The surfactant was concentrated by centrifugation. The lipids were extracted with chloroform-methanol and then acetone precipitated. To the lipids obtained in this way were added DPPC and PG (65:12). These synthetic phospholipids constituted 43% of the total. Ten milliliters of the final saline suspension, with a phospholipid concentration of approximately 60 mg/ml, were given to each infant. About 2% of the phospholipid weight was protein.

As an effective lung surfactant, Bangham et al. [40] believe that it is preferable to use a dry, protein-free powder consisting of DPPC and PG in a molar ratio of 3:1. When sprinkled on the water surface of a Wilhelmy balance, this dry phospholipid mixture adsorbed very quickly and the monolayer film was able to exert a surface pressure of about 50 $mN \cdot m^{-1}$. The PG was thought to be squeezed from the film during compression, leaving DPPC in high concentration. Following animal tests [45], this preparation was used for treating RDS in the human neonate [46].

Metcalfe et al. [27] prepared a surfactant from canine lung lavage. This had an extremely low protein content and could be sterilized by autoclaving. Tested with the pulsating bubble surfactometer and with animal experiments, it had a high adsorption rate, was able to facilitate lung aeration, and offered stability to the expanded lung [47,48]. Unfortunately, it was not possible to maintain the low protein content when the method was applied on a larger scale using calf lung lavage. The surfactant prepared from this source, used for treating infants with severe RDS, contained approximately 0.5% protein [49].

Preparations being considered as possible substitutions for pulmonary surfactant generally consist of DPPC, given a high adsorption rate by the admixture of PC with unsaturated fatty acids, or of PG. Clements [50] used another approach. He added a fatty alcohol to DPPC and found that a mixture of DPPC and hexadecanol in a ratio of 9:1 gave the required surface properties.

Some of the possible side effects of a purified animal preparation could be avoided by using surfactant originating from the mature human fetus. A recent publication [51] describes a method for isolating the surfactant from amniotic fluid, collected at cesarean sections, by nylon mesh filtration and sucrose density gradient centrifugation.

Mode of Administration

At birth, the neonate has a volume of liquid in its airways corresponding to the functional residual capacity [52], or approximately 30 ml/kg. Shortly after birth (within 30 min), and seemingly without too much difficulty, this volume is absorbed and replaced with air. From the data by Karlberg et al. [53], it can be deduced that when an infant is born vaginally in cephalic presentation, and the face has been delivered, the volume of liquid discharged through the nose and mouth due to thoracic compression can be as much as 10 ml, or one-third of the functional residual capacity that will develop. When the infant is delivered by cesarean section, or in breech presentation, this volume will not be removed, yet breathing commences, usually without difficulty.

If an effort is always made to aspirate through the nose and mouth while the chest is compressed in the vagina or is held squeezed, it would seem that depositing a volume of no more than 4 ml into the pharynx or the trachea should not jeopardize the safety of the neonate. Although the optimal time for instilling surfactant is in the immediate postnatal period, the experiences of Fujiwara and coworkers [44] make it clear that administration by instillation is possible even several hours after birth, although a larger volume will then be required (see below).

The concept that surfactant preferably should be supplied as dehydrated phospholipids [40] made it necessary to construct a special device to blow the dry powder down the airways [46]. The phospholipids are supplied in a gelatin capsule which is punctured in the device so that the powder can be blown in with an inspiration. It may be difficult to envisage how the hygroscopic lipids remain dispersed and reach the airways where they are urgently needed, i.e., the most distal cylindrical airways and the alveolar sacs. Autoradiography experiments, in animals, with labeled DPPC would allow an objective assessment of the distribution of the lipids blown down the airways as a dry powder. This technique has been used for studying dispersion of aerosolized DPPC [54].

Administering the surfactant as an aerosol spray has appeal due to its simplicity, and because the amount of water can be kept at a minimum, breathing is not disturbed. With this mode of administration, the surfactant, at least initially, would not reach the atelectatic airways, perhaps in greatest need of the surfactant. An aerosol spray of surfactant would be particularly valuable when a maintenance dose is required, preventing concentration from dropping to dangerously low levels. It is never likely to be used in the delivery room, i.e., in the initial phase just after birth.

Duration of Effect

By injecting [^{14}C]palmitic acid and [^{3}H]glucose, Tierney et al. [55] labeled the surfactant PC of the rat. They sacrificed the animals 3-43 hr after the injection and determined the biological half-life of various types of PC. They found that the half-life of the saturated variants was short, about 14 hr, but was about 20 hr for the polyunsaturated PC. Specific activity decreased at the same rate for ^{14}C in the fatty acids as for ^{3}H in the glycerol. In the last 3 years, as surfactant supplementation has become more seriously considered for prevention and treatment of neonatal RDS, there have been several reports on the turnover of tracheally instilled surfactant or components thereof [56-60]. Hallman et al. [59] found that 6 hr after instillation of phosphatidylcholine only 8% could be recovered in alveolar wash. On the other hand, there was early uptake into lamellar bodies of intact double-labeled phospholipid molecules. Also, Jacobs et al. [57] found evidence that the surfactant administered was being recycled.

The aforementioned results imply that the turnover rate for DPPC, and particularly for PG, is very high. To a large extent that turnover may be between and within the three compartments consisting of the monolayer at the air-liquid interface, the subphase, and the alveolar cells type II. Surfactant instilled into the airways is perhaps partly catabolized very rapidly, but the phospholipid molecules remaining intact, as well as the breakdown products from those catabolized, initially would be within the pool of the three compartments mentioned and should reduce the risk of a surfactant deficiency developing. The turnover rate may be high, but intact phospholipid molecules could be incorporated into the bilayers of lamellar bodies and breakdown products could serve as precursors. Even though the half-life of surfactant phospholipids is short, the recycling would help to prolong the effect of a single dose administered.

Publications by Ikegami et al. [61,62] suggest another factor limiting the value of surfactant supplementation. Natural surfactant, and even more so an artificial preparation consisting of a 9:1 mixture of DPPC and PG, was inactivated by inhibitors present in the airways. A protein with a molecular weight of approximately 110,000 daltons has been isolated from the alveolar wash and is thought to be the inhibitor [63]. Possibly this protein in itself is surface active and competes with pulmonary surfactant for the air-liquid interfaces of the alveoli. Such being the case, it would seem to be another good reason for administering the surfactant in a high dose prior to the first breath. The chances would then be in favor of the phospholipid molecules being the first to reach the air-liquid interface to form a monomolecular layer there.

The direct effect of the surfactant administered into the airways most certainly will be of limited duration and its action might be inhibited, particularly if the instillation is not immediately after birth. Nonetheless, a single dose may have a beneficial effect by preventing the start of a vicious circle of events. With a rapid lung expansion giving even and stable aeration, neither hypoxia nor acidosis may ever develop. Hyaline membranes may be forestalled as well as bronchopulmonary dysplasia. Metabolism in lung tissue may never be disturbed and synthesis, as well as release of endogenous surfactant, stimulated by lung aeration, may be able to take over as the exogenous supply becomes inadequate. In Fujiwara et al.'s series [44], a single dose was all that was needed to reverse a life-threatening RDS, and yet his treatment was not given at the optimal time—prior to the first breath.

Timing as well as the type of surfactant preparation administered could have a decisive effect on the rate of catabolism. Of special interest are the experiments by Glatz et al. [60] on newborn lambs, since they suggest that the half-life may be quite low when surfactant supplemented at birth, prior to the first breath, is retained in the lungs for a considerable time. Tritium-labeled natural surfactant was instilled into the trachea and the lamb, delivered at term by cesarean section, was stimulated to breathe. Within 1 hr, half of the labeled phosphatidylcholine could still be recovered from alveolar lavage fluid, whereas the other half was in lung tissue where it had an affinity for lamellar bodies. From the latter, the labeled phospholipid may have been released slowly into the alveolar space, explaining why it could be detected there even after 11 days. It would be of interest to ascertain the turnover rate also in the preterm lamb, using the experimental design by Glatz et al. [60].

E. Clinical Experiences

A paper by Fujiwara et al. [44], published in the *Lancet* in January 1980, was a breakthrough in the principle of treating a respiratory ailment by supplementing the lungs' surfactant stores. Ten preterm infants severely ill with RDS were treated on the average 12 hr after birth with Fujiwara's surfactant, a cow lung extract reinforced with DPPC and PG. Ten milliliters of the preparation was injected into the tracheal tube. During instillation, the infant was held in different positions to facilitate even distribution of the surfactant. The treatment took 20 sec and was followed by "bagging" with 100% oxygen. The result was immediate and unmistakable. Within 3 hr, arterial PO_2 increased from 45 ± 7 to 212 ± 46 mmHg; there was a decrease in pCO_2 and an increase in pH. As a result of the increase in arterial PO_2, it was possible to reduce the oxygen concentration in the gas mixture supplied, and peak respirator pressure could be lowered.

There were clinical signs of improvement. Peripheral circulation increased. Grunting, when present, ceased quickly. The chest radiogram improved faster than usual. Bowel sounds returned, as did diuresis. In Fujiwara's series, including more than 40 infants in October 1982, there was no mortality directly attributable to RDS or to the surfactant treatment.

A year after Fujiwara's report [44] came one from Cambridge, England, by Morley et al. [46], also published in the *Lancet.* During the first 6 hr following treatment with a dry surfactant, DPPC and PG in a ratio of 7:3 w/w, the oxygen requirement was not reduced, but otherwise this study also supported the principle of surfactant supplementation. There were no deaths in the group of 22 infants treated with a single dose of dry artificial surfactant, but eight of the 33 controls succumbed.

As Morley and his colleagues in Cambridge were assessing the value of Bangham's artificial surfactant for preventing and treating RDS, it was also being evaluated by Wilkinson et al. [64] in neighboring Oxford. Morley's enthusiasm was not shared by Wilkinson, who was unable to document a favorable effect from the treatment.

Ivey and co-workers [41] administered a nebulized suspension of DPPC and DPPG (9:1), or of saline alone. Their data do not offer convincing proof that the phospholipid treatment resulted in a reduced difference between alveolar and arterial oxygen tension ($A - aDO_2$). The final outcome was not encouraging, in that 21 infants were treated and nine died.

Stimulated by the success of Fujiwara et al. [44], a similar clinical trial was initiated by Smyth et al. [49] at the Hospital for Sick Children in Toronto, Canada. A lipid extract from calf lung wash, prepared according to Metcalfe et al. [27], was used to treat six infants with severe RDS. A total dose of 200 mg phospholipids was given in 8 ml, using a technique otherwise identical to that of Fujiwara [44]. With transcutaneous monitoring of PO_2 and PCO_2, the effect of the treatment was apparent immediately. The improved oxygenation was reflected in the increased ratio of arterial to alveolar oxygen tension (a/APO_2). That ratio rose dramatically in four of the treated infants, moderately in one, and not at all in another. It should be noted, however, that the infant receiving no benefit was not treated as were the others. Due to technical difficulties with the tracheal instillation of the surfactant, it was not given as a single 8-ml dose, but was divided into two parts; a portion of each was lost. There was no mortality in the Toronto trial.

A recent publication by Hallman et al. [51] offers further support to the principle of surfactant supplementation as treatment for severe RDS. Five infants with very low birth weights (range 850-1240 g) were treated with human surfactant obtained from amniotic fluid. A dose of 60 mg/kg was given as a single bolus in 3.5 ml of 0.6% saline. When compared with a similar group of infants receiving no surfactant supplementation, the treatment resulted in definite improvement. PaO_2 increased dramatically, permitting a lowering of FI_{O_2}, and as $PaCO_2$ dropped, pH increased. This lasted from 3 to 15 hr, and there were no adverse consequences to the treatment.

Side Effects

Only one side effect, a patent ductus arteriosus (PDA) quite likely is attributable to the treatment with surfactant. In the experiences of Morley et al. [46] and Smyth et al. [49], PDA was not a great problem, but in the series of Fujiwara et al. [44], it was noted in no fewer than nine of the 10 cases, and four infants required surgical closure of the ductus. Although indomethacin was given concurrently with the surfactant, in the series of Hallman et al. [51], at least three of the five infants treated had PDA and two were operated on. Perhaps this reflects the efficacy of the surfactant preparation administered by Fujiwara et al. [44] as well as that used by Hallman et al. [51]. This is not to say that the ductus opened as a result of the treatment. It was probably already open when therapy was instituted, but patency became apparent with the increase in left-to-right flow as a consequence of the decrease in pulmonary resistance. Also, alleviation of the symptoms of RDS may have made it easier to recognize a PDA. One would hope that the increase in arterial oxygen tension on completion of a successful treatment would act as a stimulus to spontaneous closure of the ductus arteriosus, as suggested by Born et al. [65] and Assali et al. [66].

A potential hazard with surfactant instillation into the airways is the risk of introducing pathogenic microbes, viruses in particular. Extracting the pulmonary surfactant with lipid solvents, or using the isolation technique of Hallman et al. [51], will significantly reduce the chance of infection, and adequate sterilization by autoclaving eliminates the danger.

The immune response of very preterm infants is low. Hence, the possibility of immunization with a single surfactant instillation should be minimal, but if repeated treatments are required, the risk may become real. One would hope that an artificial surfactant, an entirely synthetic preparation containing no protein, will become available. In the meantime, the protein content of the natural product should be reduced as much as is feasible.

F. Prevention of RDS Immediately After Birth

The clinical experiences with surfactant supplementation confirm the conclusions from animal experiments. Supplying a neonate suffering from severe RDS with the surfactant so desperately needed results in immediate improvement. Theoretically, it would be preferable though to administer surfactant into the upper airway prior to the first breath, i.e., before creation of air-liquid interfaces where potentially dangerous surface forces are operating. The surfactant so administered facilitates aeration, since it is concentrated in the hemispherical surfaces of the airways, exerting its effect. The surfactant automatically would be evenly distributed to all parts of the lungs, giving stability to terminal airways and alveolar sacs. Indeed, animal experiments (Fig. 3) have demonstrated that the effect is superior and longer lasting when the treatment is given at birth rather than at a later time when respiratory distress is already established. Factors supporting very early surfactant administration are listed in Table 2.

Acceptance of the concept that surfactant preferably should be instilled into the pharynx or trachea prior to the first breath gives the obstetrician the prime responsibility for prevention of RDS. He organizes the care and supervision of the pregnancy so that preterm labor can be avoided. Unfortunately, his efforts will not always be successful, and in some instances he comes to the conclusion that preterm delivery carries less risk than continued intrauterine existence. Under those circumstances or when for other reasons, such as maternal diabetes, there is an increased risk of RDS, it is up to the obstetrician, or possibly the neonatologist, to ensure that the neonate receives the surfactant it so desperately is going to need. Administration would have to be in the delivery room, or perhaps in an adjacent room for infant resuscitation. If the effect of the initial preventative administration of surfactant is successful, but not of a duration sufficient to last until endogenous synthesis is completely ready to take over, then it would be the neonatologist's responsibility to supplement the surfactant before a deficiency develops. This second supplementation, and any successive doses required for prevention of a surfactant deficiency, would be instituted while the airways are still open; hence, the surfactant could preferably be delivered as an intermittent aerosol spray.

To test the efficacy of surfactant supplementation in the immediate postnatal period, and to determine if and when a second dose is necessary, we have now started a randomized clinical trial at the University of Toronto. Pregnant women at risk of delivering prematurely are asked if they would be willing to participate in the trial. If they agree, a consent form is signed, and there is a 50% chance that their infant will receive surfactant. An autoclaved, 3% suspension of lipids extracted from calf lung wash is instilled into the tracheal tube, 3 ml for infants with a gestational age of < 27 weeks, 4 ml for infants 27–29 weeks. To ensure that the surfactant is administered prior to the first breath, the thorax is manually compressed until a tracheal tube has been inserted and the surfactant injected into the tube.

The controls are treated similarly. They are given no placebo, such as an equal amount of saline solution, which would result in an increment in the volume of pulmonary fluid and a dilution of its surfactant. This could possibly have a negative effect on the controls; however, it would make it ethically unacceptable and more difficult to interpret the outcome.

The effect is evaulated by chest radiograms, blood gases, compliance assessment, and the need for respiratory support. The trial, which started in March 1983 and was completed in June 1984, is currently being analyzed.

Table 2 Reasons for Surfactant Administration *Prior to the First Breath* Rather Than After Manifestation of RDS

	Ref. No.
Aeration would be facilitated and become more even.	8–14
Period of neonatal asphyxia with acidosis may be avoided.	13,19,20
Respiratory support, the main cause of bronchopulmonary dysplasia, can be kept to a minimum.	14,16
When surfactant is supplied as a *suspension*, deposition at an air-liquid interface, where the action is exerted, would be preferable to forcing it through air-filled bronchioli.	–
Good lung expansion promotes normal postnatal circulatory transitions. Pulmonary resistance diminishes, changing direction of flow through the ductus arteriosus. With the aeration obtained, blood flowing through the ductus from left to right would have high oxygen tension, promoting closure of the ductus.	65,66
A surfactant inhibitor may act by occupying the air-liquid interface in competition with pulmonary surfactant. Given in high dose prior to the first breath, surfactant would have a better chance of occupying the air-liquid interface, thereby inactivating the inhibitor.	61–63
Animal experiments support the concept that surfactant has a better and more prolonged effect when administered immediately after birth.	19,20

III. Summary and Conclusion

Surfactant supplementation by tracheal instillation is gradually becoming an accepted principle for treating RDS, and there are intense efforts being made in several laboratories to produce an artificial surfactant. The goal is to find a highly active, sterile preparation with low antigenicity. Presumably, such a product, consisting of synthetic ingredients only, will eventually become available. Meanwhile, surfactant prepared from human amniotic fluid [51] or extracted from bovine lungs [27,44] is an acceptable substitute. In theory, and in accordance with animal experiments, the optimal time for surfactant supplementation is immediately after birth (Table 2). Hence, the treatment is instituted as a preventative measure in the delivery room. The surfactant, suspected to be missing because of a low amniotic fluid surfactant measurement, or because delivery is at 29 weeks or earlier, is then deposited into the pharynx or trachea prior to the first breath. This should give rise to an upgraded pulmonary maturity, resulting in facilitated aeration and improved lung stability. Hypoxia and acidosis would then be avoided and surfactant synthesis and release given optimal conditions. Only clinical trials will show whether or not these expectations can be fulfilled.

References

1. Liggins, G. C., and R. N. Howie, A controlled trial of antepartum glucocorticoid treatment for prevention of the respiratory distress syndrome in premature infants, *Pediatrics,* **50**:515 (1972).
2. Howie, R. N., and G. C. Liggins, Prevention of respiratory distress syndrome in premature infants by antepartum glucocorticoid treatment. In *Respiratory Distress Syndrome.* Edited by C. A. Villee, D. B. Villee, and J. Zuckerman. New York, Academic Press, 1973, p. 369.
3. Avery, M. E., and J. Mead, Surface properties in relation to atelectasis and hyaline membrane disease, *Am. J. Dis. Child.,* **97**:517 (1959).
4. Robillard, E., Y. Alarie, P. Dagenais-Perusse, E. Baril, and A. Guilbeault, Microaerosol administration of synthetic β-γ-dipalmitoyl-L-αlecithin in the respiratory distress syndrome: A preliminary report, *Can. Med. Assoc. J.,* **90**:55 (1964).
5. Chu, J., J. A. Clements, E. K. Cotton, M. H. Klaus, A. Y. Sweet, and W. H. Tooley, Neonatal pulmonary ischemia. I. Clinical and physiological studies, *Pediatrics,* **40**:709 (1967).
6. Shannon, D. C., H. Kazemi, E. W. Merrill, K. A. Smith, and P. S. L. Wong, Restoration of volume-pressure curves with a lecithin fog, *J. Appl. Physiol.,* **28**:470 (1969).
7. Shannon, D. C., and J. B. Bunnell, Dipalmitoyl lecithin aerosol in RDS, *Pediatr. Res.,* **10**:467 (1976).
8. Enhorning, G., and B. Robertson, Lung expansion in the premature rabbit fetus after tracheal deposition of surfactant, *Pediatrics,* **50**:58 (1972).
9. Enhorning, G., G. Grossmann, and B. Robertson, Tracheal deposition of surfactant before the first breath, *Am. Rev. Respir. Dis.,* **107**:921 (1973).
10. Enhorning, G., G. Grossmann, and B. Robertson, Pharyngeal deposition of surfactant in the premature rabbit fetus, *Biol. Neonate,* **22**:126 (1973).
11. Robertson, B. and G. Enhorning, The alveolar lining of the premature newborn rabbit after pharyngeal deposition of surfactant, *Lab. Invest.,* **31**:54 (1974).

12. Enhorning, G., B. Robertson, E. Milne, and R. Wagner, Radiological evaluation of the premature rabbit neonate after pharyngeal deposition of surfactant, *Am. J. Obstet. Gynecol.,* **121**:475 (1975).
13. Enhorning. G., D. Hill, G. Sherwood, E. Cutz, B. Robertson, and C. Bryan, Improved ventilation of prematurely-delivered primates following tracheal deposition of surfactant, *Am. J. Obstet. Gynecol.,* **132**:529 (1978).
14. Cutz, E., G. Enhorning, B. Robertson, W. G. Sherwood, and D. E. Hill, Hyaline membrane disease: Effect of surfactant prophylaxis on lung morphology in premature primates, *Am. J. Pathol.,* **92**:581 (1978).
15. Rüfer, R., Der Einfluss oberflächenaktiver Substanzen auf Entfaltung und Retraktion isolierter Lungen, *Pflügers Arch.,* **298**:170 (1967).
16. Nilsson, R., G. Grossmann, and B. Robertson, Pathogenesis of neonatal lung lesions induced by artificial ventilation; evidence against the role of barotrauma. *Respiration,* **40**:218 (1980).
17. Robertson, B., Surfactant substitution: Experimental models and clinical applications, *Lung,* **158**:57 (1980).
18. Notter, R. H. and D. L. Shapiro, Lung surfactant in an era of replacement, *Pediatrics,* **68**:781 (1981).
19. Adams, F. H., B. Towers, A. B. Osher, M. Ikegami, T. Fujiwara, and M. Nozaki, Effects of tracheal instillation of natural surfactant in premature lambs: Clinical and autopsy findings, *Pediatr. Res.,* **12**:841 (1978).
20. Jobe, A., M. Ikegami, T. Glatz, Y. Yoshida, E. Diakomanolis, and J. Padbury, Duration and characteristics of treatment of premature lambs with natural surfactant, *J. Clin. Invest.,* **67**:370 (1981).
21. Ikegami, M., T. Hesterberg, M. Nozaki, and F. H. Adams, Restoration of lung pressure-volume characteristics with surfactant: Comparison of nebulization versus instillation and natural versus synthetic surfactant, *Pediatr. Res.,* **11**:178 (1977).
22. Ikegami, M., A. Jobe, H. Jakobs, and S. J. Jones, Sequential treatments of premature lambs with an artificial surfactant and natural surfactant, *J. Clin. Invest.,* **68**:491 (1981).
23. Watkins, J. C., The surface properties of pure phospholipids in relation to those of lung extracts, *Biochim. Biophys. Acta,* **152**:293 (1968).
24. Notter, R. H., and P. H. Morrow, Pulmonary surfactant: A surface chemistry viewpoint, *Ann. Biomed. Eng.,* **3**:119 (1975).
25. King, R. J., and J. A. Clements, The isolation and characterization of surface active materials from dog lung. III. Thermal analysis, *Am. J. Physiol.,* **223**:727 (1972).
26. King, R. J., The surfactant system of the lung, *Fed. Proc.,* **33**:2238 (1974).
27. Metcalfe, I. L., G. Enhorning, and F. Possmayer, Pulmonary surfactant-associated proteins: Their role in the expression of surface activity, *J. Appl. Physiol.,* **49**:34 (1980).

28. Clements, J. A., J. Nellenbogen, and H. J. Trahan, Pulmonary surfactant and evolution of the lungs, *Science*, **169**:603 (1970).
29. Hallman, M. and L. Gluck, The biosynthesis of phosphatidylglycerol in the lung of the developing rabbit, *Ref. Proc.*, **34**:274 (1975).
30. Bangham, A. D., Membrane models with phospholipids. *Prog. Biophys. Mol. Biol.*, **18**:29 (1968).
31. Chapman, D., Phase transitions and fluidity characteristics of lipids and cell membranes. *Q. Rev. Biophys.*, 8:185 (1975).
32. Phillips, M. C., The physical state of phospholipids and cholesterol in monolayers, bilayers, and membranes. *Prog. Surf. Membrane Sci.*, **5**:139 (1972).
33. Phillips, M. C. and H. Hauser, Spreading of solid glycerides and phospholipids at the air-water interface, *J. Colloid. Interface Sci.*, **49**:31 (1974).
34. Notter, R. H., S. A. Tabak, and R. D. Mavis, Surface properties of binary mixtures of some pulmonary surfactant components, *J. Lipid Res.*, **21**:10 (1980).
35. Notter, R. H., S. Holcomb, and R. D. Mavis, Dynamic surface properties of phosphatidylglycerol-dipalmitoyl phosphatidylcholine mixed films, *Chem. Phys. Lipids*, **27**:305 (1980).
36. Hawco, M. W., P. J. Davis, and K. M. W. Keough, Lipid fluidity in lung surfactant: Monolayers of saturated and unsaturated lecithins, *J. Appl. Physiol.*, **51**:509 (1981).
37. Obladen, M., F. Brendlein, and B. Krempien, Surfactant substitution. *Eur. J. Pediatr.*, **131**:219 (1979).
38. Enhorning, G., A pulsating bubble technique for evaluating pulmonary surfactant, *J. Appl. Physiol.*, **43**:198 (1977).
39. Adams, F. H. and G. Enhorning, Surface properties of lung extracts. I. A dynamic alveolar model, *Acta Physiol. Scand.*, **68**:23 (1966).
40. Bangham, A. D., C. J. Morley, and M. C. Phillips, The physical properties of an effective lung surfactant, *Biochim. Biophys. Acta*, **573**:552 (1979).
41. Ivey, H. H., J. Kattwinkel, and S. Roth, Nebulization of sonicated phospholipids for treatment of respiratory distress syndrome of infancy. In *Liposomes and Immunology*. Edited by B. H. Tom and H. R. Six. New York, Elsevier-North Holland, 1980, p. 301.
42. Papahadjopoulos, D., G. Poste, and B. E. Schaeffer, Fusion of mammalian cells by unilamellar lipid vesicles: Influence of lipid surface charge, fludity and cholesterol, *Biochim. Biophys. Acta*, **323**:23 (1973).
43. Fujiwara, T., Y. Tanaka, and T. Takei, Surface properties of artificial surfactant in comparison with natural and synthetic surfactant lipids, *I.R.C.S. Med. Sci.*, 7:311 (1979).
44. Fujiwara, T., S. Chida, Y. Watabe, H. Maeta, T. Morita, and T. Abe, Artificial surfactant therapy in hyaline-membrane disease, *Lancet*, **i**:55 (1980).

45. Morley, C., B. Robertson, B. Lachmann, R. Nilsson, A. Bangham, G. Grossmann, and N. Miller, Artificial and natural surfactant. *Arch. Dis. Child.,* **55**:758 (1980).
46. Morley, C. J., N. Miller, A. D. Bangham, and J. A. Davis, Dry artificial lung surfactant and its effect on very premature babies, *Lancet,* **i**:64 (1981).
47. Metcalfe, I. L., R. Pototschnik, R. Burgoyne, and G. Enhorning, Lung expansion and survival in rabbit neonates treated with surfactant extract, *J. Appl. Physiol.,* **53**:838 (1982).
48. Metcalfe, I. L., R. Burgoyne, and G. Enhorning, Surfactant supplementation in the preterm rabbit: Effects of applied volume on compliance and survival. *Pediatr. Res.,* **16**:834 (1982).
49. Smyth, J. A., I. L. Metcalfe, P. Duffty, F. Possmayer, M. H. Bryan, and G. Enhorning, Hyaline membrane disease treated with bovine surfactant. *Pediatrics,* **71**:913 (1983).
50. Clements, J. A., Lung surfactant compositions. U.S. Patent #4,312,860 (1982).
51. Hallman, M., T. A. Merritt, H. Schneider, B. L. Epstein, F. Mannino, D. K. Edwards, and L. Gluck, Isolation of human surfactant from amniotic fluid and a pilot study of its efficacy in respiratory distress syndrome, *Pediatrics,* **71**:473 (1983).
52. Nelson, N. M., Neonatal pulmonary function, *Pediatr. Clin. North Am., 1. The Newborn,* **13**:769 (1966).
53. Karlberg, P., R. B. Cherry, F. E. Escardo, and G. Koch, Respiratory studies in newborn infants. II. Pulmonary ventilation and mechanics of breathing in the first few minutes of life, including the onset of respiration, *Acta Paediatr.,* **51**:121 (1962).
54. Geiger, K., M. L. Gallagher, and J. Hedley-Whyte, Cellular distribution and clearance of aerosolized dipalmitoyl lecithin. *J. Appl. Physiol.,* **39**:759 (1975).
55. Tierney, D. F., J. A. Clements, and H. J. Trahan, Rates of replacement of lecithins and alveolar instability in rat lungs, *J. Appl. Physiol.,* **213**:671 (1967).
56. Young, S. L., S. A. Kremers, J. S. Apple, J. D. Crapo, and G. W. Brumloy, Rat lung surfactant kinetics: Biochemical and morphometric correlation, *J. Appl. Physiol.,* **51**:248 (1981).
57. Jacobs, J., A. Jobe, M. Ikegami, and S. Jones, Surfactant phosphatidylcholine source, fluxes, and turnover times in 3-day-old, 10-day-old, and adult rabbits, *J. Biol. Chem.,* **257**:1805 (1982).
58. Oyarzun, M. J., J. A. Clements, and A. Baritussio, Ventilation enhances pulmonary alveolar clearance of radioactive dipalmitoyl phosphatidylcholine in liposomes, *Am. Rev. Respir. Dis.,* **121**:709 (1980).

59. Hallman, M., B. L. Epstein, and L. Gluck, Analysis of labeling and clearance of lung surfactant phospholipids in rabbit, *J. Clin. Invest.,* **68**:742 (1981).
60. Glatz, T., A. Jobe, and M. Ikegami, Metabolism of exogenously administered natural surfactant in the newborn lamb, *Pediatr. Res.,* **16**:711 (1982).
61. Ikegami, M., A. Jobe, H. Jacobs, and S. J. Jones, Sequential treatments of premature lambs with an artificial surfactant and natural surfactant. *J. Clin. Invest.,* **68**:491 (1981).
62. Ikegami, M., A. Jobe, and T. Glatz, Surface activity following natural surfactant treatment in premature lambs, *J. Appl. Physiol.,* **51**:306 (1981).
63. Ikegami, M., and A. Jobe, Specific inhibitor of surfactant function and its effect on different surfactants. Paper read at NIH-sponsored meeting at Mackinac Island, October 6-8, 1982.
64. Wilkinson, A., Controlled clinical trials of dry surfactant in preterm infants. Paper read at NIH-sponsored meeting at Mackinac Island, October 6-8, 1982.
65. Born, G. V. R., G. S. Dawes, J. C. Mott, and B. R. Rennick, The constriction of the ductus arteriosus caused by oxygen and by asphyxia in newborn lambs, *J. Physiol., (Lond.),* **132**:304 (1956).
66. Assali, N. S., J. A. Morris, R. W. Smith, and W. A. Manson, Studies on the ductus arteriosus, *Circ. Res.,* **13**:478 (1963).

14

Neonatal Resuscitation

WILLIAM P. KANTO, JR., and ALEX. F. ROBERTSON, III

Medical College of Georgia
Augusta, Georgia

I. Introduction

During the past decade there has been intense interest in regionalization of perinatal care in the United States. The emphasis today is centered on our ability to recognize high-risk perinates and to transfer them to appropriate specialized facilities. These perinatal regional programs are associated with improved outcomes of pregnancies [1]. However, this emphasis on transfer tends to overlook an essential feature of regionalization, which is improvement in the quality of emergency care at the referring hospital. One must remember that it is not unusual for neonates to require resuscitation in the delivery room even though the population served is not necessarily high risk. In our survey of a general level II facility we were surprised to find that 7.6% of all newborns had Apgar scores below 7 at 1 min and 1.4% had a similar score at 5 min after birth [2]. Since scores below 7 require active resuscitation, these infants needed treatment in the delivery room. In addition, our experience suggests that stabilization of the high-risk neonate before transfer is associated with decreased morbidity and mortality, as shown by a decreased incidence of intraventricular hemorrhage [3] in appropriately managed preterm infants. Since the first efforts at stabilization begin in the delivery room, it is essential that an organized approach to resuscitation of the neonate be a part of every hospital's operating protocol. The development of an adequate resuscitation protocol is a responsibility that the tertiary center should share with the referring hospital by functioning as an educational resource within the referral area.

II. Organization of Resuscitation

A. Personnel

The first necessity is that the person(s) who will handle an emergency in the delivery room be identified prior to the occurrence of an emergency. The physician who has delivered the baby must attend the mother and precious time is lost if a harried delivery room nurse has to determine who is on call for the delivery room after an emergency has occurred. There must be a universally recognized and accepted method to communicate immediately with the responsible person. A "beeper" system with the beeper being transferred to the individual on call is one such scheme. Regardless of the method used, the same identification and communication system must be available 24 hr a day, 7 days a week.

Another prerequisite is training personnel in resuscitation methods. In many hospitals employees are required to have periodic training and recertification in cardiopulmonary resuscitation of the adult but there are no organized protocols and/or training for resuscitation of the neonate. Every hospital providing obstetrical care must ensure that personnel are available who are skilled in resuscitation of the neonate. To fail to do so is to accept preventable neonatal morbidity and mortality. There must be an accepted resuscitation protocol for the delivery room which is zealously taught to all delivery room personnel and there must be periodic training programs and practical exams. It is also important that the performance of the physician(s) responsible for resuscitation is periodically reviewed by the hospital staff to assure optimal performance. An obvious requirement for successful resuscitation practices is a medical director with the experience and knowledge to provide direction, review, and continuing education. This person must be actively supported by the obstetrical and pediatric staffs and have the authority to identify poor practices or unskilled individuals and initiate necessary changes.

B. Equipment

It is essential that the proper equipment be in the delivery room and in working order. Table 1 lists the necessary equipment and supplies. They are neither

Table 1 Resuscitation Equipment and Supplies

Equipment
Anesthesia bag
Newborn and premature masks
Plastic oropharyngeal airway
Endotracheal tubes:
Portex tubes, sizes 2.0, 2.5, 3.0, 3.5
DeLee trap and suction catheters, sizes 5, 8, 10, 12
Bulb syringe
Laryngoscope with premature and infant blades
Suction apparatus
Umbilical vessel catheters, Nos. 3 and 5 Fr
Intravenous infusion equipment
Drugs and IV Fluids
A source of 100% oxygen and capability for warming and humidifying it
Dextrose 10%
Sodium bicarbonate, 4.2%
Epinephrine 1:1000 (must be diluted to 1:10,000)
Volume expander (salt-poor albumin, plasma, O-negative whole blood)
Atropine
Calcium
Naloxone (Narcan)

extremely expensive nor particularly intricate. Despite the easy availability of these items, we were distressed to discover during a survey of community hospital delivery services that about 30% of the hospitals in one region of the state of Georgia did not have these basic items for resuscitation, and often the equipment was present but not in working order. One person should be assigned responsibility for checking the equipment daily and replenishing supplies after each use. We believe the resuscitation board described by Clark et al. [4] is a useful method of assuring easy access to the appropriate equipment and supplies, and this method or a modification of it should be used in delivery rooms and nurseries.

III. Performance of Resuscitation

A. Introduction

The first task is to determine which infants require resuscitation. Table 2 lists factors, frequently known before delivery, that increase the risk of asphyxia. Therefore, all such deliveries should be attended by a person responsible specifically for the infant's evaluation and stabilization.

Table 2 Risk Factors for Asphyxia

Maternal factors
Chronic disease, e.g., hypertensive, renal, or hematological disease
Diabetes
Preeclampsia
Rh sensitization
Drug addiction
Fever or infection
Hypotension
Fetal factors
Small for gestational age
Congenital malformations
Low maternal estriol excretion
Positive stress test
Abnormal fetal heart rate pattern or low fetal scalp blood pH
Meconium staining of amniotic fluid
Obstetrical factors
Abnormal presentations
Cesarean section
Excessive maternal sedation
Hemorrhage
Multiple gestations
Preterm delivery
Prolapsed cord
Prolonged or precipitous labor

Table 3 The Apgar Score

	Score		
Sign	0	1	2
Appearance (color)	Blue Pale	Body pink Extremities blue	Completely pink
Pulse	Absent	< 100 beats/min	>100 beats/min
Grimace (reflex irritability, response to catheter in nose)	No response	Grimace	Cough or sneeze
Activity (muscle tone)	Flaccid	Some flexion of extremities	Well flexed extremities
Respiration (respiratory effort)	None	Slow, irregular	Good; strong cry

In 1953, Dr. Virginia Apgar developed the Apgar scoring system (Table 3) in order to standardize the evaluation of the newborn infant in the delivery room [5]. The object of this standardization was to have a uniform system for predicting survival, comparing resuscitative techniques, and evaluating perinatal stress. Since the use of this system has become widespread, it has also been used to determine the infant's need for resuscitation. The score should be given at 1 min after birth of the head and feet of the infant,and, as such, is an indication of how the neonate tolerated the birth process. Further, it provides an indication of the need for resuscitation. Obviously, the birth of a depressed infant demands immediate action and does not require waiting until after a 1 min score is given. The Apgar score should be repeated at 5 min after birth. The 5-min score begins to reflect the infant's ability to survive or adapt to extrauterine life, and if resuscitation has been required, it reflects the appropriateness of the therapy. The Apgar score should continue to be given every 5 min until the score reaches 7. Although the 5-min Apgar score is strongly associated with long-term neurological dysfunction, it is not very specific. Many infants who have low Apgar scores at 5 min are normal on follow-up. The 10 and, if necessary, 20-min Apgar score, if low, appear to have better prognostic capability [6]. We urge all hospitals to change their scoring protocol to allow for extended Apgar scoring. There must also be a system of accurately notifying the attendants when the Apgar score should be assigned. A clock alone is not sufficient, since it is difficult to observe the time when one is absorbed in providing care for a depressed newborn. The delivery room should have a system which can be triggered at birth and will emit an aural signal at 1- and 5-min intervals until silenced.

Before progressing to the treatment of the infant in the delivery room, it is appropriate to reflect on an admonition that Apgar expressed in 1966 when she wrote, "Experience has demonstrated that the person delivering the infant should not be the one to assign the score" [7]. Frankly, the person who delivers the infant is usually involved in the care of the mother and is frequently too busy to devote full time to the care of the infants. Also, they are usually emotionally involved to the point of wanting the infant to have a high score and they may not be as objective as the situation demands. These are sufficient reasons to have one person available in the delivery room whose prime responsibility is the care of the newborn. Since it is impractical to have two physicians attend all deliveries, a nurse may be entrusted with this responsibility and should have sufficient training to make the first assessment of the newborn, including the Apgar scoring, and to commence necessary treatment without having to wait for a physician's order.

A low Apgar score most commonly reflects fetal asphyxia. Since the method of resuscitation depends upon the degree of asphyxia, we need to understand the physiology and biochemistry of asphyxia. Asphyxia represents a failure to provide the cell with oxygen and to remove carbon dioxide. Both ventilation and circulation are necessary to prevent asphyxia and the failure of both may be present in neonatal asphyxia. Animal studies [8] show that approximately 30 sec after the onset of asphyxia, the animal responds with rhythmic respirations lasting for about three minutes (Fig. 1). The heart rate increases initially, but then begins to decline to the range of approximately 100 beats/min. Blood pressure also begins to rise from approximately 45 to 60 mmHg at about 4 min of age. Primary apnea is the cessation of breathing that occurs at 3.0–3.5 min of age and lasts for a period of 1.0–1.5 min. Primary apnea is characterized by the ability of the animal to initiate respirations in response to tactile stimuli. During the first 5 min, extending through the period of primary apnea, the animal progressively loses muscle tone, and eventually will lie limp and flaccid. The color may at first be pink but will become cyanotic and then progressively mottled and pale, i.e., the characteristic appearance of asphyxia pallida. The pale color develops as the result of the progressive increase in acidosis and the failure of the circulatory system. At the end of 5 min, the animal may begin to make nonrhythmic gasping breaths which may last for 3.0–3.5 min. The heart rate will remain below 100 (often in the range of 40–60) and the blood pressure begins a steady decline. At approximately 8.0–8.5 min, the animal ceases to gasp and enters the stage defined as secondary or terminal apnea. The animal must be ventilated and have his circulatory system supported in order to emerge from this state. On physical exam, the heart rate will be in the range of 40–60 and

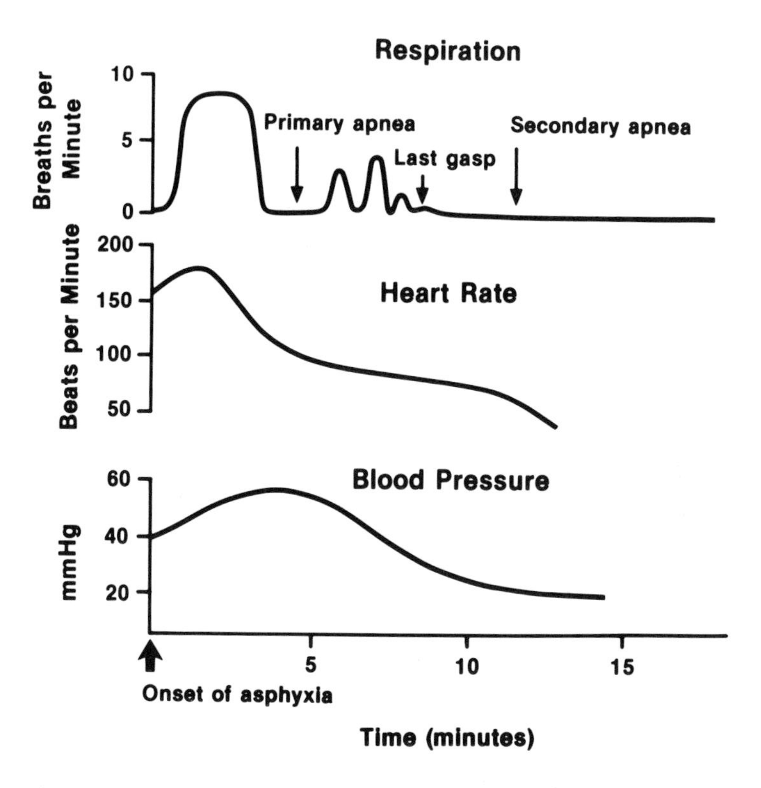

Figure 1 Physiological parameters during asphyxia.

the blood pressure will be markedly depressed below normal values. The animal will be pale, flaccid, and will not respond to noxious stimuli. It is likely that brain damage begins with the onset of secondary apnea and becomes progressively more severe as more time is spent in secondary apnea.

It is important to emphasize the major role of the cardiovascular system in asphyxia. Although hypoxia, secondary to pure hypoxemia, is a major factor in brain damage, there is increasing awareness of the impact of ischemia secondary to the impairment of blood flow. In asphyxia the brain suffers both from hypoxia and ischemia and this realization is expressed in the term hypoxic-ischemic encephalopathy. As an infant becomes progressively asphyxiated, he attempts to compensate for the drop in oxygenation by redistributing blood flow to "more critical organs", i.e., organs with a higher metabolic rate and, hence, a greater demand for oxygen. In this neonate, the critical organs which receive a greater percentage of cardiac output are the brain, heart, and adrenal glands. As asphyxia progresses, the heart becomes more hypoxic and the rate slows. Heart rate is the major determinant of cardiac output in the newborn and bradycardia reduces cardiac output, resulting in ischemia for all organs, including those which are preferentially perfused. As the hypoxic-ischemic insult progresses, there is increasing production of lactate and development of a metabolic acidosis along with the already severe respiratory acidosis.

Although the preceding description is based on asphyxia beginning at birth, in the clinical setting encountered in the delivery room the initial asphyctic episode may have started prior to delivery and have been intermittent. Therefore, the human infant may be born at any point in the asphyxial continuum. In general, the Apgar score will be 7–10 when no significant asphyxia has occurred, 4–6 during primary apnea, and 0–3 during secondary apnea. The time spent in secondary apnea can be estimated by the length of ventilation time before the reestablishment of respirations. For every minute spent in secondary apnea it will require 2 min of artificial ventilation to restore gasping efforts and 4 min of artificial ventilation to establish rhythmic breathing. The sequence of physiological changes during asphyxia is reversed during adequate resuscitation. Thus, the heart rate which declines steadily after the first few minutes of asphyxia is the first physiological parameter to improve during resuscitation. For this reason the heart rate is the best clinical indication of the progress of resuscitation. The return of muscle tone is also clinically significant. If the infant is sufficiently asphyxiated to cause changes in muscle tone, these changes will be the last to reverse and return to normal. In fact, since these changes are a reflection of central nervous system insult, their return to normal may be used as an indication of the likelihood of permanent damage. Sarnat and Sarnat [9] reported that infants with abnormal tone after 5 days are likely to have permanent neurological dysfunction.

A low Apgar score does not invariably mean asphyxia. Low Apgar scores may be associated with congenital malformations, infection, central nervous system depression, metabolic disorders, shock, and obstetrical trauma. These disorders lower the Apgar score primarily by causing apnea. Since asphyxia results in metabolic acidosis, the differentiation between asphyxia and apnea may be made by determining the umbilical artery pH shortly after delivery. Approximately 50% of newborns with an Apgar score below 7.0 will have a pH value of 7.2 or higher, indicating no significant asphyxia [10]. Determining the umbilical artery pH may be helpful in more accurately predicting long-term outcome. Of more immediate importance to the physician involved in resuscitation, the pH will reflect the degree of asphyxia and indicate the necessary steps in resuscitation.

The following cases illustrate the management plan for infants in the delivery room.

B. The Normal Infant (Apgar 7–10)

The infant with an Apgar score of 7–10 is healthy, cries shortly after delivery, maintains tone and color, and has a heart rate >100 beats/min. This is the most common situation we encounter in the delivery room. This neonate should be immediately dried and placed under a radiant warmer in order to conserve body temperature. He should be turned on his right side with the head below the level of the feet, and the head and neck extended to open the airway. Secretions in the mouth should be rapidly and gently suctioned using the bulb syringe. Vigorous suction of the hypopharynx in the first 5 min of life may result in bradycardia and should be avoided. These steps should be performed in the first minute of life and the Apgar score should then be recorded. During the next few minutes the infant should be observed closely and his body temperature maintained. If the delivery room does not have an overhead warmer, the infant should be dried with a warm blanket, which is then discarded, and wrapped in dry, warmed blankets. The stable infant may be transferred to the newborn nursery after the 5-min Apgar score is determined. Figure 2 reviews this management plan.

C. The Moderately Depressed Infant (Apgar 4–6)

The infant with an Apgar score of 4–6 is depressed and may not breathe immediately, suggesting the primary apnea stage of asphyxia. Tone is usually diminished but not absent and the infant displays slight responses to noxious stimuli.

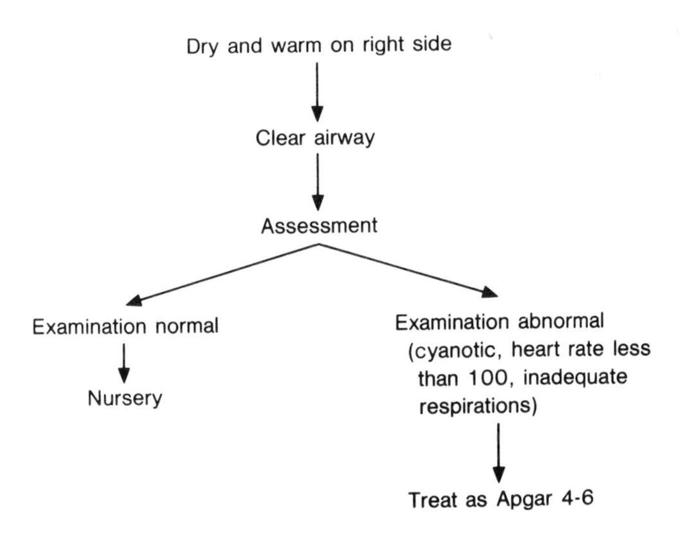

Figure 2 The normal infant (Apgar 7–10).

The initial treatment of this infant through the first minute of life includes the same treatment as described above for the normal infant. If he does not breathe immediately, and the heart rate is >100 beats/min gentle, tactile stimuli are applied to the infant and heated, humidified oxygen is supplied. Generally, these infants will make a gasping motion and then will begin rhythmic respirations. Oxygen administration should be continued until adequate respirations are established and he is pink. The oxygen is then discontinued and, if his color remains good, he may be handled as the normal infant.

If this infant does not breathe within 1 min, or if his heart rate becomes <100 beats/min, he should be ventilated with a self-inflating hand resuscitation bag and mask, using warmed, humidified oxygen at a flow rate of 5-10 liters/min, except in the case of meconium staining (discussed later). Since ventilation with oxygen stimulates breathing, the infant will usually start to gasp and then establish normal respirations. At the same time, the heart rate if depressed will accelerate. Adequacy of ventilation may be assessed by watching the movement

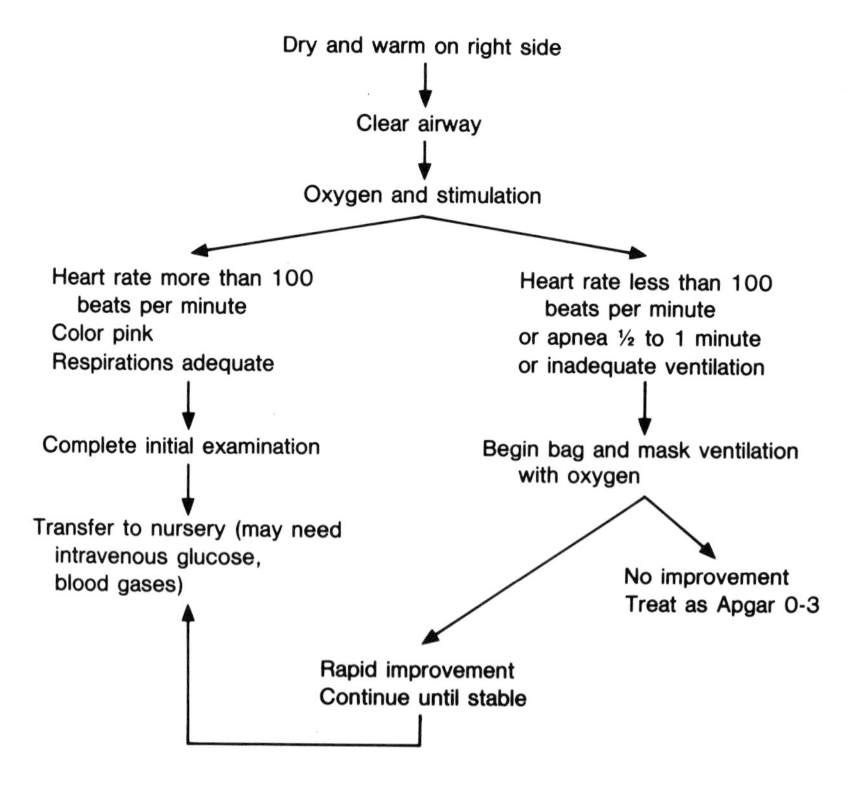

Figure 3 The moderately depressed infant (Apgar 4-6).

of the infant's chest and auscultating breath sounds in the axillae. An initial pressure as high as 50–60 cm water pressure may be required to inflate the lungs, but subsequent ventilation will usually require less pressure. Too vigorous "bagging" should be avoided because of the danger of pneumothorax. Figure 3 reviews this management plan.

D. The Severely Depressed Infant (Apgar 0–3)

The infant with an Apgar score of 0–3 is flaccid, apneic, pale, and unresponsive at birth, suggesting the secondary apnea stage of asphyxia. His heart rate is usually < 100 beats/min. This infant is a medical emergency. He presents either in the gasping stage following primary apnea or he is already in secondary apnea. He will not respond to stimuli or analeptics. He must be ventilated, and if necessary, the circulatory system must be supported. This infant should be dried immediately and placed in the supine position under an overhead warmer. The head should be lower than the feet. A small roll of towels is placed under the head and shoulders to promote extension of the head and to ensure patency of the airway. A bulb syringe should be used to rapidly clear the pharynx of secretions, except in cases of meconium staining, which will be discussed later.

This infant should be immediately intubated if the person attending the infant is skilled at intubation and if the laryngoscope and endotracheal tube are already assembled and immediately available. If a skilled person and assembled equipment are not available, it is recommended (except in cases of meconium staining) that ventilation be started with a bag and mask using warmed, humidified oxygen at a flow of 5–10 liters/min. Ventilation is gauged by observing the infant's chest movement and the response of the heart rate.

As ventilation is begun, the heart rate should be monitored. Should the heart rate respond rapidly, ventilation should be continued until the infant commences first gasping and then rhythmic respirations. Once this has occurred, the infant should be transferred to a special care nursery where arterial blood gases, glucose, and the hematocrit can be monitored and appropriate biochemical corrections made.

When ventilation with a bag and mask fails to cause heart rate acceleration, the infant must be intubated. Intubation of the right main stem bronchus can be prevented by having an assistant place his finger on the infant's suprasternal notch to feel the tube pass through the glottis. If the heart rate fails to respond to endotracheal ventilation or is < 80 beats/min, closed chest massage should be begun by placing the hands around the infant's thorax with the thumbs on the sternum or by using two fingers over the midsternum. The heart should be compressed at a rate of 100–120 beats/min with interruptions in cardiac compression every 3 sec for two inflations of the lung. If the infant's heart rate does not increase after a short period of cardiac compression, consider the possibility that the endotracheal tube may be dislodged or that a pneumothorax may have occurred. If, however, ventilation is adequate and the heart rate is not responding, the next step is to catheterize the umbilical vein. A No. 5 French, single end-hole catheter filled with 10% glucose in water should be used. Sodium bicarbonate is then infused, 1-2 mEq/kg of body weight. This volume of sodium bicarbonate should be administered as a 4.2% solution and given slowly over a period of 3-4 min through the umbilical vein while maintaining cardiac and ventilatory support. If there is no response 1-2 min after finishing the infusion, we inject 0.5-1.0 ml of 1:10,000 aqueous epinephrine. This can be given either through the umbilical vein catheter or into the endotracheal tube [11]. If there is evidence of hypoperfusion, 10-20 ml/kg of a volume expander may be given over 3-5 min. Additional treatment measures to be considered in light of the clinical situation are pressor agents, atropine, calcium, and transfusion.

It is of paramount importance that a normal body temperature be maintained during the resuscitative process. Since the needed treatment requires that the infant not be wrapped in blankets, an overhead warmer is an absolute necessity. A hospital that routinely delivers babies must anticipate and be prepared to care for asphyxiated infants; therefore, an overhead warmer is an essential part of the equipment in a delivery room. As soon as the infant is stabilized, he should be transferred to a special care unit where monitoring and biochemical correction can continue. Figure 4 reviews this management plan.

E. The Meconium-Stained Infant

The meconium-stained infant requires exception to the previously described methods. Meconium is usually passed in response to a stressful situation in utero. Asphyxia, either in utero or during the birth process, also results in gasping motions by the fetus. The combination of these two events results in aspiration of meconium into the hypopharynx and possibly the tracheobronchial tree. When the infant is born and makes his first gasping motions, any meconium in the airway may be drawn into the lungs. The resulting chemical pneumonitis causes a ventilation-perfusion imbalance and the development of respiratory and metabolic acidosis. Current evidence suggests that this disease can be prevented by immediate catheter suctioning of the hypopharynx when the head is delivered and intubation of the infant's trachea if the infant is depressed or stained with meconium. A significant number of infants who develop respiratory distress will not have obvious meconium in the mouth or larynx [12]. Therefore, all infants stained with thick meconium need endotracheal suctioning. Endotracheal suctioning should be repeated, using the endotracheal tube as the suction catheter, until no further meconium is extracted. Lavage of the trachea is not beneficial [13]. Following this treatment, any resuscitative measures needed are

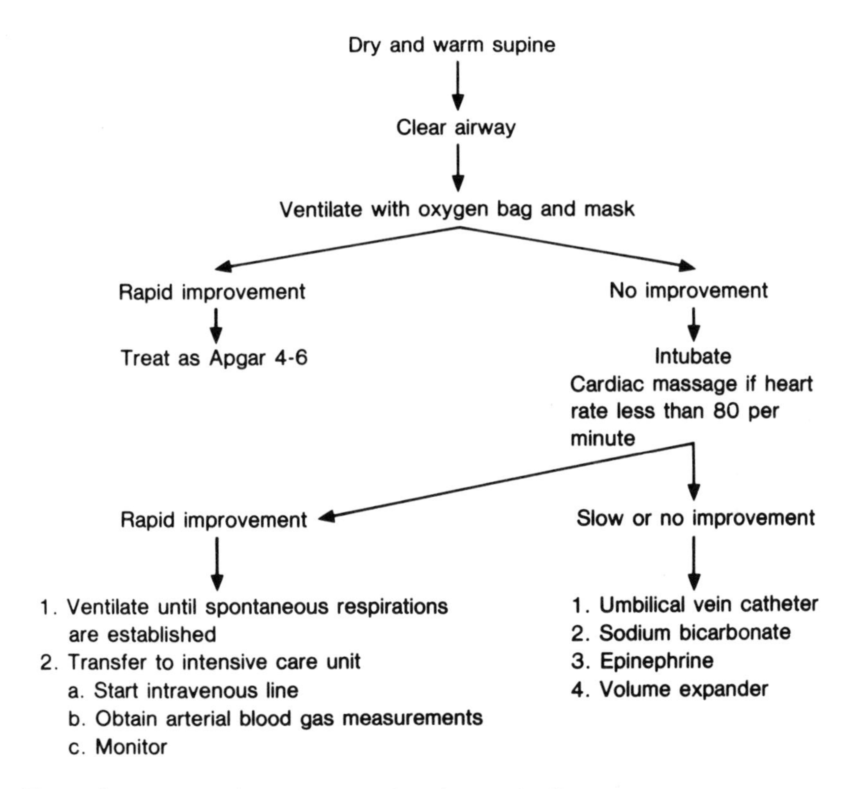

Figure 4 The severely depressed infant (Apgar 0–3).

administered as outlined. Do not use bag and mask ventilation or endotracheal ventilation before endotracheal suctioning because it will force meconium into the distal airways and facilitate the development of meconium pneumonitis. The rule to remember is: In the case of meconium staining of the neonate, intubate and remove any meconium in the trachea before ventilation.

The only other situation in which bag and mask ventilation is contraindicated is diaphragmatic hernia. Fortunately, these cases are extremely rare. If resuscitation is necessary, an endotracheal tube must be used and a gastric tube should be passed to maintain decompression of the stomach.

IV. New and/or Controversial Issues

Finally, we would like to briefly discuss several new and/or controversial issues pertaining to resuscitation.

A. Early Assisted Ventilation

In the delivery room it is frequently difficult to know if a breathing, premature infant with respiratory distress needs ventilatory assistance. Infants with hyaline membrane disease frequently require ventilatory assistance within the first 12 hr of life. The beneficial effect of continuous distending pressure begun within 3 hr of delivery has been demonstrated [14]. Over the last decade the trend has developed of intubating and ventilating more preterm infants in the delivery room. The rationale is that the early correction or prevention of any degree of hypoxia or acidosis may decrease the severity of subsequent respiratory distress. After transfer to the intensive care unit, the infants are weaned from ventilatory support as indicated by blood gases, the clinical diagnosis, and clinical condition. Comparing elective and mandatory intubation and stabilization of the airway at birth, Drew has demonstrated that mandatory intubation decreases mortality and morbidity in infants weighing < 1500 g [15]. If the intubation and ventilation are done skillfully, we feel this approach may not be harmful. In unskilled hands this approach could obviously lead to an increased incidence of tracheal injury, pneumothorax, and possibly retrolental fibroplasia. The benefits of early, skilled intubation and ventilation reinforce the need for the availability of expert personnel for resuscitation at birth and the advisability of premature deliveries being performed at a tertiary center whenever possible.

B. Narcotic Antagonists

The development of narcotic antagonists and the demonstration of opiate receptors in brain tissue led to the search for endogenous opioids. These substances, called endorphins, are peptides produced in the pituitary gland and brain. They are thought to be neuromodulators, that is, they modulate the release of neurotransmitters. Their concentration is increased by painful stimuli and their release is apparently one of the normal physiological responses to stress. Wardlaw et al. found elevated concentrations of β-endorphin in umbilical cord plasma and the higher concentrations were correlated with pH and PO_2 of the plasma [16]. This led them to suggest that perinatal hypoxia and acidosis may be major stimuli for their release. Another study found the highest concentrations of β-endorphin in cases with low Apgar scores [17]. Since opiates are known to depress the respiratory center, the question arose if these substances were contributing to the respiratory depression in asphyxia. Animal studies suggest that naloxone given before the asphyxial event ameliorates the depression resulting from asphyxia [18]. In the future, more specific antagonists of endogenous endorphins may be useful in resuscitation.

It must be emphasized that narcotic antagonists do not currently have a role in the initial management of the apneic and/or severely asphyxiated neonate. Any delay of ventilation while preparing an injection is inappropriate. Infants who have been resuscitated but remain hypotonic with poor inspiratory effort may warrant a trial of a narcotic antagonist particularly if the mother has received narcotics.

C. Correction of Metabolic Acidosis

It seemed logical, as a resuscitation technique, to correct the metabolic acidosis which results from asphyxia. This logic led to the use of bolus injections of bicarbonate in the delivery room. Soon, however, a relationship between bicarbonate injection and intracanial hemorrhage was noted [19]. It was postulated that the induced plasma hyperosmolality and resultant fluid shift were responsible for the bleeding. Although other studies suggested no unusual incidence of hemorrhage [20], there has been a marked decline in the use of bicarbonate. We recommend the use of bicarbonate for resuscitation only in the infant with an Apgar score of 0–3 whose heart rate does not rise above 100 beats/min after adequate endotracheal ventilation has been established. As mentioned before, the severely asphyxiated infant will have a mixed respiratory and metabolic acidosis. Ventilation alone will reduce the base deficit by about one-half. In addition, if ventilation is not adequate, injecting bicarbonate will elevate the PCO_2. Therefore, the use of bicarbonate is indicated only in severe asphyxia after adequate ventilation has failed to correct the hypoxemia as evidenced by a continued bradycardia. The dosage form is hyperosmolar and the danger of plasma hyperosmolality is avoided by slow infusion. Table 4 illustrates the calculation of the dosage.

D. Volume Expansion

Premature infants with respiratory distress may be hypovolemic [21]. The normal placental transfusion may be deficient due to intrapartum asphyxia [22], the position of the infant in relation to the placenta at delivery, or cord clamping before breathing begins. Clinically, it is difficult to evaluate hypovolemia, especially during resuscitation. Neither their blood pressure nor their hematocrit reflects the hypovolemia [22]. They may appear to have vasoconstriction but there is no way to measure this. Because of presumed hypovolemia early volume expansion in infants with severe cardiorespiratory distress has been advocated; however, the benefit of volume expansion is not proven and may be associated with impaired pulmonary oxygen exchange [23] and intraventricular hemorrhage [24]. If an infant remains pallid and bradycardic after adequate endotracheal ventilation has been established and especially if there is the possibility of blood loss (placenta previa, abruption), we feel a trial of volume expansion is justified after bicarbonate has been administered.

Table 4 Dosage of Sodium Bicarbonate Used in Severely Depressed Infants

Infant weight (kg)	Dosage (mEq/kg)	ml of 4.2% Solution to be infused[a]
0.6	1-2	1.2-2.4
0.8	1-2	1.6-3.8
1.0	1-2	2.0-4.0
1.2	1-2	2.4-4.8
1.4	1-2	2.8-5.6
1.6	1-2	3.2-6.4
1.8	1-2	3.6-7.2
2.0	1-2	4.0-8.0
2.2	1-2	4.4-8.8
2.4	1-2	4.8-9.6

[a]4.2% solution is marketed as "infant" sodium bicarbonate solution. It has 1 mEq/2 ml and has an osmolarity of 1000 mOsm/liter and approximately the same osmolality. "Pediatric" sodium bicarbonate solution is 8.4% and should be diluted 1:1 with distilled water prior to use.

E. When Not to Resuscitate

The final, unanswerable controversy is when to stop resuscitation measures in the delivery room. We feel this is a more accurate question than when not to resuscitate an infant. Resuscitation is a continuum beginning with suctioning the oropharynx after delivery of the head and proceeding through the previously described steps until the infant is stabilized or the resuscitation is considered a failure. Hesitancy to resuscitate an infant is usually due to the fear that we are beginning a futile, expensive effort which will only delay death. However, death is not the endpoint of resuscitation. Resuscitation can be stopped at whatever point we decide the infant has shown a physiological inability to benefit from the resuscitation. The resuscitation can then be considered unsuccessful and stopped. This process of evaluating the infant's response to resuscitation rather than predicting the response seems more rational to us. For example, in the past, we considered fused eyelids as an indication for inaction. Experience made a mockery of that as we saw infants with one lid fused and one open, or twins discordant for fusion, or shared with others [25] the experience of having such infants survive. Therefore, we proceed with resuscitation and terminate it if we are unable to adequately oxygenate the infant or unable to establish sufficient perfusion to correct a metabolic acidosis. The point at which each of us considers resuscitation a failure is still individual and arbitrary, but, at least, we have not prejudged the infant's viability.

Resuscitation of the infant with severe congenital malformations is a distressing situation. As ultrasound is used more frequently during pregnancy, we are now often able to discuss the prognosis with the parents before delivery. From that experience we realize that almost all parents, at the time of delivery, want their infant resuscitated as best we can. Therefore, when an infant is born with unexpected severe malformations, we presume a similar parental attitude and proceed with resuscitation.

References

1. Johnson, K. G., The promise of regional perinatal care as a national strategy for improved maternal and infant care, *Pub. Health Rep.*, **97**:134-139 (1982).
2. Kanto, W. P., Jr., G. Johnson, C. Sturgill, and K. West, Performance of a level II nursery in a neonatal regional program: Part I. Patient population and role of the general pediatrician, *South. Med. J.*, **75**:1043-1050 (1982).
3. Lazzara, A., W. P. Kanto, Jr., F. D. Dykes, P. A. Ahmann, and K. West, Continuing education in the community hospital and reduction in the incidence of intracerebral hemorrhage in the transported preterm infant, *J. Pediatr.*, **101**:757-761 (1982).
4. Clark, J. M., Z. A. Brown, and A. L. Jung, Resuscitation equipment board for nurseries and delivery rooms, *JAMA*, **236**:2427-2428 (1976).
5. Apgar, V., A proposal for a new method of evaluation of the newborn infant, *Curr. Res. Anesth. Anal.*, **32**:260-267 (1953).
6. Nelson, K. B., and J. H. Ellenberg, Apgar scores as predictors of chronic neurologic disability, *Pediatrics*, **68**:36-44 (1981).
7. Apgar, V., The newborn (Apgar) scoring system, *Pediatr. Clin. North Am.*, **13**:645-650 (1966).
8. Dawes, G. S., *Foetal and Neonatal Physiology. A Comparative Study of the Changes at Birth.* Chicago, Year Book, 1968.
9. Sarnat, H. B., and M. S. Sarnat, Neonatal encephalopathy following fetal distress. A clinical and electroencephalographic study, *Arch. Neurol.*, **33**:696-705 (1976).
10. Fields, L. M., S. S. Entman, and F. H. Boehm, Correlation of the one-minute Apgar score and the pH value of umbilical arterial blood, *South. Med. J.*, **76**:1477-1479 (1983).

11. Powers, R. D., and L. G. Donowitz, Endotracheal administration of emergency medications, *South. Med. J.,* 77:340–341 (1984).
12. Gregory, G. A., C. A. Gooding, R. H. Phibbs, and W. H. Tooley, Meconium aspiration in infants—A prospective study, *J. Pediatr.,* **85**:848–852 (1974).
13. Carson, B. S., R. W. Losey, W. A. Bowes, and M. A. Simmons, Combined obstetric and pediatric approach to prevent meconium aspiration syndrome, *Am. J. Obstet. Gynecol.,* **126**:712–715 (1976).
14. Tanswell, A. K., R. A. Clubb, B. T. Smith, and R. W. Boston, Individualized continuous distending pressure applied within 6 hours of delivery in infants with respiratory distress syndrome, *Arch. Dis. Child.,* **55**:33–39 (1980).
15. Drew, J. H., Immediate intubation at birth of the very-low-birth-weight infant, *Am. J. Dis. Child.,* **136**:207–210 (1982).
16. Wardlaw, S. L., R. I. Stark, L. Baxi, and A. G. Frantz, Plasma β-endorphin and β-lipotropin in the human fetus at delivery: Correlation with arterial pH and PO_2. *J. Clin. Endocrinol. Metab.,* **79**:888–891 (1979).
17. Puolakka, J., A. Kauppila, J. Leppäluoto, and O. Vuolteenaho, Elevated β-endorphin immunoreactivity in umbilical cord blood after complicated delivery, *Acta Obstet. Gynecol. Scand.,* **61**:513–514 (1982).
18. Chernick, V., and R. J. Craig, Naloxone reverses neonatal depression caused by fetal asphyxia, *Science,* **216**:1252–1253 (1982).
19. Bland, R. D., T. L. Clarke, and L. B. Harden, Rapid infusion of sodium bicarbonate and albumin into high-risk premature infants soon after birth: A controlled, prospective trial, *Am. J. Obstet. Gynecol.,* **124**:263–267 (1976).
20. Baum, J. D., and N. R. C. Roberton, Immediate effects of alkaline infusion in infants with respiratory distress syndrome, *J. Pediatr.,* **87**:255–261 (1975).
21. Brown, E. G., R. W. Krouskop, F. E. McDonnell, and A. Y. Sweet, Blood volume and blood pressure in infants with respiratory distress, *J. Pediatr.,* **87**:1133–1138 (1975).
22. Linderkamp, O., H. T. Versmold, K. Messow-Zahn, W. Müller-Holve, K. P. Riegel, and K. Betke, The effect of intra-partum and intra-uterine asphyxia on placental transfusion in premature and full-term infants, *Eur. J. Pediatr.,* **127**:91–99 (1978).
23. Barr, P. A., P. E. Bailey, J. Sumners, and G. Cassady, Relation between arterial blood pressure and blood volume and effect of infused albumin in sick premature infants, *Pediatrics,* **60**:282–289 (1977).
24. Dykes, F. D., A. Lazzara, P. Ahmann, B. Blumenstein, J. Schwartz, and A. W. Brann, Intraventricular hemorrhage: A prospective evaluation of etiopathogenesis, *Pediatrics,* **66**:42–49 (1980).
25. Antoniou, A. G., and N. McIntosh, Do fused eyelids indicate inevitable neonatal death?, *Lancet,* **i**:878–879 (1983).

Part Six

THE NEONATAL INTENSIVE CARE UNIT

15

A Modern Neonatal Intensive Care Unit and Perinatal Regionalization

GARY R. GUTCHER and ROBERT H. PERELMAN

University of Wisconsin School of Medicine
Madison, Wisconsin

I. Introduction

Intensive care of the newborn extends at least as far back as the efforts of Budin in France [1]. Though one may question their motivation for providing more than usual and customary care to those infants, Couney and Budin employed highly visible techniques in establishing a traveling exhibition of "kinderbrutanstalt" or "child hatcheries" at large expositions worldwide. Modern efforts may be traced to the establishment of a premature unit by Julius Hess in Chicago in 1922 [2]. Since then, textbooks and learned treatises on the organization and management of a neonatal intensive care unit have increased almost logarithmically in number. It is not our intent to offer yet another version of a do-it-yourself manual, but rather to review some of the salient features of extant publications, suggest some modification to their recommendations, and describe our organization as one example of a locally modified system. In addition, we will present some local and statewide data to illustrate the impact of perinatal regionalization in Wisconsin.

II. The Neonatal Intensive Care Unit

A. Organization

In August of 1968, Ross Laboratories convened its Fifty-ninth Conference on Pediatric Research [3]. Entitled *Problems of Neonatal Intensive Care Units*, the two lead papers attempted to deal with the impact of the establishment of intensive care nurseries on neonatal care as of that date. The published discussions reflect some misgivings on the part of the participants in deciding what they were talking about. What exactly is intensive care and what is the organization of a unit?

While the first question has not been and perhaps cannot be answered, numerous publications spell out each particular author's views on the proper organization of such a unit [4–7]. Indeed, these views have become incorporated into national guidelines [8,9] which are even now undergoing local modification [10]. As indicated in the introduction to this chapter, it is not our intent to reiterate these plans. Rather, we shall touch on those issues of importance in the application of the guidelines.

The critical factors involved in the establishment of a neonatal intensive care unit are the population base served, the character of population distribution, the composition of the population, and the costs of alternative means of meeting perceived needs. The *National Guidelines for Health Planning* call for a minimum of 15 beds in any single neonatal special care unit and specify that the total number of intensive and intermediate care beds should not exceed four per 1000 live births per year in a defined neonatal service area. In rural, sparsely populated regions of the country, these recommendations are difficult to achieve unless the defined neonatal service area is very large or unless modifications are made in the guidelines. The implications of either approach are clear. Large service areas impose problems of accessibility and timely response because of complicating geographical obstacles. This frequently necessitates use of high-speed transport by air with its own unique set of problems [7]. On the other hand, adjusting down to smaller service areas accessible by ground transport imposes cost/benefit problems. As outlined by Sheridan [11], Wolin has constructed cost-size curves for neonatal units to suggest that the cost per neonatal admission is minimal for a unit of 22 beds assuming 70% occupancy, while the average cost per patient day is minimal in a unit of 43 beds, again assuming 70% occupancy.

The deliberations necessary for the alternative down-sizing of a service area have also been described [10]. Specifically, when defining the boundaries for a region or the facilities within that region, one must consider the population base and its corresponding requirements for service, previously established travel and referral patterns, the availability of scarce resources, and geographical and climatic characteristics. With these factors in mind in the late 1960s, the

Wisconsin Association for Perinatal Care divided the state into six perinatal care regions after conducting a 3-year retrospective analysis of fetal and neonatal deaths and all births of < 2500 g in 35 hospitals outside the resident counties of the two medical schools in Wisconsin. Each region generally encompassed a delivery base of more than 13,000 per year, and within each one a perinatal center was organized. Supporting the efforts of these centers were the educational objectives of "needs assessment" of participating referring hospitals by a survey team of physicians and nurse practitioners. This was followed by a frank and open presentation directed to the key personnel which led to the establishment of continuing educational programs.

With the passing of time, defining personnel and equipment needs has become less important than defining the working relationship of the personnel and identifying the conditions necessary to render those individuals maximally effective. The term "intensive care nursery" is giving way to "special care nursery," reflecting a shift in emphasis with maturation. The early focus on acute care has now broadened to include the transition from acute to chronic care and the transition from hospital to home. Thus, if not physically, then functionally, special care nurseries tend to be divided into intensive care, intermediate care, and convalescent care areas – in turn, each level requiring less medical and more special intervention in efforts to aid patients and parents make the transition home easier. The need for this shift in attitude has been imposed by the changing nature of the patient population – smaller and smaller infants surviving with resulting longer hospitalizations and the emergence of chronic problems as complications of the acute care (e.g., bronchopulmonary dysplasia as a result of oxygen and respirator use in immature lungs with the respiratory distress syndrome [RDS]). This has changed the demands placed on nursery personnel, calling for mid-stride changes from the acute care sprint to the chronic care marathon.

B. Personnel

Despite the explosion in technology in the nursery, the well-trained nurse remains the single best feature in any intensive care unit. Subtle changes in a patient's state are not yet wholly amenable to electronic digitalization and microprocessing. For the intensive care areas, 1:1 or 1:2 nurse-to-patient ratios are generally recommended, and this ratio falls to 1:4 in intermediate and convalescent units. This then is clearly a labor intensive area in which a considerable investment of time and money by the hospital and management staff is necessary to produce the required degree of specialized training. Locally, formal and informal training consumes the first 6 months of a nurse's tenure. This large investment is continually threatened by the nature of working conditions in the unit. The acuity of illness, the fragility of the patient, the small margin for error in very low birth weight infants, and the stress of keeping abreast of rapidly changing approaches to care and technology tend to result in the phenomenon of "burnout" and high turnover rates [12-15]. In our own unit, turnover has averaged 39% per year since 1977, while the hospital-wide average has been 19%. In a survey conducted by Astbury and Yu [15] the issues of "personal life vs. work" and "understaffing/overwork" ranked just behind "sudden death/relapse" as the most *intense* stress, while they were ranked first and second for *frequency* of stress. Thus, the high attrition rate becomes a vicious cycle: High turnover leads to increased stress on those remaining and their excessively high expectations of the newly recruited lead to additional stress which results in additional turnover. It is in the nurses' personal interest and the hospital's financial interest for the administrative and medical staff to protect and support this group. Frequently, too little attention is paid to the creature comforts of personnel while on duty and insufficient time or space is allocated for "decompression." The organization of formal support groups has worked on occasion but tends to lose momentum unless a strong advocate exists within the system. Alternatively, provision of the time and space for informal discussion may help.

Medical personnel for intensive care nurseries have classically been supplied within the framework of the teaching hospital model: staff neonatologists who supervise individuals in training (fellows, residents, and perhaps medical students). Recently, however, nursery organizations based on the private practice model are increasing in numbers. This concept frequently displaces individuals in training with neonatal nurse clinicians or no particular group.

The teaching hospital organization imposes special problems of interpersonal relations. The classic new-intern vs. experienced-nurse confrontation potentially is a life-threatening event for the neonate because of the small margin for error. Constant surveillance is required of the system and individuals within the system to defuse problems and refocus attention on the "real" problem – the patient. Furthermore, in the past, directors of pediatric residency programs tended to overallot house-staff time to the budding neonatal intensive care units at the expense of other pediatric services. As a result, pediatric training programs now restrict all nursery time to a total of 6 months during the 3-year residency program. Since the intensive care unit provides a wealth of material to teach and reteach physiology and biochemistry with wider application and value than the neonate, this is becoming the focus of other house-staff participation. Extending this rotation in the nursery to residents in obstetrics and anesthesiology is providing valuable opportunities for enhancing communication and exchanging skills and insights.

Residents and fellows have generally served as a buffer for university-affiliated staff neonatologists. This allows the neonatologist to have more time for research and didactic teaching. In the private practice model, these elements are less demanding and more time is spent for direct patient care by the neonatologist. The private practice model may potentially degenerate into fee-for-service only, with total neglect of teaching and educational programs. On the other hand, the teaching hospital model may shift the burden of decision making too low in the hierarchy and this could result in inexperienced individuals delivering substandard care. Clearly, not all programs want to or can conduct training and research, yet those that do are the source of technical advances. Each model has its place and its potential for abuse.

C. Equipment

The equipment needs of a special care nursery and the currently available models have been recently and excellently reviewed by Y. W. Brans, and the reader is referred to that publication [16]. The major impact of this rising technology is on personnel and space. Oxygen monitoring equipment is an excellent example. The transcutaneous oxygen monitor has provided new insight into the impact of care on infants. Procedures originally designed to aid infants (chest physiotherapy, endotracheal tube suctioning, etc.) are now known to be transiently detrimental to PO_2 levels now that we possess the ability to monitor PO_2 *continuously* rather than just obtain intermittent determinations of arterial blood gases. Indwelling oxygen saturation catheters are even more sensitive in detecting changes in arterial oxygen levels. The impact of these transient events on patient outcome is unknown; hence, the response of physicians and nurses alike can only be arbitrary at present. We appear to be gluttons for data – lots of information of unknown or questionable value. Furthermore, with the advent of multiple monitoring and therapeutic devices space around the bed of a critically ill infant comes at a premium. The 10 linear feet of circumferential space around an incubator can rapidly fill with a respirator, thoracostomy tube suction devices, continuous oxygen monitors, cardiorespiratory and temperature monitors, transillumination devices, a blood pressure monitor, and an array of intravenous infusion pumps. Even more, each device is generally equipped with at least one alarm system, which means an average of five potential alarms per critically ill patient. Since there is no industry standard for the audible alarms assigned to various devices, responding appropriately to any single alarm becomes a stressful challenge. When two or three alarms are activated simultaneously, the stress on the attending nursing staff is particularly great.

D. Communications

The microcosm of the nursery frequently induces an introspective, self-serving posture that needs repeated prodding. The level of communications with referring nursing staffs and physicians tends to be the most sensitive indicator of how well a unit is maintaining its perspective. General care in a health service area is influenced most effectively by continued and close contact with those on the "front-line." The base of knowledge and behavior of a given referring physician is most amendable to change and improvement when contact is personal and nonjudgmental. Thus, maintaining regular communication with referring personnel not only enhances good public relations, but it sets the foundation for further educational endeavors.

III. Outreach Education

Educational efforts are targeted at both consumers and providers of health care. Consumer educational efforts are designed to enhance awareness of overall health promotion and prevention, or detection and management of risk situations. For the most part these efforts fall to those principally involved in the care of pregnant women, expectant fathers, and teenage siblings. Nursery personnel may also be involved in the education of parents and siblings, particularly at the time of discharge of the newborn from the nursery. *The Premature Baby Book* by Helen Harrison [17] provides excellent reading to help parents adjust to the shock of dealing with the acute illnesses of their children as well as adjust to the reality of taking their infants home as the final discharge approaches. Other modes of parental education involve the availability within the hospital complex of inexpensive or no-cost rooms for parents who have come from great distances. Moreover, "parenting" rooms adjacent to the nursery provide a safe place for parents to begin to assume care, initially with guidance and supervision of specialized tasks and eventually alone. This situation, when indicated, is welcomed by parents because of the reassurance of professional aid just outside the door.

Other educational programs are aimed at assisting hospital personnel and community professionals in providing improved primary care. In this effort, "needs assessment" plays a critical role. This can occur at the level of reviewing regional health status indicators collected by local and regional officials or it may take the form of surveys or questionnaires with institution-specific assessments. Both approaches provide valuable insight into "the problem" but the latter, more personal approach fosters an atmosphere of cooperation on the part of the recipients of the education. The "out" of "outreach," then, is not simply getting "out" there and telling folks the "right" way to do things, nor is it passive in waiting for a spontaneous generation of questions by the referring centers. Rather, it is a "reach out" to co-opt all concerned into a mutually beneficial exercise in assessing needs and responding to them. The response to identified needs is also negotiated and cooperative. A variety of educational approaches may be called upon, i.e., chart reviews, patient conferences, teaching rounds, workshops, regional conferences with or without continuing medical education credits, and hospital-specific morbidity and mortality conferences. In the educational area, more than any other, the walls of the neonatal-perinatal unit expand to encompass the entire health service area and all concerned become consumers and providers at once.

IV. Neonatal Transports

The cost incurred for specialized facilities providing high-risk perinatal care limits their number and encourages regionalization. Therefore, well-organized and controlled transport of patients has been mandatory to provide expeditious and uniform care in a given service area. Justification for the organization and initiation of neonatal transport services has been documented in numerous publications [7,18–21]. Suggestions for staffing patterns, mobile unit specifications, monitoring requirements, etc., have also been recorded [3,7,18] and for the most part are dictated by population demographics and service area size and geography. Regardless of its components, neonatal transport services must offer quickly responsive and skilled support as an integrated part of perinatal health care delivery.

Local coordination of transport services, which is depicted in Figure 1, is conducted by the clinical director of the special care nurseries in cooperation with obstetrical colleagues, nursing services, and hospital administration. As noted, each discipline maintains accountability for specific components of the system. Regionalized service areas in Wisconsin are geographically defined with the intent that transit time to a center will not exceed 2 hr; therefore, referral by ground transport has been the mode of choice since 1968. Even though distances traveled are relatively short, severe weather conditions can lengthen travel time considerably. Therefore, our transport vehicle is supplied with auxillary marine batteries and gas tanks to provide 6 hr of heat, electrical current, and blended oxygen/air mixtures even in the event of engine failure. In our center, mobilization time from referral call to team departure is expected to be between 30 and 45 min. During the interim, the attending physician is in direct contact with the referring hospital to offer telephone consultation regarding stabilization and intervening care. Communication systems required for ground transport are not complex. The mobile unit must have the capability for continued consultation prior to arrival at the referring hospital and for later notification of special care nursery personnel before return so that equipment can be readied which will permit a smooth transfer of care. Although ambulance licensing regulations in Wisconsin only require radio communication, we have found the addition of a mobile telephone system most efficatious. Upon arrival at the referring hospital the center transport team, consisting of an attending neonatologist and a transport-trained neonatal nurse, assume responsibility for the patient. The team remains at the referring hospital long enough to provide whatever medical intervention is necessary to ensure the safest and most stable return with the neonate to the perinatal center.

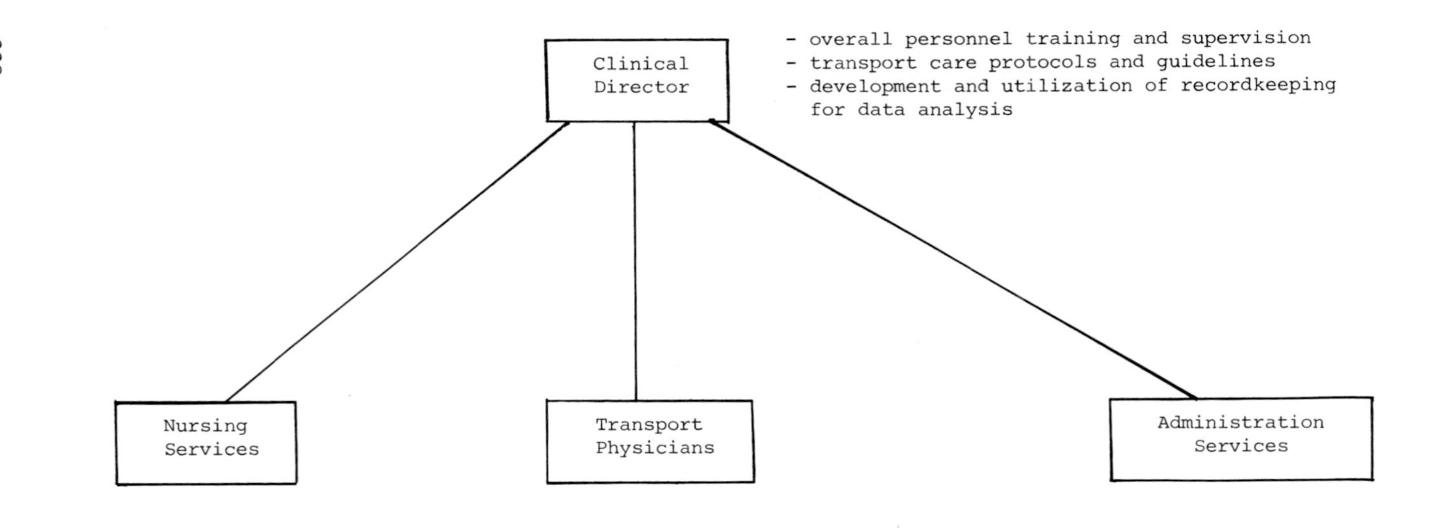

Figure 1 Organization of neonatal transport system.

As noted in the overview of the 1980 Ross Laboratories survey of perinatal health services in the United States [11], the typical transport team used an ambulance and consisted of a registered nurse, respiratory therapist, and pediatric resident. At a minimum, a nurse and respiratory therapist will accompany the neonate during transport. In contrast, all acute referral transports in our center include an attending neonatologist as the physician leader of the team. While other systems have been efficacious [7,21], we maintain this team composition to maximize patient care expertise in what may often be a difficult environment for provision of acute intensive care. Additionally, a uniform group of transport physicians offers ongoing familarity and interpersonal relationships with community health care providers and a relatively stable approach to medical and administrative procedures.

In addition to providing acute care to seriously ill newborns, the transport team has the established objective of *family support* and *local education.* In this regard, time is routinely alloted for discussions with the family concerning diagnoses, expected management and course, the differences between community hospitals and perinatal centers, and related personal concerns and questions. A pamphlet describing practice and procedure in our center and instant-developing pictures of the patient are always presented to the family. Additionally, the time during and after stabilization of the patient provides an opportunity for educational interchange with referring nursing and medical staff.

After return and admission of the patient to the special care nursery, communication with the referring medical and nursing staff and the patient's family is mandatory. During the acute phase of intensive care, the attending neonatologist updates the referring physician by telephone as frequently as is required and this is followed subsequently during convalescence by weekly calls. Likewise, the perinatal center nursing staff reports patient progress to community hospital nurses on a weekly basis.

Pre- and post-transport checklists and evaluation forms are completed by outreach education and administrative personnel to evaluate transport team performance and identify the educational needs of referring communities. Outreach educational programs have resulted in the referring physician's increased understanding of maternal/fetal pathophysiology and the technical capabilities of the perinatal centers. As a result, the referring physician now tends to anticipate and identify early pregnancy-related problems. This has resulted in more frequent maternal referral, so that transport of sick neonates now accounts for $< 20\%$ of the yearly special care nursery admissions. Return transports for convalescent care are considered when patient status and local capabilities are amenable. This not only decreases the strain on the tertiary center's staffing and space, but also brings the child closer to the family and provides experience for enhancing level I care proficiency.

V. Research

In university-based neonatal units there is usually an active clinical research program. The research projects principally involve the physician staff; however, other health professionals may also be involved. These projects or protocols may be directed at the infant, the mother, both of them, or the family as a whole. In an active center, the potential is great for multiple protocols to be applied to a given family and this may adversely affect patient care. In this regard, the establishment of an intramural perinatal research committee may be helpful. The function and purpose of such a committee are to review all protocols that utilize human subjects or medical records with respect to (1) the impact on those providing patient care (nurses, residents, ward clerks, etc.), (2) the impact on patients and their parents, (3) the impact on other on-going protocols, (4) the feasibility of the project in that perinatal center, and (5) scientific merit, when no external funding agency has provided this (i.e., the National Institutes of Health, March of Dimes, etc.).

Membership of this committee should be broad to include personnel from neonatology, obstetrics, and nursing service. It may also include ad hoc specialists when appropriate for adequate scientific review. This committee derives its authority from and is responsible to the director of the perinatal center and should provide regular reviews of the active projects (generally by requiring regular progress reports by the principal investigators).

The potential for a conflict of interest arises in research at two levels. First, the principal investigator may also be the individual providing primary care (e.g., a neonatologist). Research protocol requirements may occasionally call for procedures contrary to the patient's best interest and resolution of these conflicts needs to be anticipated and planned for. Secondly, bedside care for critically ill infants should be the primary concern of the house staff and nurses, and a mechanism is needed to decrease the demands on these individuals from research protocols. In both these instances, there should be a separation of research and clinical responsibilities. In questions of the clinical implications of research procedures, a responsible neonatologist, other than the principal investigator, should be designated to resolve the issue. The use of research nurses or other specimen and data collectors helps relieve the clinical staff of the burden of remembering timed-specimen collections.

Research is sometimes viewed as an unnecessary hindrance by the clinical staff and regular, systematic, and formal sharing of the results of protocols helps to gain acceptance of the efforts as valuable.

VI. Impact

A system for the collection of perinatal data is a basic and fundamental component of a regional perinatal program. Such a system is used to support several activities of the perinatal center at many different levels. Within the nursery the data generated help in the clinical management of patients through simple tracking of overall morbidity and mortality by weight and disease. More specific measures of outcome of morbidity and mortality help define staffing, equipment, and space needs. They also provide outcome measures for comparative analysis against published data to identify local problems. Shifting patterns of diagnoses help quantitate needs for developing new or strengthening existing programs. For instance, the well-documented increased length-of-stay of infants, the increased survival of very low birth weight infants, and a rising incidence of bronchopulmonary dysplasia (BPD) and prolonged apnea have helped us to document a need for the recruitment of a pediatric pulmonologist, the initiation of a specialized clinic for the follow-up of children with BPD, and the establishment of a comprehensive home-monitoring program.

Documenting the times of various events following requests for neonatal transport helps track response time and detect problems in mobilization. The recording of the condition and diagnosis of a potential transport on arrival at the referral hospital helps to identify hospital-specific management problems and aid in planning educational programs.

In organizing such a data collection system it is imperative that several issues be addressed:

1. Formulation of objectives: A clear statement of the purpose and goals of such a system must be made. The output must be of value to *all* participants and the system should induce cooperation among all participants and should stimulate compliance in data collection.
2. Quality control: The system must work to assure that data are accurate. This requires a consensus in terminology and definitions through initial and continuous educational and informational training.
3. Data distribution: Distribution of tabulated data must be to *all* participants and turnaround time should be as rapid as possible. Once the questions or problems to be addressed are identified, the quality of the data collected and compliance in collecting data are directly tied to a perceived need and value.

The accumulation and entry of data are time consuming, and data collection rapidly deteriorates when it fails to meet the needs of the collectors.

Through the statewide organization, the Wisconsin Association for Perinatal Care, a data collection system employing three forms was developed in 1980. One maternal and two neonatal forms (inpatient and follow-up) are used to track statewide patterns at the established level III nurseries. While initially successful, the decline in compliance in form completion and the generation of unusable data have resulted in the needs of the individual centers not being met. In retrospect, there was a lack of clearly defined objectives for the maternal and inpatient neonatal forms. However, the follow-up neonatal form was devised in cooperation with the State Bureau of Crippled Children to aid in identifying statewide, regional, and local needs for government-supported programs. Since this form clearly helps the neonatal follow-up clinics in their efforts, compliance and continuing support are much better. Indeed, the value of the data to statewide program planning and funding is such that clinics are now paid by the state to complete these forms on a capitation basis. Reevaluation and restructuring of the original maternal and inpatient neonatal forms are underway in an effort to meet the clearly identified needs of the participants.

The Wisconsin perinatal care program, now incorporating six regional centers, was initiated in 1968 after a review of community health care providers and state demographics. In spite of continuing efforts to assess the program's efficacy, numerous problems exist in attempts at serial objective evaluation. First, as noted above, early programs which were based on perceived need often did not incorporate rigid criteria for ongoing evaluation of the impact. In fact, until about 1975 there were no collaboratively developed national guidelines for initiation and comparison of regional programs for maternal and perinatal health services. Secondly, prior to 1968 when the National Center of Health Statistics adopted the eighth revision of the International Classification of Diseases, annual summaries of United States mortality data did not emphasize the neonatal period and the major etiology for death in infants < 28 days of age. Therefore, intrastate, interstate, and national comparisons could only be loosely estimated. Lastly, it is difficult to separate the effects of individual components of multifaceted programs at both the state and regional levels.

With these limitations in mind, we have analyzed obtainable data regarding neonatal mortality rates in Wisconsin and the United States. Our specific approach was to evaluate:

1. Trends in state neonatal mortality rates over the last 15 years
2. Comparison of state and national statistics
3. Objective assessments of utilization of tertiary care centers

In general, the analyses utilized disease-specific mortality because incremental weight-specific neonatal death rates have not been the norm for state or national statistical surveys until the most recent years, though they have been available locally. The birth rate of live-born infants in Wisconsin has been between 60,000 and 77,000 births per year over the last 15 years. After declining during the mid-1970s, the birth rate has gradually risen to approximately 74,000 births per year over the last 5 years. The birth rate of infants weighing <2500 g has gradually declined from approximately 7% of all births in 1968 to an average of between 5 and 6% between 1977 and 1982. These observations are similar to previously reported national trends [22].

Table 1 depicts national and Wisconsin neonatal mortality rates (deaths/1000 live births) between 1968 and 1982. In 1968, Wisconsin began 6% below the national average, and from 1968 to 1982 the death rate for neonates has decreased within the state by 60%. Although the national trends are similar, the overall neonatal mortality rate in Wisconsin has averaged 17–20% below the national norm. For all data considered herein, one should recognize that the International Classification of Disease Codes was revised between 1978 and 1979. Even though this reclassification alters the continuity of data and uniformity of trends between these 2 years, the overall effect on long-term data tracking is inconsequential. For instance, for the years 1977, 1978, and 1979, there is an anomaly in the neonatal mortality rates due to RDS (Table 2) and for all causes (Table 1). This anomaly is not reflected in the national data (Table 1). This is probably more evident for the data of Wisconsin because of the smaller absolute numbers in Wisconsin compared to those for the United States at large. In spite of the decreasing mortality trends in the intervals 1968–1978 and 1979–1982, it is not currently appropriate to incorporate all years from 1968 to present in a single longitudinal analysis.

Analysis of national statistics indicates that asphyxia, immaturity, complications of pregnancy, and hyaline membrane disease (or RDS) are the leading specific causalities for neonatal mortality. Wisconsin has maintained lower mortality rates and paralleled the almost linear decrease in national neonatal deaths due to immaturity. The state remains a significant 41% below the national norm in fatalities due to asphyxia. It is particularly interesting to note that even though Wisconsin was 39% lower than the United States in 1968, the death rate associated with asphyxia has continued to fall, most noticably after 1971, coincident with the advent of maternal antepartum referrals.

Acute complications of pregnancy include preeclampsia, ante- and intrapartum infection, difficult labor, incompetent cervix, prolonged rupture of the membranes, etc. In Wisconsin deaths attributable to this category have remained relatively constant between 1968 and 1976, while nationally complications of

Table 1 Neonatal Mortality Rates in the United States and Wisconsin Due to RDS and All Causes[a]

	All causes		RDS	
Year	USA	Wisconsin	USA	Wisconsin
1968	16.1	15.1	2.36	2.83
1969	15.6	12.8	2.48	2.10
1970	15.1	13.0	2.61	1.98
1971	15.2	11.7	2.78	1.92
1972	13.6	10.8	2.75	1.59
1973	12.9	10.4	2.73	1.53
1974	12.3	10.2	2.62	1.98
1975	11.6	9.7	2.42	1.58
1976	10.9	8.9	2.14	1.51
1977	9.9	7.5	1.86	1.17
1978	9.5	7.6	1.66	1.30
1979	8.7	7.2	1.56	1.38
1980	8.5	6.7	1.38	0.88
1981	7.9	6.9	1.16	1.10
1982	7.6	6.0	1.07	0.88

[a]Mortality rate (NNMR) = deaths/1000 live births.

pregnancy have had a declining contribution to the neonatal mortality rate. This observation has further stimulated our increasing emphasis for antepartum referral. In 1970, the respiratory distress syndrome emerged in the United States as the most frequently reported underlying cause of neonatal death. RDS accounted for 17.3% of the total deaths in that year, and nationally has been the leading total contributor to newborn deaths over the years analyzed. Again, Table 1 shows a comparison of the death rates due to the RDS between the United States and Wisconsin. The national statistics reveal a rise from 1968 to 1971 and then a gradual decline in terms of absolute numbers since that time. The trend in Wisconsin is distinctly different. Coincident with regionalization in 1968, the number of deaths per 1000 live births due to RDS began to fall rapidly while the national trend was increasing. The death rate per 1000 live births from RDS in Wisconsin for 1982 was 0.88, which represents a decline of 68.9% since regionalization of perinatal care was begun.

Table 2 Neonatal Mortality Rates in Wisconsin Due to Selected Causes[a,b]

Year	Total NNMR	RDS	Asphyxia	Immaturity	Complications of pregnancy
1968	15.1	2.83	1.79	3.11	1.31
1969	12.8	2.10	1.75	1.90	1.35
1970	13.0	1.98	1.74	2.21	1.34
1971	11.7	1.92	1.63	1.76	1.36
1972	10.8	1.59	1.08	1.45	1.44
1973	10.4	1.53	1.11	1.24	1.35
1974	10.2	1.98	0.81	1.23	1.20
1975	9.7	1.58	0.75	1.24	1.42
1976	8.9	1.51	0.80	1.00	1.39
1977	7.5	1.17	0.63	0.88	0.85
1978	7.6	1.30	0.59	0.73	1.05
1979	7.2	1.38	0.19	0.31	0.55
1980	6.7	0.88	0.28	0.36	0.43
1981	6.9	1.10	0.27	0.24	0.58
1982	6.0	0.88	0.17	0.22	0.56

[a]Mortality rate (NNMR) = deaths/1000 live births, as tabulated from resident deaths for each specific underlying cause.
[b]Although mortality rates after 1978 continue to reveal a downward trend, the International Classification of Disease Codes was revised between 1978 and 1979, which somewhat alters the baseline population.

Previous reports have noted that most neonatal deaths occurred during the first 24 hr of life and certainly within the first week. In their analysis, Manniello and Farrell [23] noted that 65% of all neonatal deaths secondary to the leading causalities occurred within 48 hr of birth. Since regionalization, Wisconsin's fatality rate during the first 24 hr following birth had declined by 50% and during the first week of life by 36% by 1978. Although firm conclusions may not be warranted, our interpretation of these data is that decreasing deaths occurring during the first week of life support the importance of perinatal rather than neonatal approach to care. Utilization of the six centers in Wisconsin during initial regionalization efforts has been evident. Approximately 60% of neonatal deaths occurred in tertiary centers in 1978 as compared to only 20% in 1968. These percentages reflect the average values for all centers with the range being somewhat wide, including one center with 75% of fatal illnesses within its region. Between 1979 and 1982 the neonatal mortality rate in Wisconsin averaged 6.7 deaths per 1000 live births. Of these 2000 total deaths, 393 succumbed to RDS. Of the latter, 52.2% were delivered in regional centers and 89.4% were cared for in regional special care nurseries.

As mentioned at the outset, it is difficult to establish the specific impact of regionalization. We conclude that the positive influence of regional care in Wisconsin is supported by the maintenance of the following: (1) low and progressively declining neonatal mortality rates, (2) consistent reduction in deaths from major treatable causes, and (3) marked shift in timing and place of death. Thus, for instance, the number of high-risk antepartum and intrapartum referrals to the Southcentral Regional Center has increased progressively in the past 5 years with 50% of resultant deliveries yielding infants requiring no special care. The trend in Wisconsin's perinatal medicine program is the prevention of serious neonatal disease. The ultimate goal is to reach a neonatal mortality rate hopefully as low as four to five deaths per 1000 live births, which presently approximates the so-called "unpreventable death rate" associated with disorders such as major congenital anomalies and extreme prematurity. As neonatal deaths resulting from the major causes discussed above continue to decline, other contributing factors such as congenital anomalies, genetic disorders, and birth injury may assume greater significance. While the absolute number of neonatal deaths is decreasing, a shift in the percent contribution of various disease states resulting in death is likely. Continued surveillance suggests a need for a shift in emphasis of outreach education for community practitioners and for early diagnostic requirements for pregnant women. Decrements in neonatal death rates cannot only be attributed in Wisconsin to a change in the incidence of deliveries of low birth weight infants. Although Lee et al. [25] have commented that the improvement in survival statistics for newborns in recent years is not derived from an altered population of disease-susceptible infants, it would be advantageous to have detailed information on very low birth weight infants inasmuch as this population has an inordinate influence on newborn mortality statistics. Although not currently available on a state by state basis, data on well-established record-keeping practices and cooperative processing of information among regionalized centers can provide invaluable information that can serve as a basis for establishing priority in perinatal health care research and services in the future.

References

1. Budin, P., *Le Nourisson, Alimentation et Hygeine des Enfants Débiles–Enfants nés à Terme.* Edited by Octane Dion. Paris, 1900.
2. Hess, J. H., *Premature and Congenitally Diseased Infants.* Philadelphia, Lea & Febiger, 1922.
3. Report of the Fifty-Ninth Ross Conference on Pediatric Research, *Problems of Neonatal Intensive Care Units.* Edited by J. F. Lucey. Columbus, Ohio, Ross Laboratories, 1969.
4. Swyer, P. R., The regional organization of special care for the neonate, *Pediatr. Clin. N. Am.,* **17**:761 (1970).
5. Swyer, P. R., The organization of perinatal care with particular reference to the newborn. In *Neonatology.* Edited by G. B. Avery. Philadelphia, Lippincott, 1975, pp. 15–34.
6. Mancianx, M., Organization of perinatal care in Europe. Methodology of evaluation. In *Perinatal Medicine.* Edited by H. Bossart, J. M. Crus, A. Huter, L. S. Prod'hom, and J. Sistek. Bern, Hans Huber, 1973, pp. 13–28.
7. Report of the Sixty-Sixth Ross Conference on Pediatric Research, *Regionalization of Perinatal Care.* Edited by P. Sunshine. Columbus, Ohio, Ross Laboratories, 1974.
8. Committee on Perinatal Health, *Towards Improving the Outcome of Pregnancy.* National Foundation – March of Dimes, 1977.
9. *Guidelines of Perinatal Care.* American Academy of Pediatrics, American College of Obstetrics and Gynecology, Evanston, Illinois, 1983.
10. Wisconsin Association for Perinatal Care. *Towards Improving the Outcome of Pregnancy in Wisconsin.* Madison, Wisconsin, 1983.
11. Sheridan, J. F., The typical perinatal center. *Clin. Perinatol.,* **10**(1):31 (1983).
12. Vreeland, R., and G. L. Lewis, Stresses on the nurse in an intensive-care unit, *J.A.M.A.,* **208**(2):332 (1969).
13. Marshall, N. E., and C. Kasmaw, Burnout in the neonatal intensive care unit, *Pediatrics,* **65**(6):1161 (1980).
14. Walker, C. H. M., Neonatal intensive care and stress, *Arch. Dis. Child.,* **57**:85 (1982).

15. Astbury, J., and V. Y. H. Yu, Determinants of stress for staff in a neonatal intensive care unit, *Arch. Dis. Child.*, **57**:108 (1982).
16. Brans, Y. W., Equipment available for nurseries. *Clin. Perinatol.*, **10**(1):263 (1983).
17. Harrison, H., *The Premature Baby Book.* New York, St. Martin's Press, 1983.
18. Feldman, B. H., and R. S. Suave, The infant transport service, *Clin. Perinatol.*, **3**:469 (1976).
19. Hood, J. L., A. Cross, B. Hulka, and E. E. Lawson, Effectiveness of the neonatal transport team. *Crit. Care Med.*, **11**:419 (1983).
20. Chance, G. W., J. D. Matthew, J. Gash, G. Williams, and K. Cunningham, Neonatal transport: A controlled study of skilled assistance. *J. Pediatr.*, **93**:662 (1978).
21. Pettett, G., G. B. Merenstein, F. C. Battaglia, L. J. Butterfield, and R. Efird, An analysis of air transport results in the sick newborn. Part I. The Transport Team, *Pediatrics,* **55**:774 (1975).
22. Perelman, R. H., and P. M. Farrell, Analysis of causes of neonatal death in the United States with specific emphasis on fatal hyaline membrane disease, *Pediatrics,* **70**:570 (1982).
23. Manniello, R. L., and P. M. Farrell, Analysis of United States neonatal mortality statistics from 1968 to 1974, with specific reference to changing trends in major causalities, *Am. J. Obstet. Gynecol.*, **129**:667 (1977).
24. Farrell, P. M., and R. E. Wood, Epidemiology of hyaline membrane disease in the United States: Analysis of national mortality statistics, *Pediatrics,* **58**:167 (1976).
25. Lee, K. S., N. Paneth, L. M. Gartner, M. A. Pearlman, and L. Gruss, Neonatal mortality: An analysis of the recent improvement in the United States, *Am. J. Public Health,* **70**:15 (1980).

16

Respiratory Distress Syndromes

ALEX. F. ROBERTSON, III

Medical College of Georgia
Augusta, Georgia

I. Introduction

Respiratory distress in the newborn is usually recognized by one or more of the following signs: tachypnea (>60 breaths/min), cyanosis in room air, retractions, and grunting. An excellent study from Sweden, which included one-third of all births in that country over a 1-year period, revealed an incidence of respiratory distress of 2.9% (1.7% in full-term infants, 28% in preterm infants) [1]. Table 1 illustrates the frequency of types of respiratory distress using nomenclature consistent with this chapter. Although respiratory distress may be the presenting sign in diseases as varied as choanal atresia and hypoglycemia, most cases of respiratory distress involve the pulmonary system and are etiologically related to alterations in fetal physiology or in the transitional physiology during and just after birth. The most common diagnoses considered are transitional respiratory distress, transient tachypnea of the newborn, hyaline membrane disease, aspiration syndromes (early-onset pneumonia and meconium aspiration), air-leak syndromes, persistent pulmonary hypertension, and pulmonary hypoplasia. These diagnoses we refer to as the respiratory distress syndromes. In this chapter we will emphasize the physiological changes which are associated with these diseases and discuss the clinical picture of each diagnosis.

Table 1 Frequency of Diagnosis of Respiratory Distress Syndromes

Diagnosis	% of Total
Transitional respiratory distress	38
Transient tachypnea of the newborn	32
Hyaline membrane disease	11
Early-onset pneumonia	6
Meconium aspiration syndrome	3
Air-leak syndromes	2
Persistent pulmonary hypertension	2
Congenital malformations (heart or diaphragm)	2
Other respiratory disorders	2
Pulmonary immaturity	1

Source: Ref. 1.

II. Transitional Respiratory Distress

We use this term to refer to the infant with mild respiratory distress beginning in the first hour of life who recovers or markedly improves by the sixth hour of life. Transition refers to the normal physiological events which begin at birth, ventilation of the lungs, progression from the fetal through the transitional circulation, and reabsorption of alveolar and interstitial lung fluid. This fleeting physiological depression, which is more common in male infants [1], may be triggered by prenatal hypoxia, maternal medications, the method of delivery, chilling, and certainly other unknown factors. Although it may occur at all gestational ages, the condition is more likely at or after 30 weeks' gestation [1], since the inciting event, occurring earlier in gestation, would likely lead to more severe maladaptation such as transient tachypnea or hyaline membrane disease. The infant with transitional respiratory distress may have tachypnea, retractions, grunting, and mild cyanosis. Auscultation may reveal crackling rales and a systolic ductus arteriosus murmur, both normal findings in the first hours of life. The chest x-ray will be normal for that age (Fig. 1), although we are tempted to overinterpret the fluid in the fissures and the prominent vascular markings. An immediate hematocrit level is necessary to rule out polycythemia or blood loss and a glucose level to rule out hypoglycemia. The immediate treatment should include a neutral thermal environment, and if cyanosis is present, an FI_{O_2} of 0.30–0.40. Whether oxygen is supplemented or not, the arterial blood gases are

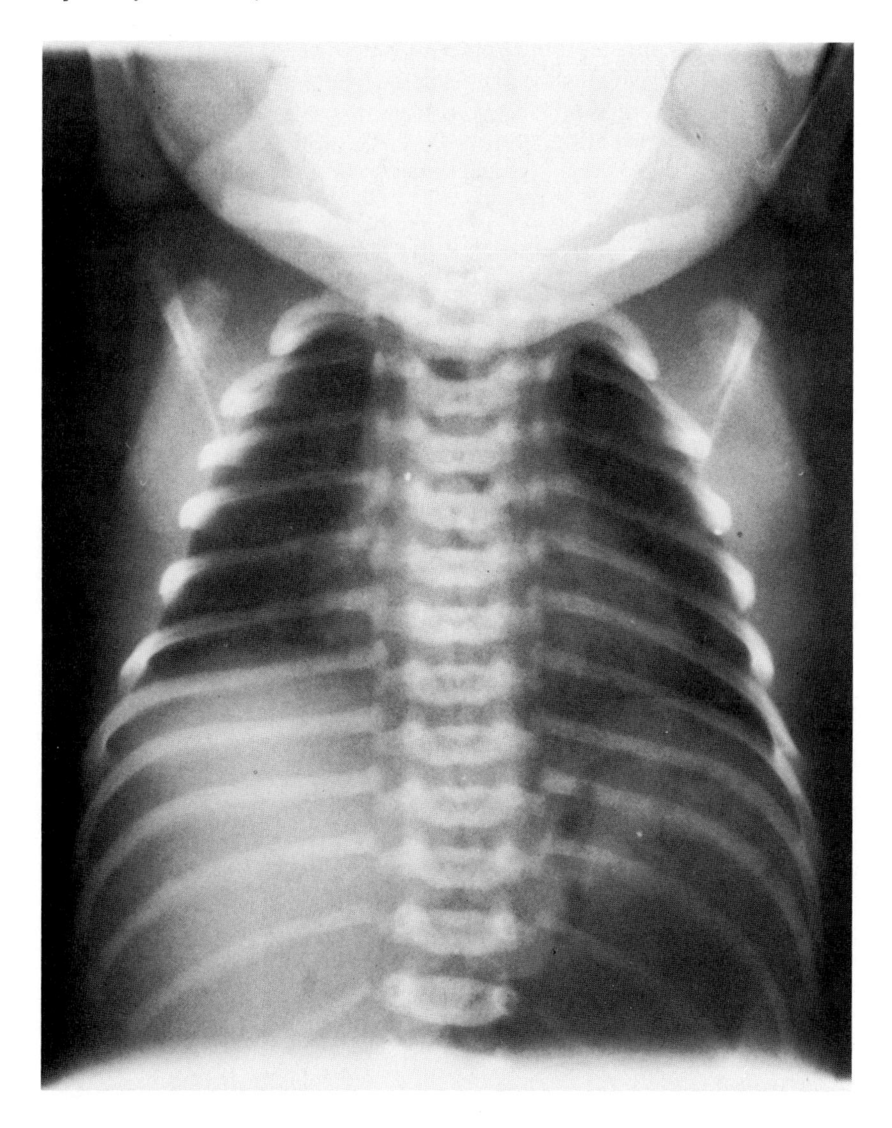

Figure 1 Normal newborn x-ray.

determined shortly after admission. Presuming a normal physical exam, x-ray, blood glucose level, and hematocrit level, and no evidence of airway obstruction, we should observe this infant for up to 6 hr of age if the arterial PO_2 can be maintained above 50 mmHg with an FI_{O_2} below 0.40. Often, in that time the infant will recover, and his difficulties may then be called transitional respiratory distress. If improvement is not marked within 6 hr or if over 0.40 FI_{O_2} is required, this condition is no longer considered transitional respiratory distress and the infant is sent to the intensive care nursery for closer monitoring and further diagnostic procedures.

III. Transient Tachypnea of the Newborn

Transient tachypnea of the newborn is a frequent diagnosis referring to respiratory distress lasting beyond the postnatal adjustment period of 6 hr and characterized primarily by tachypnea [2]. It is probably the same disease as the previously described respiratory distress syndrome type II [3], which was earlier thought to be caused by aspiration of amniotic fluid. Transient tachypnea is

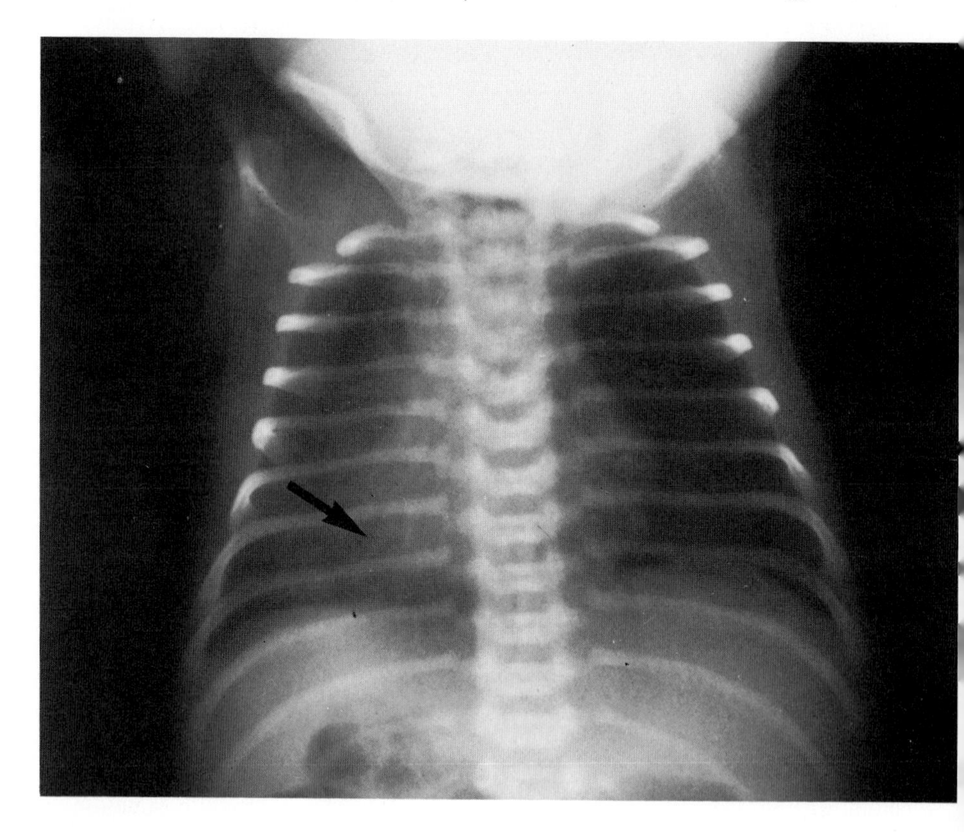

Figure 2 Transient tachypnea of the newborn. The arrow points to prominent, ill-defined vascular markings.

also referred to as wet-lung disease. Because the x-ray shows prominent vascular markings and small effusions in the fissures, a suggested etiology has been delayed resorption of alveolar fluid.

The fetal lungs are partially distended by fluid produced within the airways. Adaptation to air breathing requires that the production of this fluid be diminished and that the fluid present in the lungs be eliminated. It is possible that fetal catecholamine production, stimulated by labor, suppresses this fluid production [4]. A similar role for vasopressin has been suggested. Part of the fluid present at birth is extruded through the nasopharynx [5], and this extrusion is facilitated by uterine pressure on the thorax after delivery of the head. Alveolar fluid also enters the pulmonary interstitial space aided first by the subatmospheric pressure of that space with inspiration, and then by the positive pressure of expiration [6]. Subsequently, reabsorption may proceed from the interstitial space via the lymphatics and/or pulmonary capillaries. Humidification of inspired air also accounts for some fluid removal. A delay in the suppression of fluid production or in its reabsorption could lead to decreased lung compliance and respiratory distress, and this may explain the apparent increase in cases of transient tachypnea of the newborn when the infant is delivered by cesarean section [7]. Infants born by cesarean section have decreased pulmonary compliance for up to 48 hr which is less marked when labor has begun prior to the operative delivery [8].

Most descriptions of transient tachypnea of the newborn mention mild cardiomegaly. Echocardiographic studies in sick infants [9] suggest that transient tachypnea of the newborn may result from transient ventricular failure as a result of birth asphyxia. Previous studies had shown no evidence of heart failure [7]. This disaccord probably results from the inclusion of several different diseases of varying etiologies in our diagnosis of transient tachypnea of the newborn. As an example, simple hypervolemia may resemble transient tachypnea of the newborn [10]. Also, what we described as transitional respiratory distress, resolving itself by 6 hr of age, would be considered by many as an extremely mild form of transient tachypnea of the newborn.

The first infants described as cases of transient tachypnea were usually born at term, but it is now known that the incidence of transient tachypnea increases with decreasing gestational age. No specific antenatal events have been clearly associated with transient tachypnea of the newborn, but transient tachypnea seems more frequent in diabetic progeny and infants born by cesarean section [11]. Other risk factors mentioned are prenatal asphyxia and excessive maternal sedation.

In cases of transient tachypnea, the onset of respiratory distress is at or shortly after birth. The common findings upon physical examination are tachypnea without significant retractions or rales and relatively normal alveolar ventilation as measured by blood pH and PCO_2. Oxygen requirements vary, but 0.40

FI_{O_2} suffices to maintain an adequate arterial PO_2 in most cases. In cases requiring a very high FI_{O_2}, there may well be persistent pulmonary hypertension resulting from hyperinflation secondary to air trapping [12]. The typical chest radiograph shows prominent, ill-defined vascular markings (Fig. 2), edematous interlobar septa, and pleural effusions. There is usually mild to moderate hyperaeration and mild cardiomegaly [13]. Since many asymptomatic infants have these radiological features in the first 2 hr of life, the early x-ray is not diagnostic [14]. A more remarkable but relatively uncommon picture consisting of partial or complete opacification of the right lung has also been described [15]. The respiratory distress has usually stabilized by 12-24 hr, and the chest radiographs are improved within 24 hr. In a premature infant with respiratory distress it is sometimes difficult to differentiate transient tachypnea of the newborn from hyaline membrane disease if the initial x-ray is not diagnostic of either. Usually at 24 hr, the stabilization of the clinical course and improvement in the x-ray clarifies a diagnosis of transient tachypnea of the newborn, although in occasional cases the question remains. The clinical picture may take 3-7 days to clear up, with recurring episodes of tachypnea. Recovery is complete, and there are no sequelae.

IV. Hyaline Membrane Disease

Hyaline membrane disease (also known as idiopathic respiratory distress syndrome and type I respiratory distress syndrome) is best described as progressive atelectasis with surfactant deficiency, occurring almost exclusively in premature infants. The reliability of amniotic fluid lecithin levels in predicting the absence of hyaline membrane disease establishes surfactant as a key factor in the syndrome [16]. The surfactant system is discussed at length in other chapters. The clinical risk factors for hyaline membrane disease are less clear, but include gestational age, perinatal asphyxia, route of delivery, and previous delivery of a premature infant with hyaline membrane disease.

Prematurity is a necessity for an unequivocal diagnosis of hyaline membrane disease. The incidence and severity of hyaline membrane disease increases with decreasing gestational age [17] (see Table 2).

Perinatal asphyxia is a clear risk factor [18,19] and may explain the higher incidence of hyaline membrane disease in the second-born infant of twins [20].

Another clear risk is cesarean section delivery [21]. Even though much controversy surrounds the question of the risk from elective vs. emergency cesarean section, our current opinion is that abdominal delivery increases the incidence of hyaline membrane disease. Although the incidence of hyaline membrane disease is not clearly lessened by the onset of labor prior to cesarean

Table 2 Incidence of Hyaline Membrane Disease in Vaginal Deliveries

Gestation (completed weeks)	Incidence
37-40	.9
35-36	5.4
33-34	20.5
31-32	35.0
29-30	64.3

Source: Ref. 17.

section [22], the incidence of death from hyaline membrane disease is apparently lessened by the onset of labor prior to cesarean section [23].

After the delivery of an infant with hyaline membrane disease, subsequent premature infants born to that mother have a greater than 90% incidence of hyaline membrane disease. The incidence of hyaline membrane disease after the delivery of a premature infant without hyaline membrane disease is only 3% [24]. That these incidences may represent a maternal genetic factor is suggested by the equal incidence of hyaline membrane disease in both maternal half siblings and full siblings of the affected infants [25].

An iatrogenic risk related to gestational age, the unintentional premature delivery of infants due to obstetrical intervention, represents 12-15% of the cases of hyaline membrane disease in the United States and Canada [26]. Male sex increases both the incidence of hyaline membrane disease [25] and the mortality rate from the disease [27]. Diabetes is frequently mentioned as a risk factor, but reports which control the effect of gestational age and route of delivery conflict in their conclusions [17,28].

Some factors apparently reduce the risk of hyaline membrane disease. Prolonged rupture of the membranes was reported as one such factor [29], but subsequent studies have not resolved the question of whether it does reduce the risk of hyaline membrane disease [30]. Other forms of chronic stress such as maternal hypertension are more convincing [31]. Maternal heroin addiction may also be protective [32].

The clinical picture is characterized by the early onset (< 6 hr of age) of progressively worsening respiratory distress with physical findings of decreased lung compliance (poor air exchange), increased work of breathing (retractions, nasal flaring, "seesaw" respirations), and grunting respirations. Hypoxia results from right-to-left shunting through the foramen ovale and ductus arteriosus due

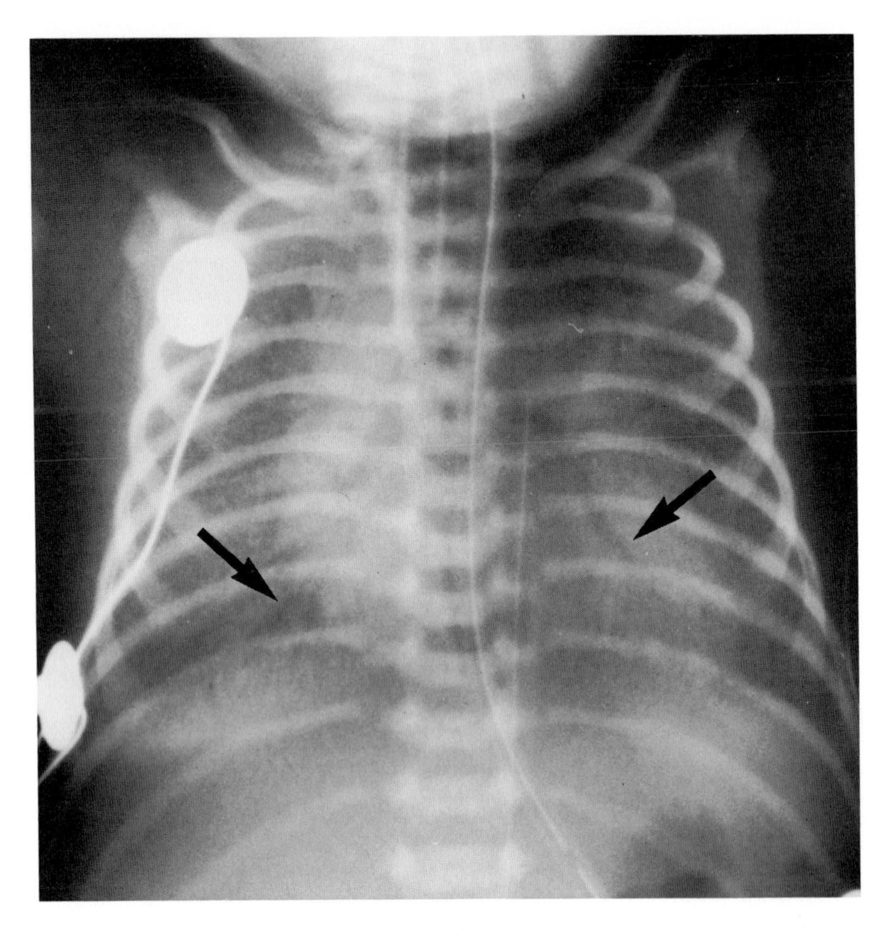

Figure 3 Hyaline membrane disease. The arrows point to air bronchograms. The reticulogranular pattern is most obvious throughout the right lung.

to pulmonary hypertension and from perfusion of unventilated, atelectatic areas of the lung. CO_2 retention occurs later as the infant tires from the work of breathing. At about 72 hr, the problem reaches a peak, and recovery usually occurs within the next 7 days.

In the typical case of hyaline membrane disease with progressive distress and an x-ray showing a fine reticulogranular pattern with air bronchograms (Fig. 3), the diagnosis is clear. Two situations can make this diagnosis difficult. In the first 24 hr, the x-ray may not be diagnostic and, thus, the differentiation from transient tachypnea of the newborn is impossible. This uncertainty is usually resolved in the second and third day of life, since hyaline membrane disease tends to worsen, whereas transient tachypnea of the newborn peaks in severity between 12-24 hr of age. A second diagnostic problem is the question of pneumonia. The early onset form of group B streptococcal pneumonia may result in an x-ray picture consistent with a diagnosis of hyaline membrane disease [33]. In most cases where this question arises, systemic antibiotics are given until blood and cerebrospinal fluid culture results are known.

The treatment of hyaline membrane disease is directed toward minimizing those factors which promote pulmonary hypertension such as hypoxia, acidosis, systemic hypotension, and cold stress. Aside from advances in assisted ventilation technology, the use of continuous distending pressure is the most notable advance in the treatment of hyaline membrane disease [34]. In theory, this method prevents alveolar collapse, thereby improving oxygenation and may also preserve available surfactant [16]. In practice, continuous distending pressure improves oxygenation and the main question is how early to institute it [35]. The decision to place an infant on intermittent mandatory ventilation is reached on the basis of the clinical course and arterial blood gases. An excellent text on assisted ventilation in newborns was published in 1981 [36].

There are numerous areas of uncertainty in regard to treatment of hyaline membrane disease. Several studies have shown a decreased red blood cell volume in infants with hyaline membrane disease [37,38]. The blood volume changes seen in conjunction with hyaline membrane disease are not reflected by change in the systemic blood pressure, although some of these infants appear peripherally vasoconstricted. The common use of volume expanders shortly after birth is controversial, since studies have suggested that this practice impairs pulmonary oxygen exchange [39], and they may be related to the occurrence of subependymal hemorrhages [40,41]. We use volume expanders only when the infant is clinically vasoconstricted and the blood pressure is >2 standard deviations below the published figures for premature infants [42].

It is also unclear at what level the hematocrit should be maintained to facilitate oxygenation during the most severe phase of the disease. Since assisted ventilation may decrease cardiac output, it is probably wise to maintain an hematocrit >40% [43]. Since hypoxia is caused partially by right-to-left shunting, some authors suggest a trial of tolazoline in severe hyaline membrane disease to lower the pulmonary resistance [44].

A frequent concern in the care of infants with severe hyaline membrane disease is the effect of a patent ductus arteriosus. The occurrence of a patent ductus arteriosus is clearly related to gestational age and the presence of hyaline membrane disease, occurring in about one-third of the infants < 1500 g birth weight with hyaline membrane disease. Over half of these infants with a patent ductus arteriosus and hyaline membrane disease develop congestive cardiac failure [45]. As recovery from hyaline membrane disease begins at 3-4 days of life and the pulmonary vascular resistance falls, left-to-right shunting through the patent ductus arteriosus increases. The increased pulmonary blood flow, pulmonary vascular congestion, and increased interstitial water result in the increased work of breathing, a rise in the PCO_2, and continued or increased ventilator dependency. The heart may be enlarged, the pulse pressure widened, and a systolic or continuous murmur present. An increase in the left atrium/aorta width ratio on echocardiography is helpful in assessing the significance of the ductal shunt. Both the occurrence and the morbidity of a patent ductus arteriosus are probably affected by the level of fluid intake [46]. This association between hyaline membrane disease and fluid intake has led to fluid restriction in small infants with severe hyaline membrane disease. If the patent ductus arteriosus is associated with signs of heart failure, the treatment is further fluid restriction, diuretics, and digoxin. Closure of the ductus, if not spontaneous, will occur in about one-half of the infants treated with indomethacin, a prostaglandin synthetase inhibitor [47]; otherwise surgical ligation may be necessary.

The prognosis in hyaline membrane disease is excellent when tertiary level care is available. In cases of extreme prematurity, death usually occurs in the first 3 days of life as a result of ventilation failure. In more mature infants, death may occur later due to complications of assisted ventilation, primarily pulmonary interstitial emphysema and bronchopulmonary dysplasia.

Bronchopulmonary dysplasia is the term used to describe a spectrum of chronic lung changes which may develop during the treatment of hyaline membrane disease. Eleven to 21% of premature infants with severe hyaline membrane disease who have been treated with intermittent mandatory ventilation and oxygen for >24 hr will develop this condition [48]. Although each of these factors (prematurity, hyaline membrane disease, intermittent mandatory ventilation, and supplemental oxygen) apparently contributes to the development of bronchopulmonary dysplasia, the most important single factor is probably high-pressure ventilation [49]. The risk of bronchopulmonary dysplasia is increased in infants with pulmonary interstitial emphysema [50] and patent ductus arteriosus [51].

The condition is considered when there is an unusually slow, or arrested, recovery from hyaline membrane disease at 4–14 days of age. The infant requires unusually high or increasing ventilator settings and supplemental oxygen. In addition, CO_2 retention may be the first sign of pulmonary insufficiency.

The diagnosis is made by x-ray, and is characterized by the appearance of translucent cystic areas and dense bands of fibrosis (Fig. 4).

These pulmonary abnormalities may clear up over the ensuing weeks or months but about 40% of the infants with this complication of therapy will die [52]. Death usually results from progressive pulmonary insufficiency and cor pulmonale.

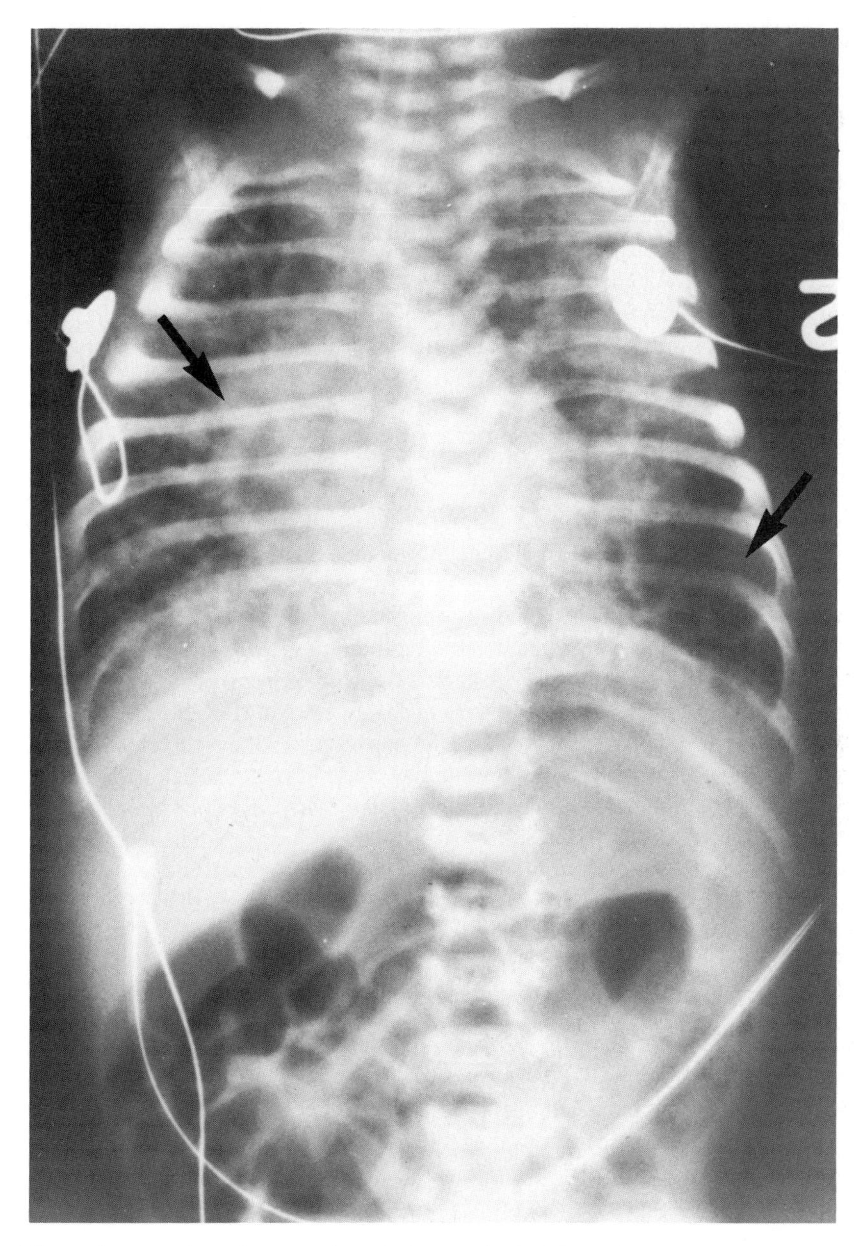

Figure 4 Bronchopulmonary dysplasia. In the left lung the arrow points to a translucent cystic area. In the right lung the arrow points to dense bands of fibrosis.

There is no clearly effective therapy for bronchopulmonary dysplasia. The possible role of oxygen toxicity in the etiology of the disease led to the consideration of using the antioxidant vitamin E [53]. Subsequent investigation has shown that vitamin E is not effective in preventing bronchopulmonary dysplasia [54]. The high incidence of patent ductus arteriosus in infants developing bronchopulmonary dysplasia led to the consideration of fluid overload and chronic pulmonary edema as contributing factors [55]. Preliminary studies suggest that administration of the diuretic furosemide (Lasix) may ameliorate the disease [56]. Bronchopulmonary dysplasia is one of the most discouraging results of our treatment methods. The use of high-frequency ventilation, resulting in lower peak inspiratory pressure, may in the future decrease the incidence of bronchopulmonary dysplasia.

V. Aspiration Syndromes

The aspiration of amniotic fluid and its contents by the fetus may lead to respiratory distress. Normal fetal breathing movements, as observed in animals, will not introduce amniotic fluid into the lungs [57], but if the fetus is provoked (e.g., by asphyxia) to make gasping movements, it will inhale amniotic fluid. The aspiration of uncontaminated amniotic fluid, prenatally or intrapartum, probably causes little respiratory distress. The clinical pictures previously attributed to amniotic fluid aspiration were probably cases of transitional respiratory distress or transient tachypnea of the newborn. The two common situations in which amniotic fluid aspiration may cause respiratory distress are the meconium aspiration syndrome and congenital or early-onset pneumonia. A very unusual relationship of respiratory distress and the aspiration of amniotic fluid contents is the respiratory difficulty seen in newborns with congenital ichthyosis. This respiratory distress is presumably due to increased amniotic fluid debris from excessive fetal skin desquamation [58].

A. Meconium Aspiration Syndrome

The presence of meconium-stained amniotic fluid occurs in 10–20% of deliveries. The passage of meconium is probably a response to hypoxia. Since the majority of infants with meconium-stained amniotic fluid do not show either meconium aspiration syndrome or other signs of asphyxia, the risk of aspiration is difficult to assess in the delivery room. Table 3 presents a classification of meconium passage in labor from a prospective study [59]. Using this classification, over 50% were categorized as I-A (early-light), and had a neonatal course with few problems. Two-thirds of the cases of meconium aspiration syndrome came from the I-B (early-heavy) category and one-third from the II (late) category.

Table 3 Classification of Meconium Passage in Labor

A. Early: Noted on rupture of the fetal membranes prior to or during the active phase of labor.
   1. Light meconium: lightly stained amniotic fluid, yellow or greenish in color.
   2. Heavy meconium: darkly stained amniotic fluid, dark green or black, usually thick and tenacious.

B. Late: Meconium-stained fluid noted in the second stage of labor after clear fluid had been noted previously.

Source: Ref. 59.

Although alveolar meconium has been found in stillborn infants [60] and in infants well-suctioned before the delivery of the body [61], it is likely that most of the aspiration occurs after delivery of the chest. Therefore, the accepted practice is to suction the nasopharynx before the chest is delivered. Experimental work indicates that catheter suction is far better than bulb suction [62]. A significant number of infants who develop respiratory distress will not have obvious meconium in the mouth or larynx [63]. Therefore, the trachea should be examined as soon as possible in all infants with early-heavy meconium-stained amniotic fluid and suctioned until no more meconium is visible. The efficacy of suctioning the trachea as a preventive and ameliorative measure is well established [64]. Tracheal lavage is not beneficial [65]. It is advisable to aspirate the stomach soon after birth to prevent further meconium aspiration.

The clinical picture of meconium aspiration syndrome is depression at birth due to asphyxia, and immediate respiratory distress after resuscitation. If the infant and/or placenta are meconium stained, it indicates that the hypoxic episode occurred at least 4–6 hr before delivery, and in this instance the mortality rate is higher, although not necessarily from the result of aspiration [66]. Meconium leads to air trapping by a ball-valve mechanism; overdistention of the chest is obvious. The x-ray shows multiple patchy areas of decreased aeration mixed with hyperlucent areas (Fig. 5). As a result of the preceding asphyxia, the peripheral blood count frequently shows an abnormal number of immature neutrophils [67]. There is an interesting clinical association between thrombocytopenia and meconium aspiration, especially in those cases that develop persistent pulmonary hypertension. It is suggested that amniotic fluid constituents may cause platelet aggregation and release of pulmonary vasoconstrictors [68]. The seriousness of the disease varies with the degree of chemical pneumonitis caused by the meconium, the occurrence of air-leak syndrome in about 40% of cases [69], and the presence of persistent pulmonary hypertension. For these

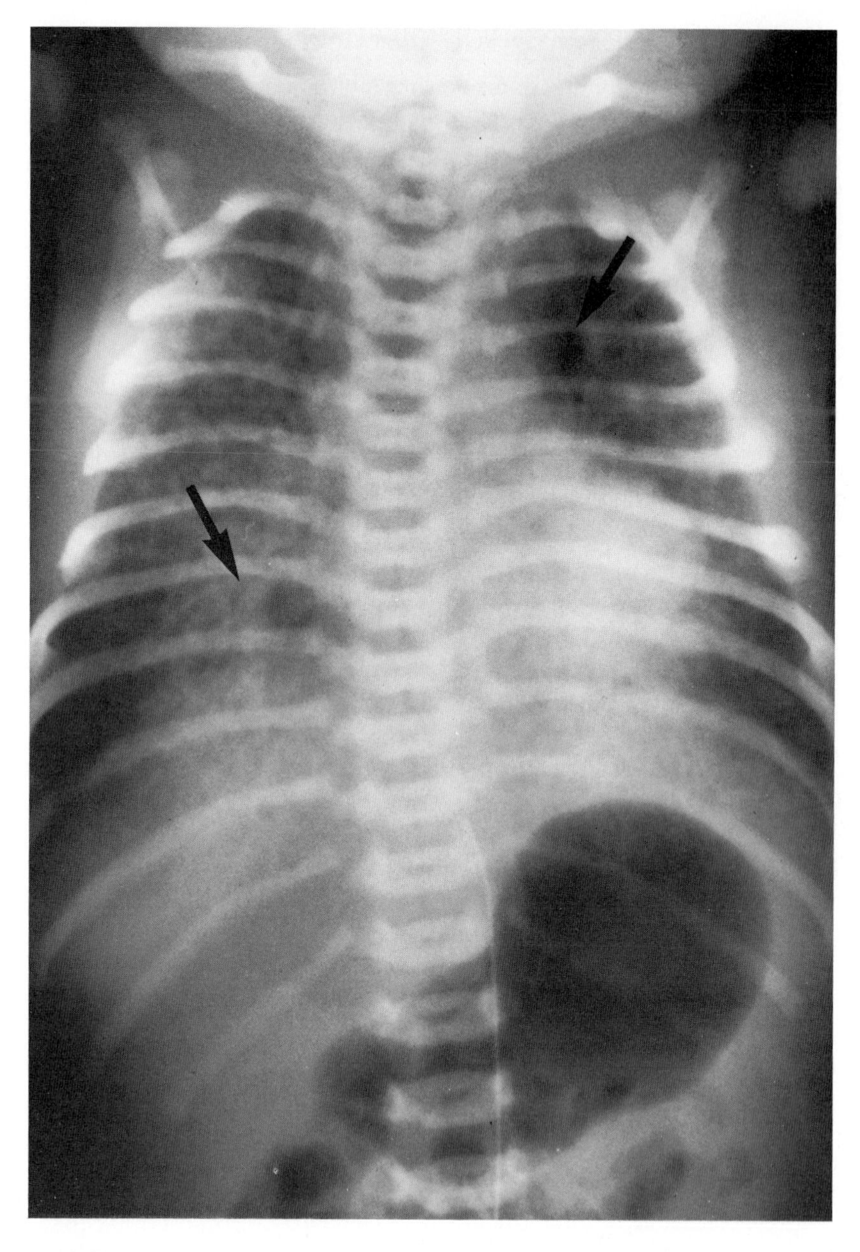

Figure 5 Meconium aspiration syndrome. In the right lung the arrow points to a patchy area of decreased aeration. In the left lung the arrow points to a hyperlucent area.

reasons, it is difficult to predict the outcome of meconium aspiration until several days after birth except in mild cases. Other complications, which are less frequent, are bacterial pneumonia, subglottic stenosis in those requiring intermittent mandatory ventilation, and pulmonary hemorrhage [70].

Aside from the preventive measures mentioned earlier, chest physiotherapy and postural drainage may help to remove residual meconium. Ventilatory therapy consists of supplementary oxygen, continuous distending airway pressure, and intermittent mandatory ventilation. These infants frequently require high peak inspiratory pressures. Because of the high ventilatory pressures required, their restlessness, and their tendency toward air leak many centers use neuromuscular blockade for the first day or two of intermittent mandatory ventilation. There is no clinical evidence that antibiotics are of value prophylactically. The use of steroids apparently retards recovery [71]. Remembering that many of these infants have had a severe prenatal asphyxial event, the neonatologist must be alert to the possibilities of severe metabolic acidosis, transient myocardial ischemia, persistent pulmonary hypertension, anuria, hyperglycemia, and encephalopathy.

About one-third of the cases of meconium aspiration syndrome die. There are no apparent pulmonary sequelae among the survivors. Most worrisome is the high incidence of psychomotor retardation among those infants with meconium aspiration syndrome and seizures during the neonatal period [72], presumably due to hypoxemic-ischemic encephalopathy.

B. Early-Onset Pneumonia

Another possible aspiration syndrome is congenital or early-onset pneumonia. In the last 75 years, the predominant disease-producing organisms in neonates have varied between group A β-hemolytic streptococcus, staphylococcus aureus, gram-negative organisms, and group B β-hemolytic streptococcus [73]. Most organisms cause a similar clinical picture in the neonate, but since our experience is so much greater with group B streptococcal infections, we will discuss group B streptococcal pneumonia as characteristic of most types of early-onset pneumonia. It is difficult to determine if the pneumonia truly arises from aspiration of contaminated amniotic fluid. In favor of this theory are the following facts: Respiratory distress with pneumonia is the predominant clinical picture at birth, similar serotypes are in the vagina of mothers with affected babies, prolonged rupture of the membranes is a risk factor, and the majority of the mothers are not clinically ill [74]. However, group B streptococcal infection may also begin as a bloodstream infection in the fetus. Arguments for this theory are that infants may have positive blood cultures without pneumonia and that the respiratory distress may result from the effects on the pulmonary microvasculature of a toxin produced by group B streptococcus [75].

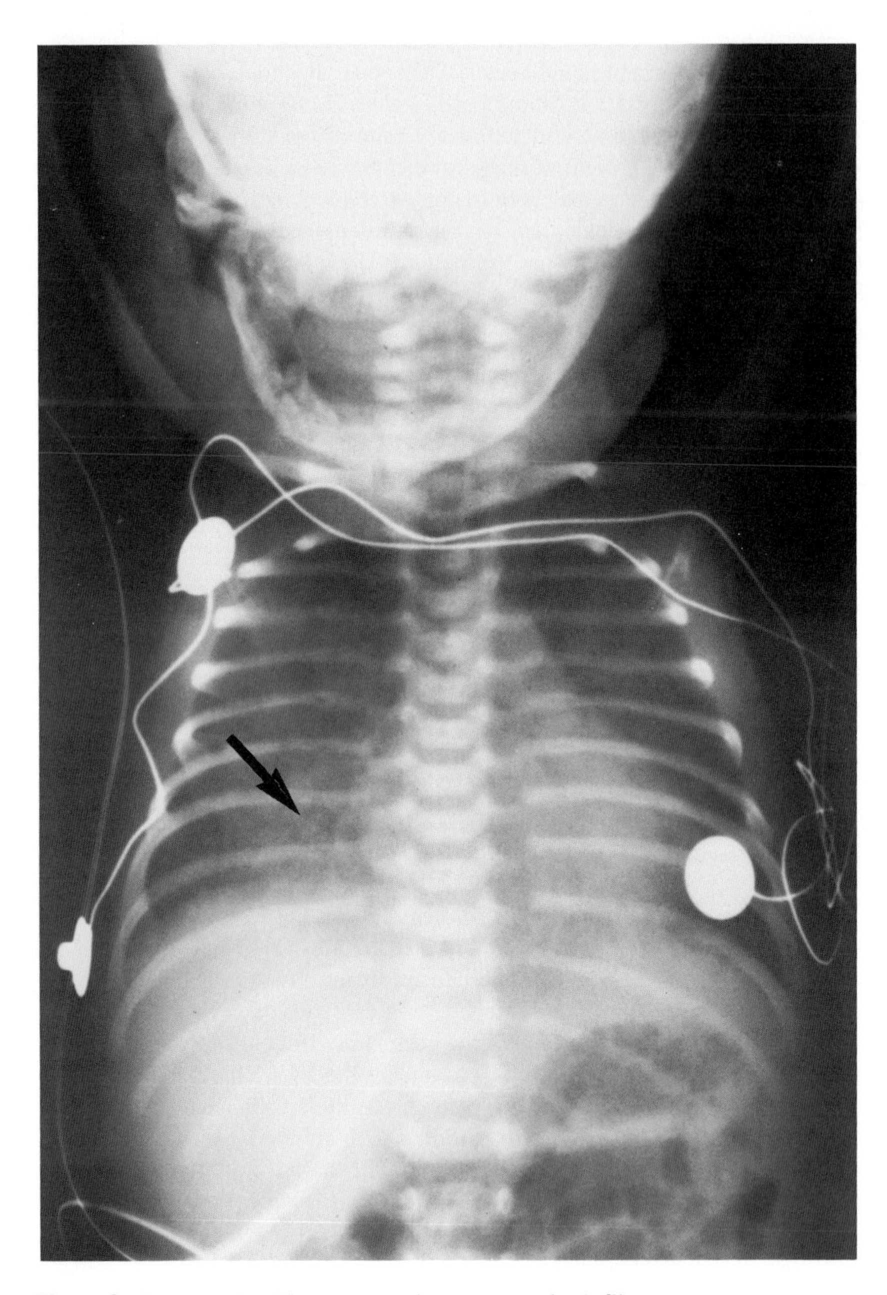

Figure 6 Pneumonia. The arrow points to a patchy infiltrate.

The clinical risk factors are prematurity and prolonged rupture of the membranes. The disease is more common in male infants. Although most colonized mothers are asymptomatic, a fair number will have postpartum endometritis after cesarean section [76]. Of the mothers colonized with group B streptococcus, over one-half of their infants will be colonized and 1–2% of colonized infants will develop clinical disease [74]. The susceptibility of the infant to infection is related to the absence of maternal antibodies which would otherwise cross the placenta and protect the infant [77].

The clinical picture shows respiratory distress at or shortly after birth. The x-ray may show patchy infiltrates (Fig. 6) typical of pneumonia, but many infants have a radiological picture indistinquishable from hyaline membrane disease. The clinical differentiation of pneumonia from hyaline membrane disease is difficult. Although some reports stress that early-onset pneumonia is more frequently associated with hypotension and apnea in the first 24 hr of life [33, 78], others have found no clinical difference [79]. It is now common practice to do a sepsis workup and begin antibiotics on all infants with a radiological picture of hyaline membrane disease, especially if there is a history of maternal chorioamnionitis and/or prolonged rupture of the membranes. The clinical disease varies from mild respiratory distress to overwhelming infection and death in the first day or two. The treatment is cardiorespiratory support and antibiotics. It is unlikely that the antibiotics administered shortly after birth affect the course of the disease in the first 48 hr of life and, therefore, their prophylactic use is not generally recommended. Prophylactic antibiotics are recommended in multiple births when one sibling is infected, since the risk of occurrence in the apparently healthy sibling is so high [80]. The mortality of early-onset infection is about 50% [74]. In survivors, recovery is usually complete, especially in the absence of meningitis. However, there are reports of subsequent right diaphragmatic hernias developing in the course of the disease and persisting after recovery. The hernia, presumably, results from involvement of the diaphragm by the etiological organism [81,82].

VI. The Air-Leak Syndromes

The air-leak syndromes are pneumothorax, pneumomediastinum, and pulmonary interstitial emphysema. The basic anatomical mechanism is rupture of the alveolus with dissection of the air along the vascular sheaths to the lung root. This perivascular air is referred to as pulmonary (or intrapulmonary) interstitial emphysema. At the lung root, rupture of the mediastinal wall may lead to the accumulation of air in the mediastinal compartments (pneumomediastinum) and in the interpleural space (pneumothorax) [83]. Alternately, the interstitial air can penetrate directly into the pleural cavity after rupture of a subpleural bleb.

Direct penetration may explain why pneumomediastinum does not always accompany pneumothorax [84]. The predisposing factors relate to alveolar pressure and unequal alveolar ventilation. The first breaths of an infant may generate negative interpleural pressures of up to -70 cmH_2O [85], and these pressures may explain the air-leak syndromes in otherwise normal infants. Also, any uneven inflation of parts of the lung would result in the already open alveoli being exposed to all the pressure applied to the unopen alveoli. This excessive pressure could result from collapsed alveoli in hyaline membrane disease, small airway plugs in the aspiration syndromes, or fluid-filled alveoli in transient tachypnea of the newborn. Aspiration of material such as blood and meconium may result in a ball-valve action, leading to alveolar rupture [86]. Any decreased volume of the lung causing hypoxia leads to enhanced respiratory efforts which produce unusually large negative pressures, and for this reason atelectasis and pulmonary hypoplasia increase the risk of air-leak syndromes.

The incidence of air leak in routine deliveries, cesarean section, and delivery of normal premature infants is 1–2% [87]. Most air leaks in term infants are not symptomatic; the incidence of symptomatic cases is about one in 1000 deliveries. Usually, the term infant with symptomatic air leak has been meconium stained and/or required resuscitation. The occurrence of air leak increases in premature infants with hyaline membrane disease primarily due to an increase in widespread interstitial emphysema. With the use of continuous distending pressure and intermittent mandatory ventilation, the incidence of air leak rises to around 25% [88].

The diagnosis of air leak should be considered in any newborn infant with respiratory distress. The physical exam of an infant with pneumothorax may show bulging of one side of the chest, decreased respiratory movements on one side, and decreased breath sounds. However, none of these signs are consistently present. In premature infants, the signs are even less reliable, and the main clinical indicators are abrupt changes in the vital signs and blood gases [89,90]. Depending upon the severity of the clinical signs, diagnosis can be made by x-ray (Fig. 7), transillumination [91], or needle aspiration. Occasionally, a small pneumothorax may not be easily seen on an AP film of a supine infant. A lateral decubitus view will help reveal small air collections.

Treatment is not necessary in mildly symptomatic cases. In full-term infants, not seriously distressed, the administration of 100% oxygen will result in more rapid resolution of the pneumothorax by washing out the nitrogen and the oxygen being absorbed into the tissues and blood. If needle aspiration has to be repeated or if the infant is on intermittent mandatory ventilation, a chest tube and water-sealed suction are needed. Aside from cardiorespiratory complications, pneumothorax has also been associated with inappropriate antidiuretic hormone secretion [92], subependymal hemorrhage [93], and both pneumoperitoneum and pneumopericardium [94,95].

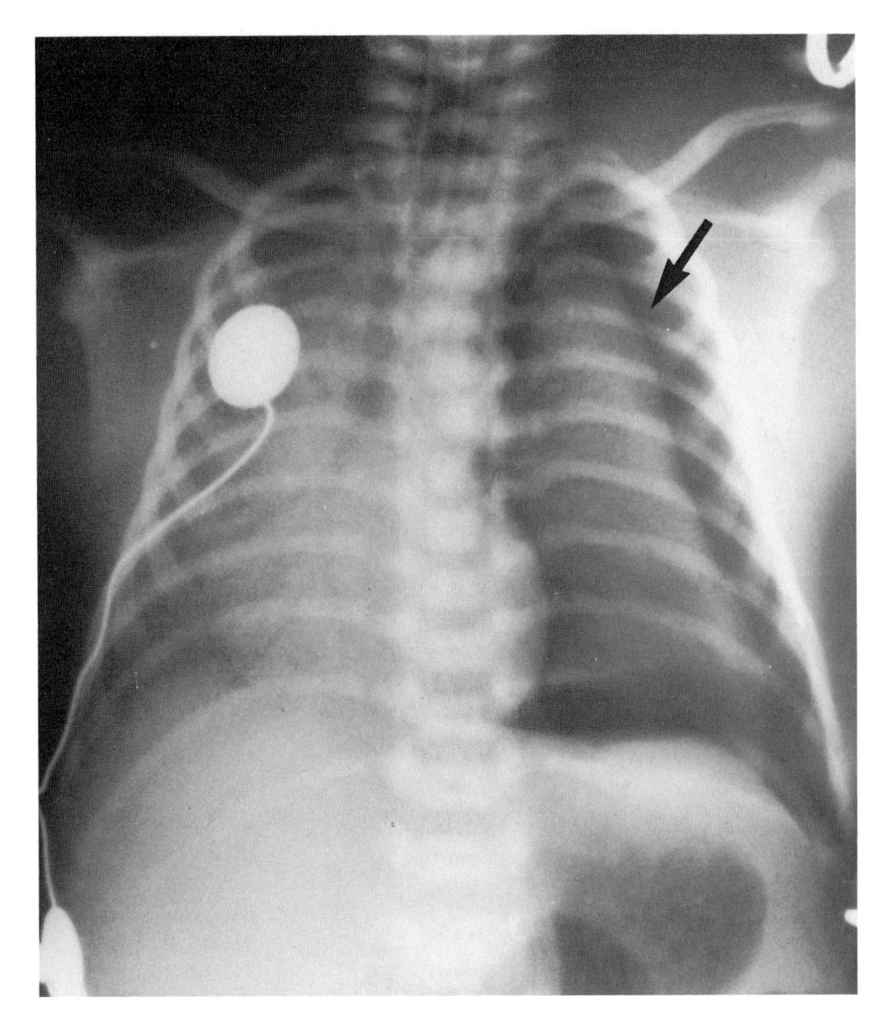

Figure 7 Pneumothorax. The arrow points to the interpleural collection of air.

Pneumomediastinum physiologically usually precedes pneumothorax, and the two are usually coexistent. In isolated pneumomediastinum the physical exam shows respiratory distress and only rarely a bulging sternal area and/or a shift of the heart sounds to the right side of the chest. The diagnosis is made using x-ray or transillumination. The PA view will show air adjacent to the border of the heart and, frequently, elevation of the thymus (Fig. 8). The lateral view will show air replacing the normal thymic shadow (Fig. 9). Treatment is

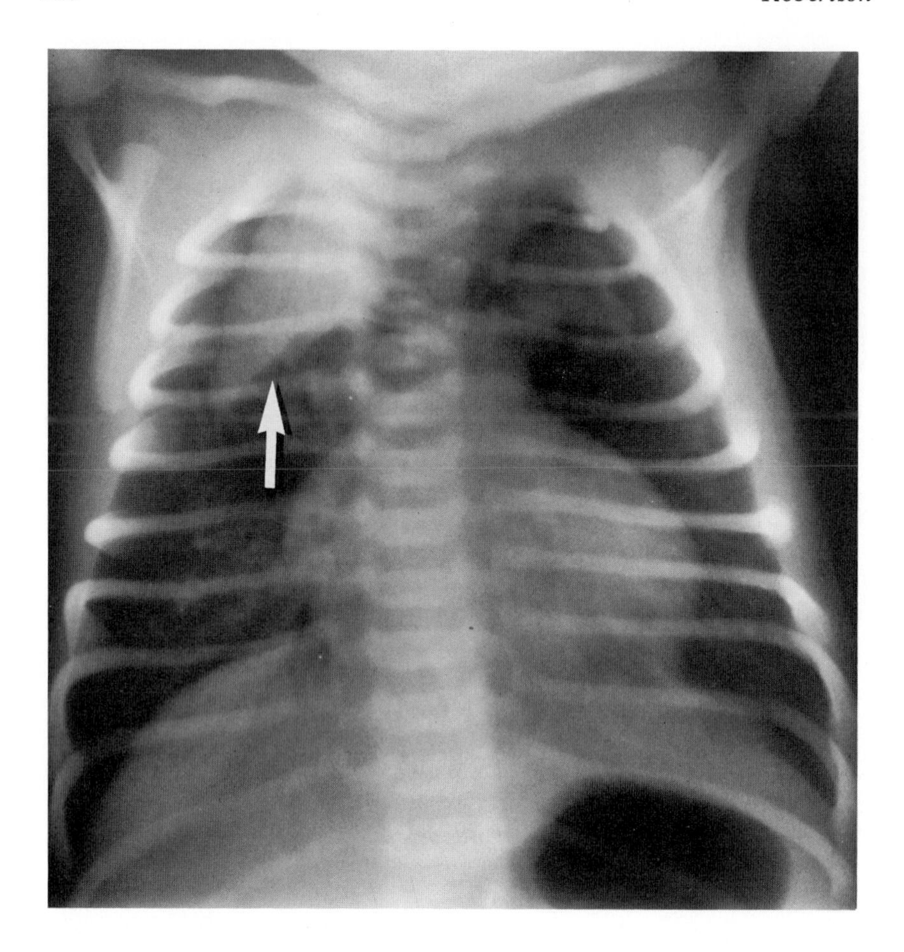

Figure 8 Pneumomediastinum. The arrow points to the elevated thymus.

usually limited to 100% oxygen in full-term infants, and in premature infants supplemental oxygen can be used if the arterial oxygen levels are being monitored. Needle aspiration generally is not advisable, since it is not therapeutic due to the loculation of air in separate, small compartments of the mediastinum. Aspiration of air is sometimes attempted and successful when severe cardiovascular signs result from compression of the superior vena cava and pulmonary veins [96]. When and if the mediastinal air ruptures into the interpleural space, the pneumomediastinum either resolves spontaneously or the pneumothorax may be treated.

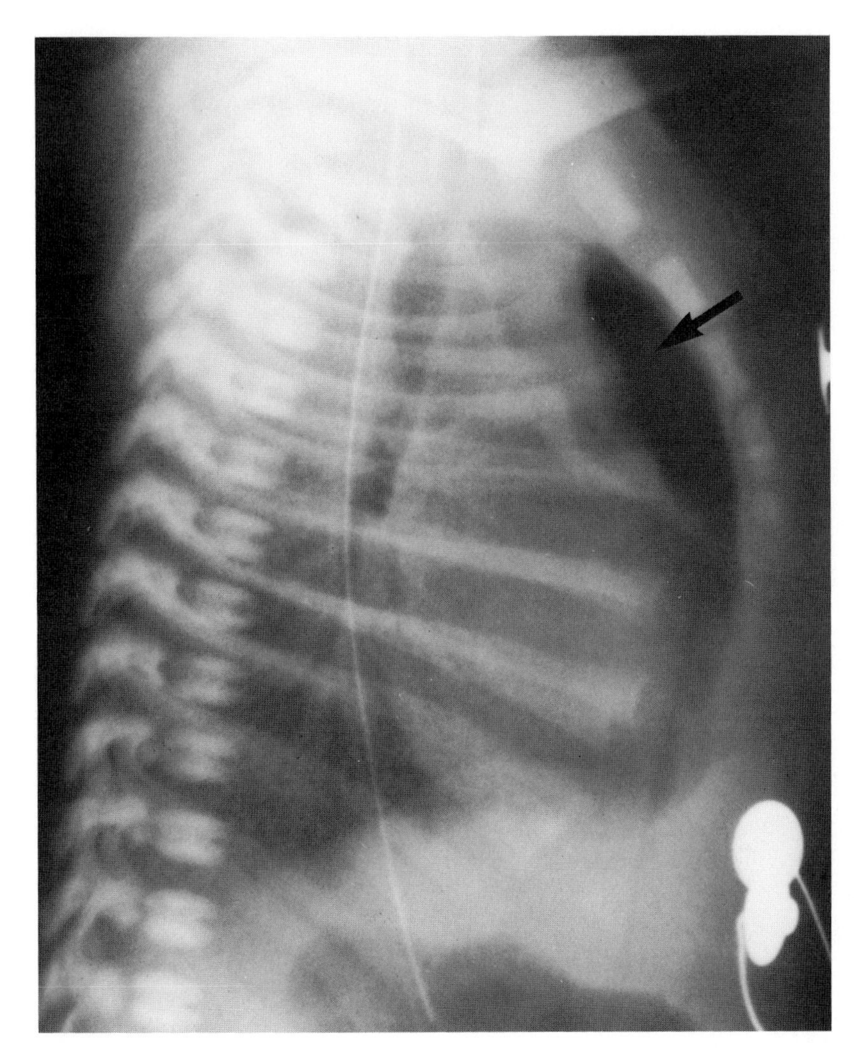

Figure 9 Pneumomediastinum. The arrow points to air replacing the normal thymic shadow.

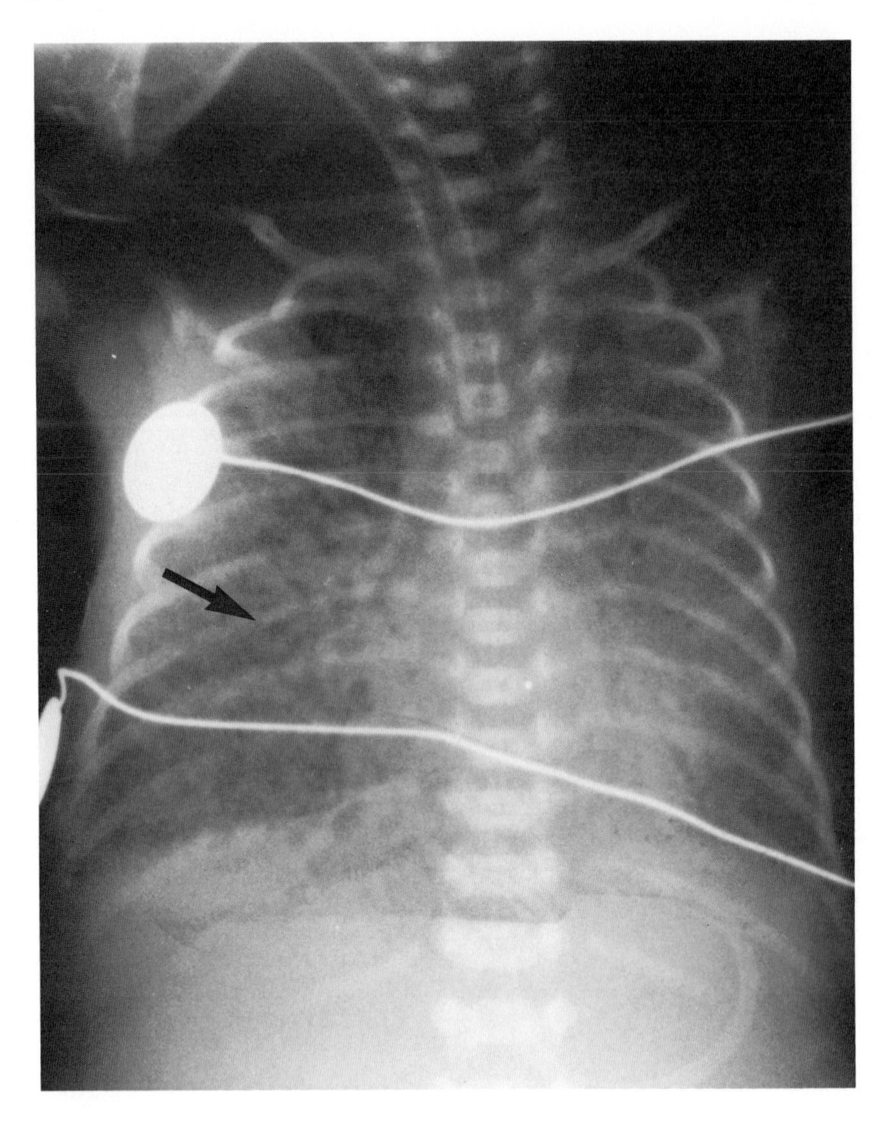

Figure 10 Pulmonary interstitial emphysema. The arrow points to a typical "bubbly" area.

Pulmonary interstitial emphysema, the presence of air in the perivascular interstitium, precedes the development of most cases of pneumomediastinum and pneumothorax, but the picture of generalized pulmonary interstitial emphysema is usually associated with hyaline membrane disease and intermittent mandatory ventilation. It is suggested that after the rupture of the alveolus with air entering the perivascular space, if the perivascular planes are easily cleaved, then pneumomediastinum and pneumothorax occur without radiological evidence of pulmonary interstitial emphysema. Prematurity and hyaline membrane disease presumably increase the resistance to cleavage and result in more frequent generalized pulmonary interstitial emphysema [97]. The generalized dissection of air in the perivascular space leads to a marked decrease in pulmonary compliance and may compromise the pulmonary circulation. Generalized pulmonary interstitial emphysema occurring in an infant with hyaline membrane disease gives a "bubbly" appearance on x-ray (Fig. 10) and is usually an ominous development, especially since it is frequently a precursor of bronchopulmonary dysplasia [50]. Interstitial emphysema has on occasion been treated successfully with very rapid ventilatory rates allowing a lower peak inspiratory pressure [98].

VII. Persistent Pulmonary Hypertension

The fetal circulation is characterized by low systemic vascular resistance due to the ease of flow through the placenta, and high pulmonary vascular resistance due to the vasoconstriction of the pulmonary arterioles. This resistance difference leads to shunting of blood right-to-left through the foramen ovale and the ductus arteriosus. The transitional circulation is characterized by elevation of the systemic vascular resistance with clamping of the umbilical cord and lowering of the pulmonary vascular resistance as the pulmonary arterioles dilate with the onset of ventilation. These changes in resistance result in changes in pressure and flow which lead to functional closure of the foramen ovale. The postnatal elevation of arterial PO_2 leads to functional closure of the ductus arteriosus. Thus, the right-to-left shunting normally decreases markedly with the first breaths and then declines more gradually until it usually ceases 12-24 hr after birth. Any alteration of this sequence may lead to continued or renewed right-to-left shunting and the clinical picture referred to as persistent fetal circulation (a misnomer, since the placenta is absent), persistent transitional circulation, or persistent pulmonary hypertension. Right-to-left shunting may result from alteration in the systemic vascular resistance (e.g., hypovolemia from blood loss or decreased left ventricular output from myocardial ischemia) [99], but is more frequently due to persistence or recurrence of elevated pulmonary vascular resistance. The pulmonary arterioles are quite reactive, especially to low pH, low PO_2, and, possibly, elevated PCO_2 at the alveolar level [100]. Other factors that may affect pulmonary arteriolar tone are sympathetic nervous system stimulation, main pulmonary artery distention [101], and hyperinflation of the lungs [12].

Therefore, persistent pulmonary hypertension is seen in association with perinatal asphyxia resulting in early systemic hypoxia, pulmonary parenchymal disease (especially the perinatal aspiration syndromes) [102], polycythemia (the hyperviscosity syndrome), and hypoglycemia [103]. Recent studies [104] show a relationship between maternal ingestion of prostaglandin synthetase inhibitors, including aspirin, and persistent pulmonary hypertension. This association is presumably due to prenatal constriction of the ductus arteriosus, resulting in increased pulmonary artery pressure which leads to increased muscle development in the pulmonary vessels [105].

There is an interesting clinical association of nonbacterial endocardial thrombosis, thrombocytopenia, and persistent pulmonary hypertension [106]. It is suggested that the endocardium is damaged by asphyxia and that aggregating platelets on the endocardium and in the pulmonary arterial bed may release vasoactive substances, leading to pulmonary hypertension. As previously mentioned, thrombocytopenia is often associated with persistent pulmonary hypertension in the fetal aspiration syndromes [68].

The most common precursor in our experience is perinatal asphyxia, often associated with the meconium aspiration syndrome. The clinical picture is varied, depending on whether persistent pulmonary hypertension is accompanied by myocardial dysfunction, pulmonary disease, or simply reflex pulmonary vasoconstriction. In the absence of myocardial or pulmonary disease, the picture is that of a full-term infant with a history of perinatal complications such as prolonged gestation or maternal hypertension [107]. The infant is cyanotic shortly after birth and has only mild respiratory distress with tachypnea, without grunting or retractions, similar to an infant with cyanotic congenital heart disease. Air exchange is adequate, and there are no signs of congestive heart failure. A murmur of atrioventricular valve insufficiency may be present [108]. The chest x-ray reveals mild "streaky" densities and no significant pulmonary parenchymal disease; hyperinflation may be present. The echocardiogram shows a large right ventricular dimension and increased right and left ventricular pre-ejection period to ejection time ratios. These echocardiographic findings may precede clinical deterioration [109]. The blood gases are characterized by hypoxemia without retention of CO_2 unless severe lung disease is present, as in the meconium aspiration syndrome. The diagnosis is suggested by the history, by the absence of severe pulmonary disease, and by the demonstration of normal cardiac anatomy by by echocardiography. A significant difference (>10 mmHg) in the right radial (preductal) and umbilical artery (postductal) PO_2 verifies a ductal right-to-left shunt. The absence of a difference implies that a major right-to-left shunt is occurring at the atrial level through the formen ovale.

The treatment is aimed at correction of the causes, i.e., hypoglycemia, hyperviscosity, depressed PO_2, and/or depressed pH. If this specific therapy does not quickly improve the baby's state, we proceed to endotracheal hyperventilation to elevate the pH [110]. Tolazoline may subsequently be used for its pulmonary vasodilating effect. If myocardial dysfunction accompanies the persistent pulmonary hypertension, the concomitant use of dopamine is suggested to increase myocardial contractility and to reduce afterload by capillary dilation [111]. Prostaglandin E_2 decreases the pulmonary vascular resistance in animal studies and may be of future use upon humans [112].

The clinical course is characterized by extreme swings in PO_2 [100]. The mortality rate is high in infants with concomitant lung disease (~ 50%) and low (~ 15%) in those without lung disease [113]. Alternately, resolution may occur in 3-7 days, although occasionally a protracted course occurs [114].

VIII. Pulmonary Hypoplasia

The anatomical development of the lung is discussed in Chapter 2. The growth of the lung is primarily affected by volume or distention in fetal life [115], and pulmonary hypoplasia may result from either external compression of the lung or lack of distention. Obvious examples are the association of pulmonary hypoplasia with diaphragmatic hernia, membranous diaphragm, ascites, and large abdominal masses. Table 4 categorized the causes of pulmonary hypoplasia. Lack of distention of the fetal lung, due to absent or decreased fetal breathing movements, may explain the association between fetal neurological disorders (e.g., myotonic dystrophy) and pulmonary hypoplasia [116]. This hypothesis is also suggested by animal experiments [117].

The mechanism by which oligohydramnious causes pulmonary hypoplasia is not completely clear. Thoracic cage compression is a likely explanation, especially when other pressure deformities are seen. Another suggestion is that the decreased amniotic fluid volume may lead to an inability to retain liquid within the fetal airways and that this fluid is necessary for adequate pulmonary growth and maturation [118]. An alternative theory is that the inspiration of amniotic fluid during fetal life is partially responsible for pulmonary growth. The occasional coexistence of polyhydramnios and pulmonary hypoplasia suggests that the fetal lung may be an important absorptive surface for amniotic fluid [119].

Cases of primary pulmonary hypoplasia have been reported [120,121]. With refinement of the pathological assessment at autopsy [122] and higher clinical suspicion, it is likely that this diagnosis will include a spectrum of degrees of hypoplasia and become more commonly recognized. The etiology of primary pulmonary hypoplasia is unknown. It is possible that pulmonary hypoplasia relates to decreased fetal respiratory activity [117], which may be caused by intrauterine hypoxemia [123] and probably other unrecognized causes.

Table 4 Causes of Pulmonary Hypoplasia

A. Extrathoracic compression
  1. Oligohydramnios with renal disease
     - Potter's syndrome
     - Bilateral cystic kidneys
     - Obstructive uropathy
  2. Oligohydramnios without renal disease
     - Prolonged amniotic fluid leakage
     - Fetal development in amniotic fluid-deficient uterine saccules
  3. Chronically elevated diaphragm – no oligohydramnios
     - Large abdominal masses
     - Massive ascites
     - Membranous diaphragm

B. Thoracic cage compression
  1. Thoracic dystrophies
     - Asphyxiating thoracic dystrophy
     - Achondrogenesis
     - Thanatophoric dwarfism
     - Severe achondroplasia
     - Congenital osteogenesis imperfecta
     - Ellis-van Creveld syndrome
     - Short limb polydactyly syndrome
     - Metatrophic dwarfism
  2. Muscular disease with "functional" compression
     - Myotonic dystrophy?
     - Amyotonia congenita?
     - Myasthenia gravis?
     - Arthrogryposis multiplex congenita [119]

C. Intrathoracic compression
  1. Diaphragmatic defects
     - Congenital diaphragmatic hernia
     - Agenesis of diaphragm
  2. Excess pleural fluid
     - Chylohydrothorax
     - Fetal hydrops
  3. Large intrathoracic tumor or cyst

D. Primary hypoplasia – no cause of compression demonstrable

Source: Ref. 111.

Infants with pulmonary hypoplasia have respiratory distress within minutes after delivery, and most require assisted ventilation. The chest x-ray will show small clear lungs, but their size is often overlooked or attributed to the film being taken at expiration. There are three clinical clues of value. The first clue is the inability to ventilate the infant adequately, demonstrated by hypercapnia in the presence of clear lung fields. The second clue is the occurrence of multiple and refractory pneumothoraces. The third clue is the presence of persistent pulmonary hypertension, which occurs in most cases. In all cases of persistent pulmonary hypertension without an obvious cause, pulmonary hypoplasia should be considered. In the absence of congenital malformations or diseases known to be associated with pulmonary hypoplasia, the diagnosis is usually made after several x-rays reveal diminished lung volume.

The treatment involves ventilatory support and treatment of persistent pulmonary hypertension. In the few surviving cases, artificial ventilation was unnecessary beyond 1 week. All infants with lungs weighing 50% below normal or less have died [116].

References

1. Hjalmarson, O., Epidemiology and classification of acute neonatal respiratory disorders, *Acta Paediatr. Scand.*, **70**:773 (1981).
2. Avery, M. E., O. B. Gatewood, and G. Brumley, Transient tachypnea of newborn, *Am. J. Dis. Child.*, **111**:380 (1966).
3. Smith, C. A., Respiratory physiology and respiratory distress in the newborn infant, *Int. Anesthesiol. Clin.*, **3**:209 (1965).
4. Walters, D. V., and R. E. Olver, The role of catecholamines in lung liquid absorption at birth, *Pediatr. Res.*, **12**:239 (1978).
5. Saunders, R. A., and A. D. Milner, Pulmonary pressure/volume relationships during the last phase of delivery and the first postnatal breaths in human subjects, *J. Pediatr.*, **93**:667 (1978).
6. Vyas, H., A. D. Milner, and I. E. Hopkin, Intrathoracic pressure and volume changes during the spontaneous onset of respiration in babies born by cesarean section and by vaginal delivery, *J. Pediatr.*, **99**:787 (1981).
7. Sundell, H., J. Garrott, W. J. Blankenship, F. M. Shepard, and M. T. Stahlman, Studies on infants with type II respiratory distress syndrome, *J. Pediatr.*, **78**:754 (1971).
8. Boon, A. W., A. D. Milner, and I. E. Hopkin, Lung volumes and lung mechanics in babies born vaginally and by elective and emergency lower segmental cesarean section, *J. Pediatr.*, **98**:812 (1981).
9. Halliday, H. L., G. McClure, and M. McC. Reid, Transient tachypnea of the newborn: Two distinct clinical entities?, *Arch. Dis. Child.*, **56**:322 (1981).

10. Richardson, D. W., Transient tachypnea of the newborn associated with hypervolemia, *Can. Med. Assoc. J.,* **103**:70 (1970).
11. Wesenberg, R. L., S. N. Graven, and E. B. McCabe, Radiological findings in wet-lung disease, *Radiology,* **98**:69 (1971).
12. Bucciarelli, R. L., E. A. Egan, I. H. Gessner, and D. V. Eitzman, Persistence of fetal cardiopulmonary circulation: One manifestation of transient tachypnea of the newborn, *Pediatrics,* **58**:192 (1976).
13. Swischuk, L. E., Transient respiratory distress of the newborn (TRDN). A temporary disturbance of a normal phenomenon, *Am. J. Roentgenol. Rad. Ther. Nucl. Med.,* **108**:557 (1970).
14. Rimmer, S., and J. Fawcitt, Delayed clearance of pulmonary fluid in the neonate, *Arch. Dis. Child.,* **57**:63 (1982).
15. Swischuk, L. E., C. K. Hayden, Jr., and C. J. Richardson, Neonatal opaque right lung: Delayed fluid resorption, *Radiology,* **141**:671 (1981).
16. Farrell, P. M., and M. E. Avery, Hyaline membrane disease, *Am. Rev. Resp. Dis.,* **111**:657 (1975).
17. Usher, R. H., A. C. Allen, and F. H. McLean, Risk of respiratory distress syndrome related to gestational age, route of delivery, and maternal diabetes, *Am. J. Obstet. Gynecol.,* **111**:826 (1971).
18. Jones, M. D., Jr., L. I. Burd, W. A. Bowes, Jr., F. C. Battaglia, and L. O. Lubchenco, Failure of association of premature rupture of membranes with respiratory-distress syndrome, *New Engl. J. Med.,* **292**:1253 (1975).
19. Caspi, E., P. Schreyer, R. Reif, and M. Goldberg, An analysis of the factors associated with respiratory distress syndrome in premature infants whose mothers had been given dexamethasone therapy, *Br. J. Obstet. Gynaecol.,* **87**:808 (1980).
20. Rokos, J., O. Vaeusorn, R. Nachman, and M. E. Avery, Hyaline membrane disease in twins, *Pediatrics,* **42**:204 (1968).
21. Usher, R., F. McLean, and G. B. Maughan, Respiratory distress syndrome in infants delivered by cesarean section, *Am. J. Obstet. Gynecol.,* **88**:806 (1964).
22. Goldberg, J. D., W. R. Cohen, and E. A. Friedman, Cesarean section indication and the risk of respiratory distress syndrome, *Obstet. Gynecol.,* **57**:30 (1981).
23. Fedrick, J., and N. R. Butler, Hyaline membrane disease, *Lancet,* **ii**:768 (1972).
24. Graven, S. N., and H. R. Misenheimer, Respiratory distress syndrome and the high risk mother, *Am. J. Dis. Child.,* **109**:489 (1965).
25. Lankenau, H. M., A genetic and statistical study of the respiratory distress syndrome, *Eur. J. Pediatr.,* **123**:167 (1976).
26. Chance, G. W., Elective delivery, premature rupture of the membranes and the respiratory distress syndrome, *Can. Med. Assoc. J.,* **122**:265 (1980).

27. Shanklin, D. R., The sex of premature infants with hyaline membrane disease, *South. Med. J.,* **56**:1018 (1963).
28. Robert, M. F., R. K. Neff, J. P. Hubbell, H. W. Taeusch, and M. E. Avery, Association between maternal diabetes and the respiratory-distress syndrome in the newborn, *New Engl. J. Med.,* **294**:357 (1976).
29. Bauer, C. R., L. Stern, and E. Colle, Prolonged rupture of membranes associated with a decreased incidence of respiratory distress syndrome, *Pediatrics,* **53**:7 (1974).
30. Taeusch, H. W., Jr., and D. Tulchinsky, Obstetric factors affecting risk of respiratory distress syndrome. In *Premature Labor.* Mead Johnson Symposium on Perinatal and Developmental Medicine, No. 15, 1979.
31. Yoon, J. J., S. Kohl, and R. G. Harper, The relationship between maternal hypertensive disease of pregnancy and the incidence of idiopathic respiratory distress syndrome, *Pediatrics,* **65**:735 (1980).
32. Glass, L., B. K. Rajegowda, and H. E. Evans, Absence of respiratory distress syndrome in premature infants of heroin-addicted mothers, *Lancet,* **ii**:685 (1971).
33. Ablow, R. C., S. G. Driscoll, E. L. Effmann, I. Gross, C. J. Jolles, R. Uauy, and J. B. Warshaw, A comparison of early-onset group B streptococcal neonatal infection and the respiratory-distress syndrome of the newborn, *New Engl. J. Med.,* **294**:65 (1976).
34. Gregory, G. A., J. A. Kitterman, R. H. Phibbs, W. H. Tooley, and W. K. Hamilton, Treatment of the idiopathic respiratory-distress syndrome with continuous positive airway pressure, *New Engl. J. Med.,* **284**:1333 (1971).
35. Tanswell, A. K., R. A. Clubb, B. T. Smith, and R. W. Boston, Individualised continuous distending pressure applied within 6 hours of delivery in infants with respiratory distress syndrome, *Arch. Dis. Child.,* **55**:33 (1980).
36. Goldsmith, J. P., and E. H. Karotkin (Eds.), *Assisted Ventilation of the Neonate.* Philadelphia, Saunders, 1981.
37. Brown, E. G., R. W. Krouskop, F. E. McDonnell, and A. Y. Sweet, Blood volume and blood pressure in infants with respiratory distress, *J. Pediatr.,* **87**:1133 (1975).
38. Linderkamp, O., H. T. Versmold, H. Fendel, K. P. Riegel, and K. Betke, Association of neonatal respiratory distress with birth asphyxia and deficiency of red cell mass in premature infants, *Eur. J. Pediatr.,* **129**:167 (1978).
39. Barr, P. A., P. E. Bailey, J. Sumners, and G. Cassady, Relation between arterial blood pressure and blood volume and effect of infused albumin in sick preterm infants, *Pediatrics,* **60**:282 (1977).
40. Goldberg, R. N., D. Chung, S. L. Goldman, and E. Bancalari, The association of rapid volume expansion and intraventricular hemorrhage in the preterm infant, *J. Pediatr.,* **96**:1060 (1980).

41. Dykes, F. D., A. Lazzara, P. Ahmann, B. Blumenstein, J. Schwartz, and A. W. Brann, Intraventricular hemorrhage: A prospective evaluation of etiopathogenesis, *Pediatrics,* **66**:42 (1980).
42. Versmold, H. T., J. A. Kitterman, R. H. Phibbs, G. A. Gregory, and W. H. Tooley, Aortic blood pressure during the first 12 hours of life in infants with birth weight 610 to 4,220 grams, *Pediatrics,* **67**:607 (1981).
43. Roberton, N. R. C., Management of hyaline membrane disease, *Arch. Dis. Child.,* **54**:838 (1979).
44. McIntosh, N., and R. O. Walters, Effect of tolazoline in severe hyaline membrane disease, *Arch. Dis. Child.,* **54**:105 (1979).
45. Obeyesekere, H. I., S. Pankhurst, and V. Y. H. Yu, Pharmacological closure of ductus arteriosus in preterm infants using indomethacin, *Arch. Dis. Child.,* **55**:271 (1980).
46. Stevenson, J. G., Fluid administration in the association of patent ductus arteriosus complicating respiratory distress syndrome, *J. Pediatr.,* **90**:257 (1977).
47. Alpert, B. S., M. J. Lewins, D. W. Rowland, M. J. A. Grant, P. M. Olley, S. J. Soldin, P. R. Swyer, F. Coceani, and R. D. Rowe, Plasma indomethacin levels in preterm newborn infants with symptomatic patent ductus arteriosus—Clinical and echocardiographic assessments of response, *J. Pediatr.,* **95**:578 (1979).
48. Northway, W. H., Jr., Observations on bronchopulmonary dysplasia, *J. Pediatr.,* **95**:815 (1979).
49. Milner, A. D., Bronchopulmonary dysplasia, *Arch. Dis. Child.,* **55**:661 (1980).
50. Watts, J. L., R. L. Ariagno, and J. P. Brady, Chronic pulmonary disease in neonates after artificial ventilation: Distribution of ventilation and pulmonary interstitial emphysema, *Pediatrics,* **60**:273 (1977).
51. Brown, E. R., Increased risk of bronchopulmonary dysplasia in infants with patent ductus arteriosus, *J. Pediatr.,* **95**:865 (1979).
52. Edwards, D. K., W. M. Dyer, and W. H. Northway, Jr., Twelve years' experience with bronchopulmonary dysplasia, *Pediatrics,* **59**:839 (1977).
53. Ehrenkranz, R. A., R. C. Ablow, and J. B. Warshaw, Prevention of bronchopulmonary dysplasia with vitamin E administration during the acute stages of respiratory distress syndrome. *J. Pediatr.,* **95**:873 (1979).
54. Saldanha, R. L., E. E. Cepeda, and R. L. Poland, The effect of vitamin E prophylaxis on the incidence and severity of bronchopulmonary dysplasia, *J. Pediatr.,* **101**:89 (1982).
55. Brown, E. R., A. Stark, I. Sosenko, E. E. Lawson, and M. E. Avery, Bronchopulmonary dysplasia: Possible relationship to pulmonary edema, *J. Pediatr.,* **92**:982 (1978).

56. Kao, L. C., et al., Effect of oral diuretics on pulmonary mechanics in infants with chronic bronchopulmonary dysplasia: Results of a double-blind cross-over sequential trial. *J. Pediatr.,* **74**:37 (1984).
57. Dawes, G. S., Revolutions and cyclical rhythms in prenatal life: Fetal respiratory movements rediscovered, *Pediatrics,* **51**:965 (1973).
58. Perlman, M., and J. Bar-Ziv, Congenital ichthyosis and neonatal pulmonary disease, *Pediatrics,* **53**:573 (1974).
59. Meis, P. J., M. Hall, III, J. R. Marshall, and C. J. Hobel, Meconium passage: A new classification for risk assessment during labor, *Am. J. Obstet. Gynecol.,* **131**:509 (1978).
60. Brown, B. L., and N. Gleicher, Intrauterine meconium aspiration, *Obstet. Gynecol.,* **57**:26 (1981).
61. Turbeville, D. F., M. A. McCaffree, M. F. Block, and H. F. Krous, *In utero* distal pulmonary meconium aspiration, *South. Med. J.,* **72**:535 (1979).
62. Gage, J. E., H. W. Taeusch, Jr., S. Treves, and W. Caldicott, Suctioning of upper airway meconium in newborn infants, *J.A.M.A.,* **246**:2590 (1981).
63. Gregory, G. A., C. A. Gooding, R. H. Phibbs, and W. H. Tooley, Meconium aspiration in infants—A prospective study, *J. Pediatr.,* **85**:848 (1974).
64. Ting, P., and J. P. Brady, Tracheal suction in meconium aspiration, *Am. J. Obstet. Gynecol.,* **122**:767 (1975).
65. Carson, B. S., R. W. Losey, W. A. Bowes, Jr., and M. A. Simmons, Combined obstetric and pediatric approach to prevent meconium aspiration syndrome, *Am. J. Obstet. Gynecol.,* **126**:712 (1976).
66. Fujikura, T., and B. Klionsky, The significance of meconium staining, *Am. J. Obstet. Gynecol.,* **121**:45 (1975).
67. Merlob, P., J. Amir, R. Zaizov, and S. H. Reisner, The differential leukocyte count in full-term newborn infants with meconium aspiration and neonatal asphyxia, *Acta Paediatr. Scand.,* **69**:779 (1980).
68. Segall, M. L., B. W. Goetzman, and J. B. Schick, Thrombocytopenia and pulmonary hypertension in the perinatal aspiration syndromes, *J. Pediatr.,* **96**:727 (1980).
69. Hoffman, R. R., Jr., R. E. Campbell, and J. P. Decker, Fetal aspiration syndrome. Clinical, roentgenologic and pathologic features, *Am. J. Roentgenol. Rad. Ther. Nucl. Med.,* **122**:90 (1974).
70. Bancalari, E., and J. A. Berlin, Meconium aspiration and other asphyxial disorders, *Clin. Perinatol.,* **5**:317 (1978).
71. Yeh, T. F., G. Srinivasan, V. Harris, and R. S. Pildes, Hydrocortisone therapy in meconium aspiration syndrome: A controlled study, *J. Pediatr.,* **90**:140 (1977).
72. Marshall, R., E. Tyrala, W. McAlister, and M. Sheehan, Meconium aspiration syndrome. Neonatal and follow-up study, *Am. J. Obstet. Gynecol.,* **131**:672 (1978).

73. Wilson, H. D., and H. F. Eichenwald, Sepsis neonatorum, *Pediatr. Clin. North Am.*, **24**:571 (1974).
74. Baker, C. J., Group B streptococcal infections in neonates, *Pediatr. Rev.*, **1**:5 (1979).
75. Rojas, J., R. S. Green, C. G. Hellerqvist, R. Olegard, K. L. Brigham, and M. T. Stahlman, Studies in group B β-hemolytic streptococcus. II. Effects on pulmonary hemodynamics and vascular permeability in unanesthetized sheep, *Pediatr. Res.*, **15**:899 (1981).
76. Faro, S., Group B beta-hemolytic streptococci and puerperal infections, *Am. J. Obstet. Gynecol.*, **139**:686 (1981).
77. Baker, C. J., D. L. Kasper, I. R. Tager, A. Paredes, S. Alpert, W. M. McCormack, and D. Goroff, Quantitative determination of antibody to capsular polysaccharide in infection with type III strains of group B streptococcus, *J. Clin. Invest.*, **59**:810 (1977).
78. Modanlou, H. D., S. K. Bosu, and M. H. Weller, Early onset group B streptococcus neonatal septicemia and respiratory distress syndrome: Characteristic features of assisted ventilation in the first 24 hours of life, *Crit. Care Med.*, **8**:716 (1980).
79. Ingram, D. L., E. L. Pendergrass, P. I. Bromberger, J. D. Thullen, C. D. Yoder, and A. M. Collier, Group B streptococcal disease–Its diagnosis with the use of antigen detection, Gram's stain, and the presence of apnea, hypotension, *Am. J. Dis. Child.*, **134**:754 (1980).
80. Edwards, M. S., C. V. Jackson, and C. J. Baker, Increased risk of group B streptococcal disease in twins, *J.A.M.A.*, **245**:2044 (1981).
81. McCarten, K. M., H. K. Rosenberg, S. Borden, IV, and G. A. Mandell, Delayed appearance of right diaphragmatic hernia associated with group B streptococcal infection in newborns, *Radiology*, **139**:385 (1981).
82. Harris, M. C., W. B. Moskowitz, W. D. Engle, H. Rosenberg, J. Templeton, and S. Kumar, Group B streptococcal septicemia and delayed-onset diaphragmatic hernia, *Am. J. Dis. Child.*, **135**:723 (1981).
83. Macklin, C. C., Transport of air along sheaths of pulmonic blood vessels from alveoli to mediastinum, *Arch. Intern. Med.*, **64**:913 (1939).
84. Monin, P., and P. Vert, Pneumothorax, *Clin. Perinatol.*, **5**:335 (1978).
85. Karlberg, P., R. B. Cherry, F. E. Escardo, and G. Koch, Respiratory studies in newborn infants. II. Pulmonary ventilation and mechanics of breathing in the first minutes of life, including the onset of respiration. *Acta Paediatr.*, **51**:121 (1962).
86. Mandansky, D. L., E. E. Lawson, V. Shernick, and H. W. Taeusch, Jr., Pneumothorax and other forms of pulmonary air leak in newborns, *Am. Rev. Resp. Dis.*, **120**:729 (1979).
87. Steele, R. W., J. R. Metz, J. W. Bass, and J. J. DuBois, Pneumothorax and pneumomediastinum in the newborn, *Radiology*, **98**:629 (1971).

88. Yu, V. Y. H., S. W. Liew, and N. R. C. Roberton, Pneumothorax in the newborn. Changing pattern, *Arch. Dis. Child.,* **50**:449 (1975).
89. Ogata, E. S., G. A. Gregory, J. A. Kitterman, R. H. Phibbs, and W. H. Tooley, Pneumothorax in the respiratory distress syndrome: Incidence and effect on vital signs, blood gases, and pH, *Pediatrics,* **58**:177 (1976).
90. Goldberg, R. N., Sustained arterial blood pressure elevation associated with pneumothoraces: Early detection via continuous monitoring, *Pediatrics,* **68**:775 (1981).
91. Kuhns, L. R., F. J. Bednarek, M. L. Wyman, D. W. Roloff, and R. C. Borer, Diagnosis of pneumothorax or pneumomediastinum in the neonate by transillumination, *Pediatrics,* **56**:355 (1975).
92. Stern, P., F. T. LaRochelle, Jr., and G. A. Little, Vasopressin and pneumothorax in the neonate, *Pediatrics,* **68**:499 (1981).
93. Lipscomb, A. P., R. J. Thorburn, E. O. R. Reynolds, A. L. Stewart, R. J. Blackwell, G. Cusick, and M. D. Whitehead, Pneumothorax and cerebral haemorrhage in preterm infants, *Lancet,* **i**:414 (1981).
94. Kirkpatrick, B. V., A. H. Felman, and D. V. Eitzman, Complications of ventilator therapy in respiratory distress syndrome. Recognition and management of acute air leaks, *Am. J. Dis. Child.,* **128**:496 (1974).
95. Burt, T. B., and P. D. Lester, Neonatal pneumopericardium, *Radiology,* **142**:81 (1982).
96. Reiffel, R. S., and C. J. Priebe, Jr., Evacuation of pericardial, anterior mediastinal, and peripleural air collections in neonatal respiratory distress, *J. Thorac. Cardiovasc. Surg.,* **73**:868 (1977).
97. Thibeault, D. W., R. L. Lachman, V. R. Laul, and M. S. Kwong, Pulmonary interstitial emphysema, pneumomediastinum, and pneumothorax. Occurrence in the newborn infant, *Am. J. Dis. Child.,* **126**:611 (1973).
98. Ng, K. P. K., and D. Easa, Management of interstitial emphysema by high-frequency low positive-pressure hand ventilation in the neonate, *J. Pediatr.,* **95**:117 (1979).
99. Riemenschneider, T. A., H. C. Nielsen, H. D. Ruttenberg, and R. B. Jaffe, Disturbances of the transitional circulation: Spectrum of pulmonary hypertension and myocardial dysfunction, *J. Pediatr.,* **89**:622 (1976).
100. Peckham, G. J., and W. W. Fox, Physiologic factors affecting pulmonary artery pressure in infants with persistent pulmonary hypertension, *J. Pediatr.,* **93**:1005 (1978).
101. Baylen, B. G., G. C. Emmanouilides, C. E. Juratsch, Y. Yoshida, W. J. French, and J. M. Criley, Main pulmonary artery distention: A potential mechanism for acute pulmonary hypertension in the human newborn infant, *J. Pediatr.,* **96**:540 (1980).
102. Fox, W. W., M. H. Gewitz, R. Dinwiddie, W. H. Drummond, and G. J. Peckham, Pulmonary hypertension in the perinatal aspiration syndromes, *Pediatrics,* **59**:205 (1977).

103. Gersony, W. M., Persistence of the fetal circulation: A commentary, *J. Pediatr.,* 82:1103 (1973).
104. Rudolph, A. M., The effects of nonsteroidal anti-inflammatory compounds on fetal circulation and pulmonary function, *Obstet. Gynecol.,* **58**:63S (1981).
105. Levin, D. L., D. E. Fixler, F. C. Morriss, and J. Tyson, Morphologic analysis of the pulmonary vascular bed in infants exposed *in utero* to prostaglandin synthetase inhibitors, *J. Pediatr.,* **92**:478 (1978).
106. Morrow, W. R., J. E. Haas, and D. R. Benjamin, Nonbacterial endocardial thrombosis in neonates: Relationship to persistent fetal circulation, *J. Pediatr.,* **100**:117 (1982).
107. Drummond, W. H., G. J. Peckham, and W. W. Fox, The clinical profile of the newborn with persistent pulmonary hypertension, *Clin. Pediatr.,* **16**: 335 (1977).
108. Levin, D. L., M. A. Heymann, J. A. Kitterman, G. A. Gregory, R. H. Phibbs, and A. M. Rudolph, Persistent pulmonary hypertension of the newborn infant, *J. Pediatr.,* **89**:626 (1976).
109. Valdes-Cruz, L. M., G. G. Dudell, and A. Ferrara, Utility of M-mode echocardiography for early identification of infants with persistent pulmonary hypertension of the newborn, *Pediatrics,* **68**:515 (1981).
110. Drummond, W. H., G. A. Gregory, M. A. Heymann, and R. A. Phibbs, The independent effects of hyperventilation, tolazoline, and dopamine on infants with persistent pulmonary hypertension, *J. Pediatr.,* **98**:603 (1981).
111. Fiddler, G. I., R. Chatrath, G. J. Williams, D. R. Walker, and O. Scott, Dopamine infusion for the treatment of myocardial dysfunction associated with a persistent transitional circulation, *Arch. Dis. Child.,* **55**:194 (1980).
112. Soifer, S. J., F. C. Morin, III, and M. A. Heymann, Prostaglandin D_2 reverses induced pulmonary hypertension in the newborn lamb, *J. Pediatr.,* **100**:458 (1982).
113. Goetzman, B. W., P. Sunshine, J. D. Johnson, R. P. Wennberg, A. Hackel, D. F. Merten, A. L. Bartoletti, and N. H. Silverman, Neonatal hypoxia and pulmonary vasospasm: Response to tolazoline, *J. Pediatr.,* **89**:617 (1976).
114. Levin, D. L., L. Cates, E. A. Newfeld, A. J. Muster, and M. H. Paul, Persistence of the fetal cardiopulmonary circulatory pathway: Survival of an infant after a prolonged course, *Pediatrics,* **56**:58 (1975).
115. Liggins, G. C., and J. A. Kitterman, Development of the fetal lung. In *The Fetus and Independent Life.* London, Pitman, Ciba Foundation, 1981, pp. 308–330.
116. Swischuk, L. E., C. J. Richardson, M. M. Nichols, and M. J. Ingman, Bilateral pulmonary hypoplasia in the neonate, *Am. J. Roentgenol.,* **133**:1057 (1979).

117. Wigglesworth, J. S., R. M. L. Winston, and K. Bartlett, Influence of the central nervous system on fetal lung development. Experimental study, *Arch. Dis. Child.,* **52**:965 (1977).
118. Wigglesworth, J. S., R. Desai, and P. Guerrini, Fetal lung hypoplasia: Biochemical and structural variations and their possible significance, *Arch. Dis. Child.,* **56**:606 (1981).
119. Mendelsohn, G., and G. M. Hutchins, Primary pulmonary hypoplasia. Report of a case with polyhydramnios, *Am. J. Dis. Child.,* **131**:1220 (1977).
120. Swischuk, L. E., C. J. Richardson, M. M. Nichols, and M. J. Ingman, Primary pulmonary hypoplasia in the neonate, *J. Pediatr.,* **95**:573 (1979).
121. George, P., C. R. Handorf, and E. A. Suttle, Primary pulmonary hypoplasia, *South. Med. J.,* **74**:884 (1981).
122. Askenazi, S. S., and M. Perlman, Pulmonary hypoplasia: Lung weight and radial alveolar count as criteria of diagnosis, *Arch. Dis. Child.,* **54**:614 (1979).
123. Dawes, G. S., Breathing before birth in animals and man. An essay in developmental medicine, *Physiol. Med.,* **290**:557 (1974).
124. Leichman, L. G., B. Say, and N. Barber, Primary pulmonary hypoplasia and arthrogryposis multiplex congenita, *J. Pediatr.,* **96**:95 (1980).

Part Seven

THE NONSURVIVORS AND THE SURVIVORS

17

Pathological Observations on Infants Who Do Not Survive the Respiratory Distress Syndrome

JOSEPH F. TOMASHEFSKI, JR.,* GORDON F. VAWTER, and LYNNE M. REID

The Children's Hospital
and Harvard Medical School
Boston, Massachusetts

I. Introduction

The reasons that an infant does not survive the respiratory distress syndrome (RDS) or hyaline membrane disease (HMD) include: the degree of immaturity of the lung; the severity of pathological changes associated with the RDS; the complications of its evolution, such as infection, acidosis, and disseminated intravascular coagulation (DIC); and the effect of treatment that, while necessary to maintain life, leaves its quota of injury, particularly damage from oxygen toxicity and barotrauma. The degree to which growth then occurs is also critical to survival. The lungs of an infant who does not survive RDS are like a pentimento that must be scanned for signs of the presence and significance of these various features.

This chapter, therefore, calls for consideration of the development of the lung to its stage of viability, although this cannot yet be defined precisely.

**Present affiliation*: Case Western Reserve University School of Medicine and Cleveland Metropolitan General Hospital, Cleveland, Ohio

Prematurity—birth before the end of 37 weeks' gestation—means that intrauterine development is cut short. However, a premature lung is not necessarily an immature one and vice versa, since immaturity is not proportional to gestational age. A full-term infant may have an immature lung and a premature lung may be more mature than expected for age. Although we know something of how such a lung is deficient, we know little of how the premature lung adapts to postnatal development, and to what extent it adopts the postnatal growth timetable of the term infant.

The structural findings in RDS and HMD are described for both early and late stages. The isolated injury of high FI_{O_2} and barotrauma are considered, but of course in the RDS patients these interact with a sick and immature lung. The effects of treatment offer a bridge to discussion of bronchopulmonary dysplasia (BPD), the term that seems now to encompass all long-term injury and fatality from RDS. This calls for consideration also of resolution, of scarring that is part of the healing process, and of the compensatory catch-up growth in the residual lung tissue.

II. General Development of the Lung

The embryonic and fetal development of the lung have been described in detail (see Chaps. 1–3). Worthy of reemphasis is the fact that normal lung development requires interaction of epithelium and mesenchyme. In microscopic sections of developing lung, three stages affecting the future alveolar or respiratory region are identified (Table 1) [1–3]. It is at the end of the canalicular period that vascularization of the future alveolar or respiratory region occurs, associated with localized thinning of the epithelium, so that a continuous epithelial lining no longer is apparent by light microscopy. Electron microscopy is necessary for its identification. Part of the alveolar wall now has the structure of the adult blood-gas barrier and also the same thickness [4]. Such is one mature feature of the premature lung. In the canalicular and alveolar stage the lung has air spaces resembling alveoli, but since the individual air space is larger and more primitive than the alveolus of the adult, Boyden preferred to call these spaces "primitive saccules" [1].

To understand lung growth, in addition to examination of random cross sections of lung, it is necessary to consider each structural component (airways, alveolar region, and vascular constituents) of the mature lungs separately, since each develops by a different time table.

The development of these is summarized conveniently in the following three laws of lung development. Although these take us beyond the perinatal period, postnatal growth is relevant to our discussion of recovery and catch-up growth.

Table 1 Previous Descriptions of Stages of Intra-uterine Lung Development

Dubreuil, Lacoste, and Raymond	*Loosli and Potter*	*Boyden*
Glandular Up to 6 months	Glandular 5 weeks–4 months	Pseudo-glandular 5–17 weeks
Canalicular 7 months to birth	Canalicular 4–6 months	Canalicular 13–25 weeks
Alveolar After birth	Alveolar 6 months to birth	Terminal-sac period 24 weeks to birth

Source: Refs. 130–132.

A. Law 1, Airways

All airways are present by the sixteenth week of intrauterine life [5]. This means that at this early time all bronchi and preacinar bronchioli are present, perfect, but miniature. The premature lung has its normal complement of airways, but the appearance of normal alveoli at the periphery does not necessarily mean that airway number is normal. The number of airways can be reduced—one sort of hypoplasia—and yet the alveolar growth and differentiation appear relatively normal. The development program can switch to alveolar multiplication before the airway program is fulfilled. If airway number is reduced, certainly total alveolar number can be expected to be also reduced, but in this case the number of alveoli distal to a terminal bronchiolus is often nearly normal for age, as judged by the Emery-Mithal count [1,6,7]. This count is a way of estimating the number of alveoli distal to the terminal bronchiolus, that is, the alveoli included within an acinus [7]. The acinus is the respiratory unit of lung. It is supplied by a terminal bronchiolus and includes respiratory bronchioli, alveolar ducts, and alveoli. In the normal term infant the terminal bronchiolus is present, but the respiratory bronchiolar region is still relatively incomplete and is an extremely short segment [8].

B. Law 2, Alveoli

The alveoli develop mainly after birth. In the term infant it is not until the seventh or eighth week of life that a burst of alveolar multiplication occurs in the region of the respiratory bronchiolus, thereby increasing its length [8]. It is at this time that alveoli with a more adult configuration first appear.

Between 28 and 40 weeks in utero, there is an increase in the radial-alveolar count. Whereas Emery and Mithal give an average of 2.8 at 28 weeks' gestation, their figure for term is 4.4 [7]. The premature lung, whether or not its surfactant system is mature, will be certain to have a reduced number of alveolar units and a reduced surface area compared with the normal for term.

Alveolar multiplication continues until the age of about 8 years when the adult complement is reached [9,10]. The figures reported from one or two studies suggest that about 20 million air spaces are present at birth, and about 200 million alveoli at the age of 8 [9,10]. While there is some debate as to when the multiplication of alveoli ceases and what is the normal range for the adult, there seems little doubt that during the first 4 or so years of life there is a dramatic multiplication of alveoli.

C. Law 3, Blood Vessels

The pulmonary artery branches running with preacinar airways develop as the airways develop; whereas, the intra-acinar arteries develop as alveoli multiply [2,3,11,12].

The pulmonary artery branches multiply so that their density, relative to alveoli, increases in the first few years of life but muscularization of their walls lags behind. In the infant lung relatively large arteries have no muscle in their walls as identified by light microscopy [12]. A pulmonary artery gives off many more branches than the airways it accompanies. Those arteries running with airways we call "conventional" branches, and those that run independently we call "supernumerary" [13]. The supernumerary arteries run a short course that supplies the alveoli immediately adjacent to the bronchoarterial sheath. They represent a type of collateral circulation. Between the hilum and the acinus the pulmonary artery has first an elastic structure, then, more peripherally, a transitional, and finally a muscular one. These terms are based on the relative proportion of elastic laminae and muscle fibers, with elastic laminae reducing in number progressively to the periphery. If the position of the artery is related to the accompanying airway ("landmarking" an artery), the level at which these transitions occur is fixed in fetal life. The structural type, therefore, of the preacinar artery is programmed before birth and is based on position within the pattern of branching of the artery rather than on the arterial size.

The fetal arteries are relatively more muscular than the adult if wall thickness is considered in relation to external diameter. We have little knowledge, however, as to the reactivity of the human arteries in the prenatal period. Before birth and at term in the normal infant, the muscular arteries are virtually all proximal to the respiratory or future alveolar surface. This is a major difference between the newborn lung, be it immature or mature, and the adult [14] in which muscular arteries are found in alveolar walls throughout the acinus.

The wall thickness of the small resistance arteries falls rapidly within minutes to hours of birth. An increase in compliance occurs, which is evidence that some mediator is capable of influencing all coats within the wall of the small muscular artery [12]. Wall thickness of the larger arteries takes some months to drop to adult levels, indicating that here "thinning" occurs by increase in diameter of the artery without proportional increase in muscle coat. It seems that certainly in some patients the premature lung shows the same drop in wall thickness of the muscular small arteries as the mature lung. The arteries before birth are relatively thicker walled than in the mature term or adult lung and the veins show a similar wall thickness for size and position within the lung throughout fetal life, childhood, and adulthood [15].

Recent studies in the piglet have indicated that if the vasopressor effect of hypoxia is expressed as a percent change on baseline, it is less in the young than in the older and adult lung [16]. The absolute increase in pulmonary artery pressure with hypoxic vasoconstriction may be larger in the young animal, but because the resting values are higher in the newborn, the increase as a percentage change in baseline is less than in the adult.

III. Hyaline Membrane Disease

Our main focus will be that form of respiratory distress of the newborn known as hyaline membrane disease (HMD). The disease occurs spontaneously in nonhuman primates, but since no satisfactory animal model of HMD has been developed experimentally, this description of the evolution of the pathological changes is constructed from interpretation of autopsy findings in fatal cases. The story is probably true; at least it provides a framework for our discussion.

Respiratory distress in the very immature infant (one weighing 500 g or less at birth) is reflected anatomically by an immature lung that is either atelectactic or expanded by low protein-containing fluid, and without obvious cell death or hyaline membrane formation. Thus, structural pulmonary immaturity alone can be lethal by causing a decrease in ventilatory surface, difficulty in ventilation, and reduced perfusion with decreased pulmonary compliance. The problem these infants have with volume expansion is illustrated in Figure 1. The graph compares gestational age and percent potential air space in stillborn fetuses. It is obvious that the more immature the infant the less potential airspace it has. If such infants die after a week or so, the alveoli of the respiratory portion of the lung are characteristically thick walled and hypercellular with little evidence of differentiation of alveolar wall structure, of scar, or of other changes of BPD. A variety of terms has been suggested for this condition, the most recent being chronic pulmonary insufficiency of prematurity [17]. It may occur in infants up to about 1200 g birth weight. Ultrastructural, biochemical, and

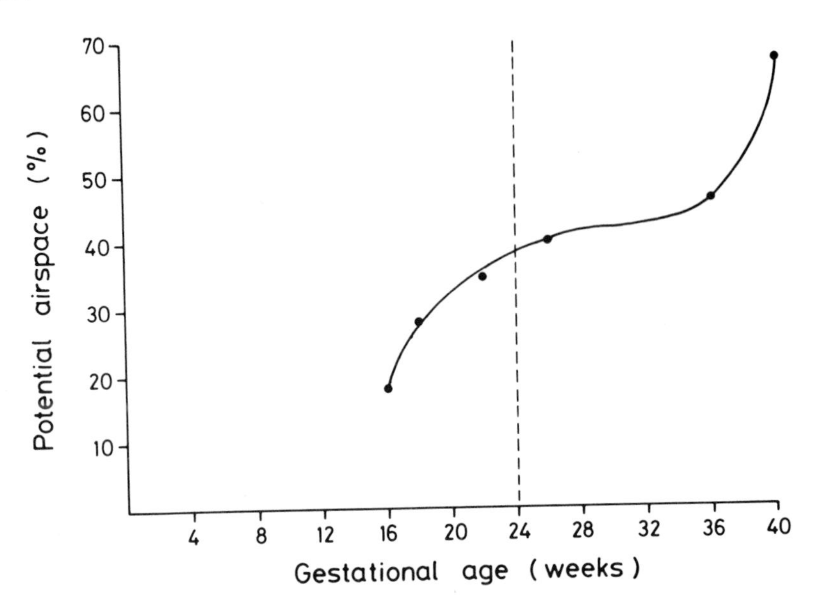

Figure 1 Correlation of gestational age with the percent of peripheral lung represented by potential air space. Based on measurements of fluid-filled lungs from stillborn infants.

mediator studies are badly needed in such patients. In such infants, the processes characteristic of HMD are the consequences of complications of structural prematurity, albeit life threatening and serious in themselves.

Clinical experience and physiological studies suggest that HMD starts at birth and runs most of its course over the first 3–5 days of life. The pathological findings are consistent with decreased tidal volume, decreased compliance, decrease in respiratory surface, intrapulmonary vascular shunting with ventilation-perfusion imbalance, and perhaps obstruction to peripheral air flow [18].

The pathological findings are conveniently discussed as representing four stages, although three of these stages overlap in time: (1) *prodrome*, birth to 8 hr; (2) *HM stage,* 4 hr to 5 days; (3) *complications,* at any time; and (4) *resolution and repair,* 2 days to 2 weeks. Features of each stage may be investigated by cytological studies of tracheal aspirates as previously suggested by D'Ablang et al. [19] and, more recently, by Merritt and colleagues [20].

A. Prodrome

If infants die of respiratory distress before hyaline membranes are formed, the lung has a normal weight [21] and macroscopically is dusky pink in color. The greater the immaturity, the thicker appear the edematous connective tussue septa with their dilated lymphatics [22]. The acini show as small punctate dots.

Microscopically, centroacinar spaces usually contain a pale eosinophilic and faintly PAS-positive granular material, which could be either retained lung fluid or edema. In utero the alveoli and airways are expanded by lung fluid, much of which is normally cleared during or immediately after vaginal delivery.

B. Hyaline Membrane Stage

In HMD the atelectasis is the central pathological feature for many pathologists. It evidently results from clearance of fluid without its replacement by air. This is most obvious at the periphery of the acinus [18,22-25]. It is the central acinar air spaces that receive air and in which subsequently the hyaline membranes develop. Even if air reaches the peripheral alveoli they are not stable and collapse on expiration because surfactant is absent or deficient there; thus, the alveolar volume decreases and the alveoli again become airless. Effective vascular supply may be related to this distribution. If vascular leak first occurs centrally, blood flow to the periphery could be less and/or it may be that the supply of blood is greater centrally, being from both pulmonary and bronchial arteries, and so favors leak at this level. These are only speculations on the reason for the central distribution of air and membranes and the increasing airlessness at the acinar periphery.

Ultrastructurally cellular damage is seen as vacuolization of capillary endothelium with sloughing of epithelium [26] and hyperchromatism. That epithelial desquamation, which is considered artifact by some [22], is an essential feature is suggested by cytological studies of tracheal aspirates [19,20]. Thus, in the early stage, there is evidence for loss of epithelial and capillary integrity and of disordered fluid transport. Epithelial necrosis is centroacinar, with less, if any, being seen at the periphery [24-27].

The hyaline membrane (HM) consists of layers of eosinophilic material coating the walls of primitive alveoli. Meticulous search has demonstrated rare wispy HM material as early as half an hour after birth, but well-established, although thin, membranes are seldom found diffusely until 4-6 hr later. Figures 2 and 3 illustrate hyaline membranes from two newborns who died at 18 and 84 hr of age, respectively. Early in the process the membranes may be patchy in distribution and even confined to one lobe. Epithelium of respiratory bronchioli is sloughed or necrotic [24-27], and cell lysis may contribute to faint hematoxylophilia (bluish granular or globular deposits) sometimes seen relatively early in the diffuse HM stage. HMs are deposited along surfaces of respiratory bronchioli and of the centroacinar air space, and the more peripheral air spaces are increasingly collapsed. When it is poorly perfused with blood, the tissue seems solid. Watery edema fluid is usually present in small airways, but it may

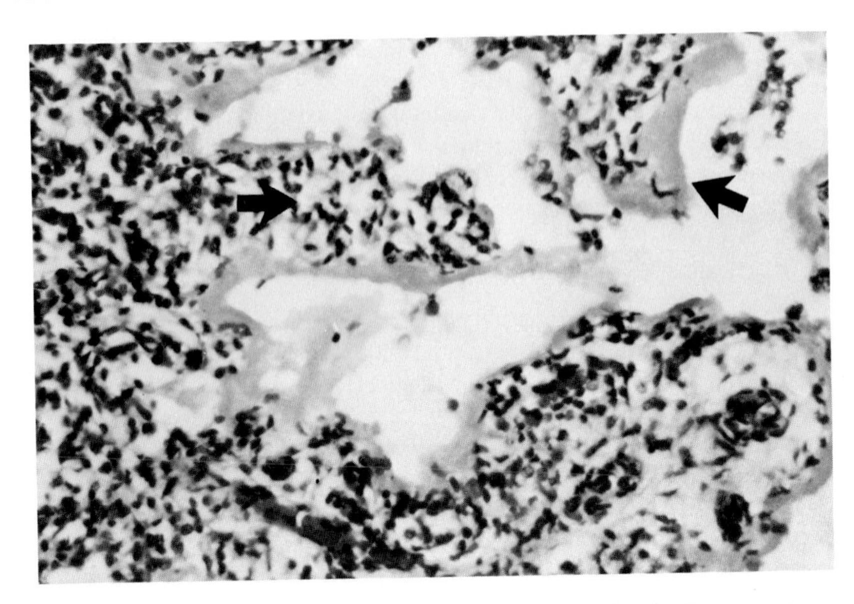

Figure 2 Photomicrograph of hyaline membrane formation in the premature lung showing the homogeneous membranes against the alveolar wall (upper right arrow). Alternately airless, cellular alveoli are seen (upper left arrow). Alveolar expansion and hyaline membrane formation both show central acinar distribution. From a newborn weighing 1750 g at birth who died 18 hr after birth (X 200).

require special techniques for demonstration [22]. The capillary bed appears congested as it usually does in acutely collapsed lung. In necropsy studies resistance to pulmonary artery perfusion is increased [21], and arteriograms, in which radiopaque material demonstrates pulmonary arteries down to about 0.2 mm internal diameter, show decreased peripheral filling [22].

Recent vascular morphometric studies of HMD in four neonates who died 4-72 hr after birth indicate greater dilatation of small pulmonary arteries (below 0.1 mm internal diameter) than occurs in age-matched control infants [28]. This dilation involves both preacinar (extraparenchymal) muscular arteries and intraparenchymal nonmuscular arteries. How this dilatation occurs in the face of stimuli such as hypoxia, which in the mature lung cause pulmonary arterial vasoconstriction, is not clear. Perhaps the receptors that mediate vasoconstriction [29] are not yet present or are blocked or destroyed, or a dilator mediator may be active.

Sloughing and necrosis of epithelium could arise from different mechanisms, although they are often both attributed to the effect of anoxia, or ischemia, or both. The reason for cellular necrosis needs further reevaluation. Clinical trials suggest that vitamin E therapy has no beneficial effect upon established RDS or its complications [30], but it is still possible that necrosis is worse in infants who have vitamin E deficiency.

With longer survival the hyaline membranes become thicker, to as much as 20 μm. The membranes contain plasma proteins, including fibrinogen and incompletely stabilized fibrin [31,32], nucleic acids (early), lipids, including neutral fat, bound carbohydrates [25], and iron, which may be the result of diapedesis of red blood cells [27] or it may be of cytochrome origin.

Occasionally HMs are yellow (yellow HMD) [33] and evidence indicates that unconjugated bilirubin is responsible for the color [34]. Whether the course of the disease is modified by the presence of bilirubin remains to be established. Although virtually all neonates with yellow HMs are jaundiced, there is poor correlation between degree of membrane staining and the level of hyperbilirubinemia.

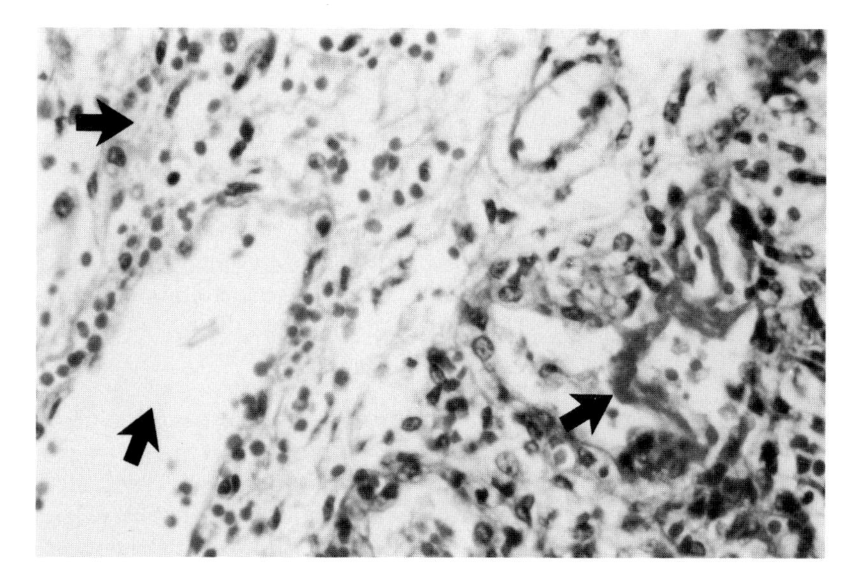

Figure 3 Photomicrograph of several alveoli adjacent to a connective tissue septum (upper left arrow) that is thickened by edema and inflammatory cell infiltration and contains a dilated lymphatic (lower left arrow). The alveoli show a hyaline membrane (lower right arrow) that seems to be lifted from the alveolar wall by the regenerating epithelial cells. From an infant at 28 weeks' gestational age who died 84 hr after birth (X 200).

Macroscopically, at this stage, the lungs are heavy and increased in volume, feel rubbery but not hard, are uniformly dull red in color, usually do not float in water [22], cannot be inflated with air under normal transbronchial pressure [23], and closely resemble shock lung of children and adults. The seeming paradox of microscopical collapse and airlessness in a lung of increased resting volume and weight doubtless reflects both fluid translocation into extravascular compartments and cellular infiltration.

C. Complications

Pulmonary microvascular thrombi are rare in early and untreated cases of HMD. This does not support the hypothesis that a major or sustained necrotizing endothelial injury is a primary process. Thrombi are more common later, especially in the presence of acidosis or a vascular catheter, or as part of DIC. While infarction is virtually never found, petechial hemorrhages are common (30-50%) [35]. Interstitial hemorrhages are seen early and are thought to reflect asphyxia or venous hypertension. Intra-acinar hemorrhages become more frequent with longer survival [27]. Massive pulmonary hemorrhage of the newborn has occasionally complicated HMD and probably indicates a serious form of hemorrhagic diathesis or infection [36].

Before modern aggressive therapy became common, interstitial emphysema occurred in perhaps 5% of cases, but now the incidence of this complication is much higher (see section on interstitial emphysema, p. 402). It is a particular hazard for the more immature infant. Pneumothorax, mediastinal emphysema, pneumopericardium, and air embolism may follow. Subcutaneous emphysema indicates large airway rupture. If unilateral pneumothorax occurs, it is likely it will spread and become bilateral, both because interstitial emphysema tends to occur at many sites and because the rupture from one pleural space to the other is common. The mediastinal tissues are especially delicate in the premature infant.

The HMD found in infants with *Rhesus* isoimmunization (associated with pulmonary hypoplasia) [37], or in prematures born to diabetic mothers (associated with particular vascular lesions) [38] has not been shown to be different pathologically from that seen in newborns with similar degrees of lung immaturity. However, HMD has been reported to be associated with normal pulmonary surfactant in some mature or postmature infants born to diabetic mothers [39]. Here the peripheral air space collapse may not occur and HMs are found throughout the acinus. This disease should be clearly separated from usual HMD and definitely needs more study.

D. Resolution and Repair

Clinical improvement in the respiratory function begins by the third or fourth day of illness. It is accompanied or sometimes heralded by a dramatic improvement in the chest radiograph. Surfactant, characteristically low in HMD, has been shown to increase as early as day 3.

For the pathologist, processes of repair may begin as early as the second day [40] when cells with eosinophilic cytoplasm appear and spread over denuded alveolar surfaces beneath the HM, first as single cells, then as a confluent monolayer of squamous cells, and ultimately as rows of plump cells producing an almost glandular appearance. It is almost as if the epithelium lyses the junction between the HM and lung tissue and lifts the HM free (Fig. 3).

Cytologically, the regenerative alveolar epithelium resembles that seen after the administration of steroids in pharmacological doses [41] or of folate or vitamin B_{12} deficiency. The eosinophilic cytoplasm, reflecting numerous organelles, is often interrupted by tiny, clear refractile vacuoles that indicate lipid-rich accumulation. Such cells frequently contain diastase-resistant, periodic acid Schiff-positive material that is characteristic of the type II pneumocyte, the cell thought to synthesize and discharge pulmonary surfactant.

Factors which may interfere with normal repair include: (1) continuing primary injury, (2) iatrogenic causes (oxygen toxicity, fluid overload, and barotrauma), and (3) reduction in cell proliferation (e.g., caused by cortisol administration or by vitamin B_{12} or folate deficiency). Administration of steroids, besides promoting maturation, suppresses cellular proliferation. Trials of folic acid therapy have not clearly shortened the duration or reduced the complications of HMD. Other factors include: (1) interference with maturation of epithelial cells (as is seen with acidosis or prolonged deficiency of protein or trace metals), (2) secondary infection, and (3) interference with mucociliary clearance.

Pathological analysis of the lungs of many patients dying from hyaline membrane disease demonstrates that some patients show evidence of considerable epithelial repair, while in others it is lacking [40] (Figs. 4-7). The reason for this lack of repair in some patients needs to be addressed.

Within 24 hr or so after birth scattered neutrophils and mononuclear cells thought to be histiocytes appear. It is suggested that the lung of sick immature infants is relatively deficient in protease activity [42], so that it is enzymes from these leukocytes that digest the membranes. In any case, the membranes do become fragmented and lie free in air spaces. Whether these masses cause obstruction to air flow and predispose to interstitial emphysema is not clear (Fig. 8). Tracheal aspirates sometimes contain coagulated protein, suggesting that at least some membrane is removed by the mucociliary escalator.

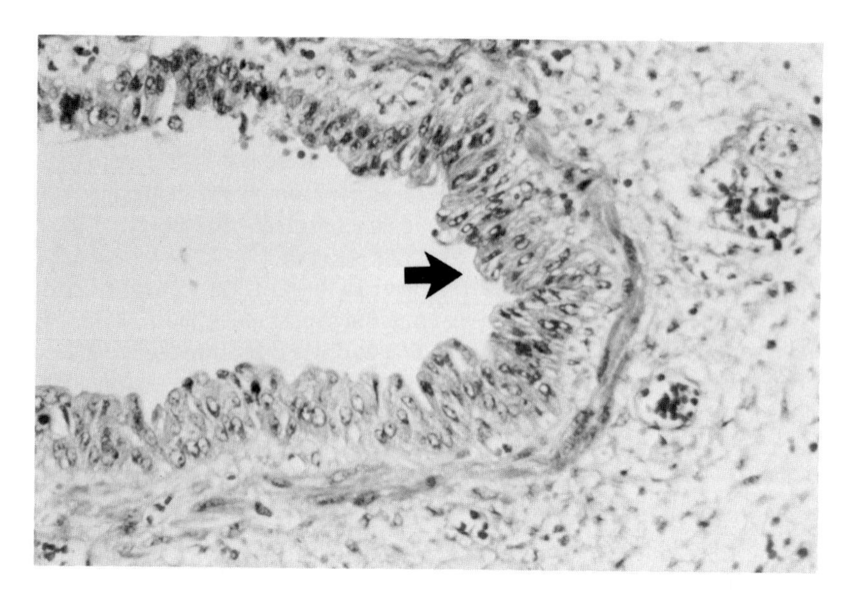

Figure 4 Photomicrograph of a small bronchiolus showing a thickened wall that includes blood vessels and smooth muscle; its epithelium is replaced by a non-ciliated and multicellular layer of epithelium (arrow) (X 200).

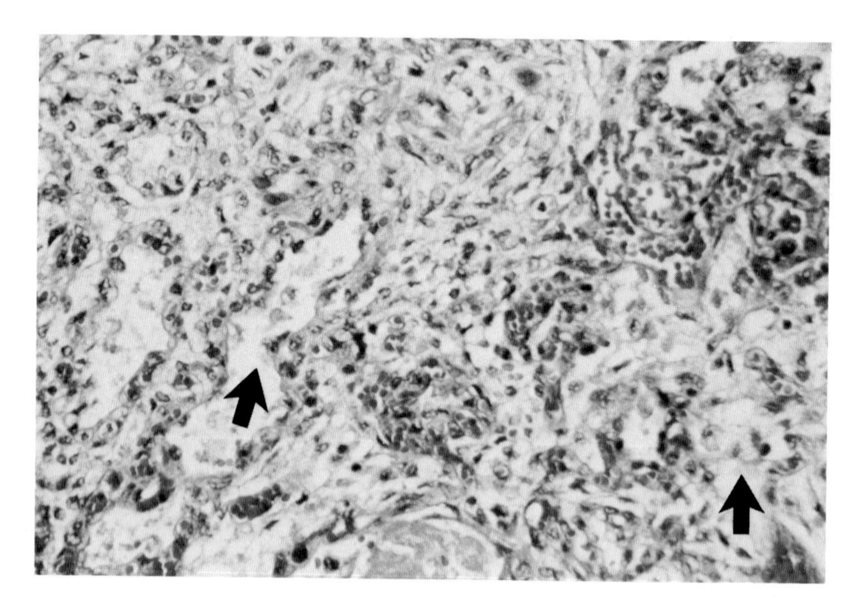

Figure 5 Photomicrograph of the alveolar region of the lung of an infant following hyaline membrane disease. Alveolar structure (left arrow) is still apparent and the walls are thickened and the alveolar space lined by cuboidal epithelium; to the right the alveolar architecture (right arrow) is obliterated by intra-alveolar organization (X 200).

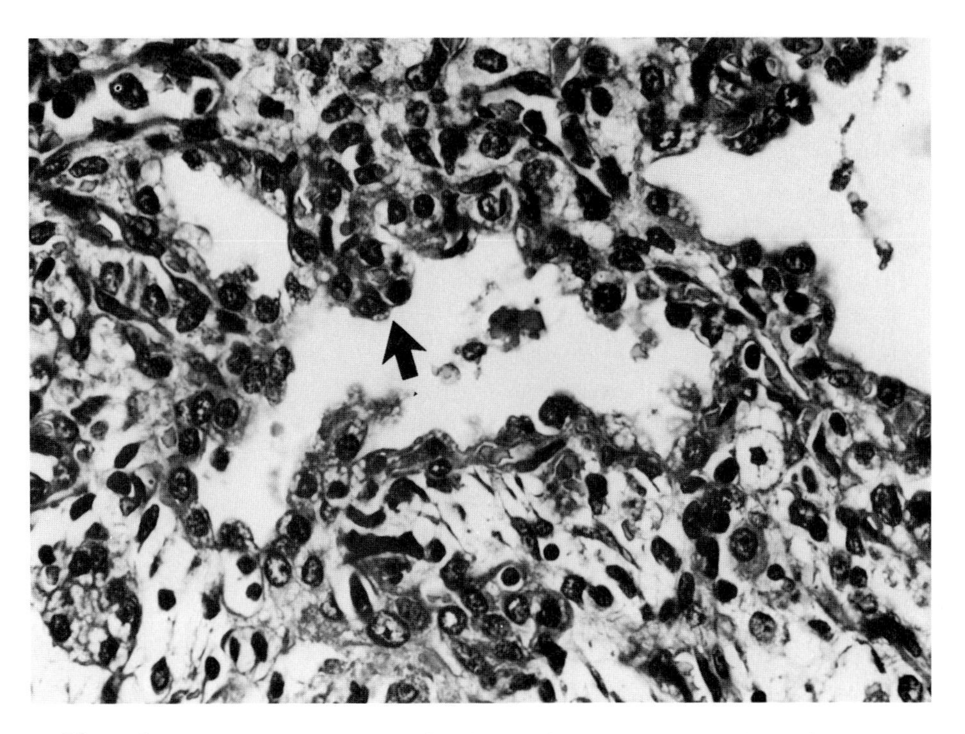

Figure 6 Photomicrograph of an alveolus in which the epithelial lining is seen as hyperthrophied and cuboidal (arrow). The alveolar wall consists of loose granulation tissue (X 400).

Protease and fibrinolysin deficiency can have effects other than failure to prevent or digest hyaline membranes; e.g., angiotensin II is destroyed by proteases which in normal lung are particularly rich in pulmonary veins. Pulmonary venous constriction could result from excess of this mediator and be the cause of the increased pulmonary vascular resistance associated with the collapse of the peripheral alveoli. This concept is in contrast to the previously held postulate that the alveolar collapse is associated with low vascular flow or left ventricular failure.

In those rare instances of death 2 or 3 weeks after clinical healing, lung structure has usually been reported to be normal, although sometimes scattered residues of hyaline material remain.

We have studied three sudden infant deaths occurring at 6-8 weeks of age. All infants were prematurely born and had been treated for 4-8 days for mild respiratory distress syndrome. On routine study the lungs were essentially normal in two, but in the lung of one patient, goblet cell hyperplasia was widespread.

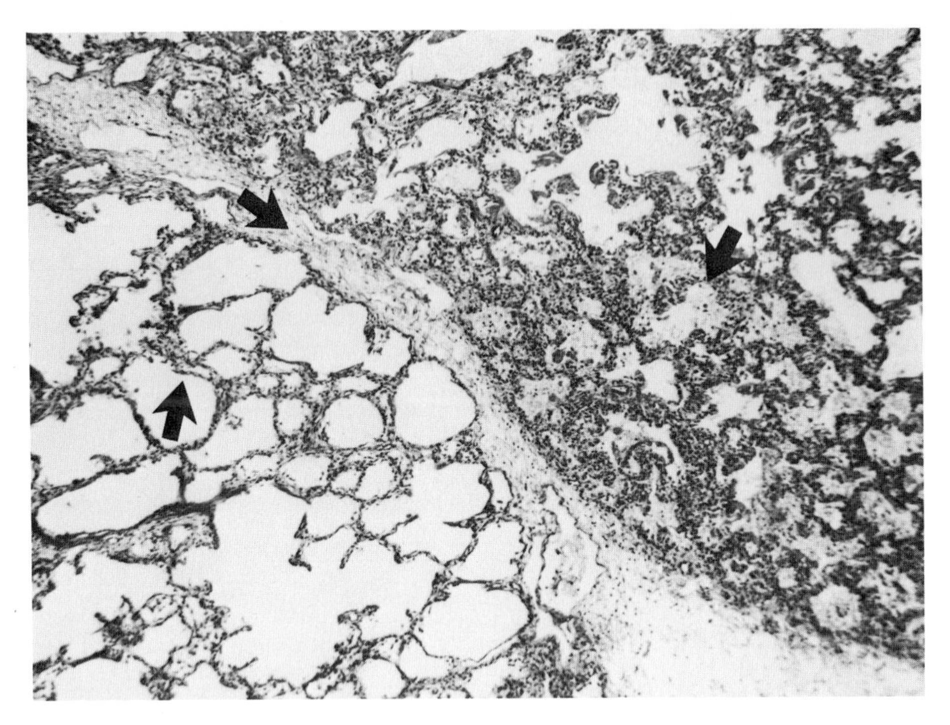

Figure 7 Photomicrograph of section of lung showing to the right small alveoli containing hyaline membranes (right arrow) and to the left larger and better aerated alveoli (lower left arrow). The focally irregular changes are apparent in this picture. The two areas of lung are separated by a connective tissue septum (upper left arrow) (X 16).

IV. Complications of Treatment

In infants who do not survive RDS the effects of treatment and superimposed infection make a significant contribution to the pathological changes. Advances in ventilatory care of the newborn, including application of continuous positive airway pressure (CPAP) and positive end-expiratory pressure (PEEP), have increased survival of premature infants with RDS. But while these techniques have brought benefits, they also have their complications.

Injury to the respiratory and digestive tracts may occur during insertion of endotracheal tubes or from continuous pressure during prolonged intubation. Barotrauma, implicated as a cause of BPD [43], can also produce potentially fatal pulmonary air leaks. The adverse effects of high levels of inspired oxygen are discussed later with BPD. Additional lung injury can be caused by the presence of intravascular catheters or from fluids given as parenteral alimentation.

A. Mechanical Injury to the Upper Airway

During insertion endotracheal tubes can lacerate or perforate the mucosa of the nasopharynx, oropharynx, or esophagus [44]. Insufflation of the stomach following accidental esophageal intubation has also been reported [44]. More commonly seen at autopsy is injury to the vocal cords following long-term tracheal intubation with pressure necrosis of the cords and subglottic stenosis due to organized granulation tissue [44].

Exposure laryngotracheobronchitis, long known to respiratory therapists, is characterized by loss of epithelium, by necrosis of superficial stroma, and

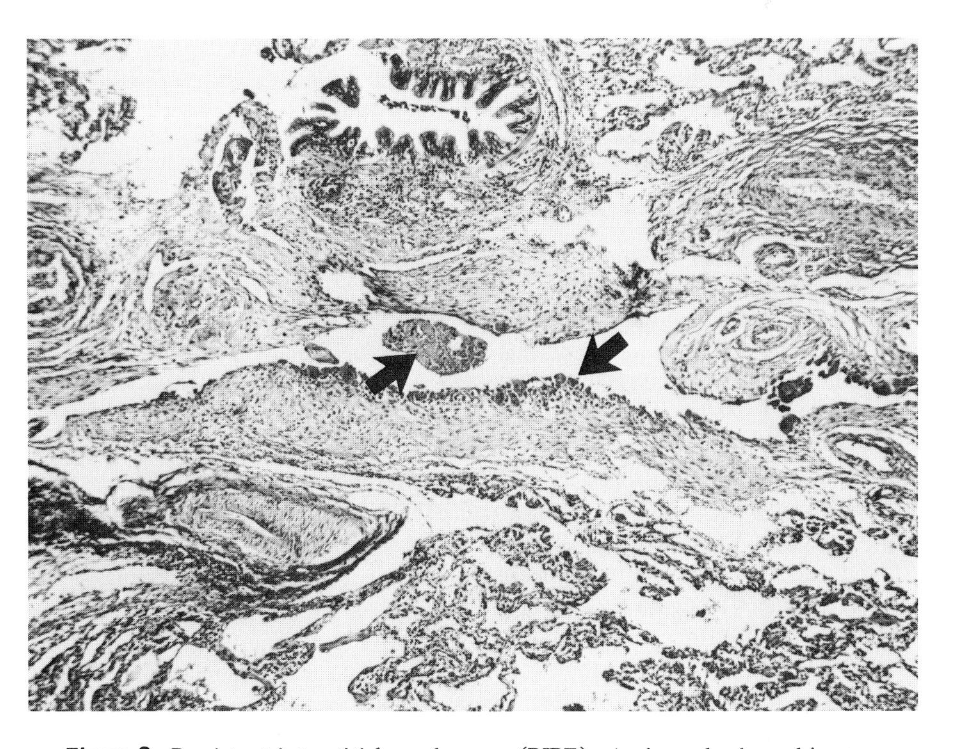

Figure 8 Persistent interstitial emphysema (PIPE). An irregular branching space lined by giant cells (right arrow). The space lies in the periacinar connective tissue that includes, in this case, a fibrinous mass (left arrow) (X 63).

sometimes by a meager inflammatory cell infiltrate. When the process involves airway cartilage, airway stenosis is likely to develop as a late sequela. Rapid healing of surface epithelium depends upon sparing of submucosal gland ducts from which regeneration occurs, much like a second-degree thermal burn. This lesion impairs mucociliary clearance and can provide a portal of entry for secondary bacterial invaders. It has become less common now that smaller endotracheal catheters are used, nitrous oxide sterilization of cannulae has been discontinued, cleanliness and sterility of respiratory equipment are more meticulous, and humidification and filtration of the oxygen supply are more careful.

In the lower tracheobronchial tree, unilateral ventilation of a lung or lobe follows cannulation of a mainstem or lobar bronchus. Less frequently, the endotracheal tube perforates the carina, or suction catheters damage the segmental bronchi [45]. Repeated injury to the bronchial mucosa from suction catheters can produce polypoid masses of granulation tissue which, by obstructing the bronchial lumen, cause lobar hyperinflation, described particularly in the right middle and lower lobes [46]. Lobar emphysema of undetermined etiology has also been described in the right lower lobe of patients with BPD [47,48]. The role of bronchial obstruction in these cases is unclear. Such acquired neonatal lobar emphysema should be distinguished radiologically and pathologically from the interstitial emphysema due to barotrauma.

B. Interstitial Emphysema and Air Leaks from the Lung

A premature and surfactant-deficient newborn lung, with its irregular zones of hyperaeration and collapse and its increased airway pressures, is prone to alveolar rupture and interstitial air dissection (Fig. 8). Air leaks have been reported in up to 41% of premature infants managed with mechanical ventilators [49]. In animal experiments, Macklin and Macklin showed that increased intra-alveolar pressure, stretching of alveolar walls, and decreased intrapulmonic blood volume caused rupture at the junction of alveolar walls with subsequent dissection along perivascular sheaths [50,51]. Interstitial air dissects either centrally toward the hilum to produce pneumomediastinum or pneumopericardium, or peripherally toward the pleura to produce pneumothorax [49-53]. Dissection of air into the soft tissues of the neck gives rise to subcutaneous emphysema, while extension along the para-aortic or paraesophageal connective tissue produces pneumoperitoneum [49,51].

After air has ruptured the alveolar walls, within the interlobular connective tissue septa cystlike spaces or dilated lymphatics are present often accompanied by fresh hemorrhage [51]. Interstitial emphysema can be either localized or diffuse within the lung. In the localized type, large cysts up to 3 cm in diameter are found and are sometimes confined to one or a few lobes. This form is amenable to surgical resection and survival of 70% of cases so treated has been reported [54]. When it is diffuse, persistent interstitial pulmonary emphysema is commonly fatal and cysts in this type are usually < 0.3 cm in diameter [54]. When interstitial air persists for more than 5 days, large pseudocysts rimmed by foreign body giant cells and hemosiderin-filled histiocytes widen the interstitium and compress pulmonary lobules, lymphatics, and blood vessels ("air block") [51,54]. The characteristic giant cells probably represent a reaction to persistent gas [54]. Interstitial air perhaps persists because it is within lymphatics [55,56].

Stocker and Madewell [54] reported that five of 10 patients with localized persistent interstitial emphysema and nine of 12 patients with the diffuse form developed pneumothorax. Decreased pulmonary venous return associated with pneumothorax is accompanied by increased systemic venous pressure and decreased cardiac output. This, along with acidemia and hypercarbia, probably increases flow in the anterior cerebral arteries and elevates pressure in the germinal matrix capillaries [57], contributing to the high incidence of associated intraventricular hemorrhage.

Systemic air embolism, recognized in < 1% of mechanically ventilated newborns, is another fatal complication of pulmonary air leak [58]. Air probably enters through tears opening into the connective tissue septa. Other ways that gas may become intravascular are by accidental injection of air during intravenous infusion or by its entry around an umbilical vein catheter [59]. Postmortem radiographs of patients with systemic air embolism show air within the cardiac chambers as well as in systemic arteries and veins [58] (Fig. 9).

C. Chest Tube Insertion

The treatment of pulmonary air leaks is itself associated with serious, life-threatening complications. In one series, the alarming figure is given that in 25% of neonates needing percutaneous drainage of a pneumothorax, the chest tube perforated their lung during its insertion [60]. Patients with RDS or BPD are especially susceptible to this complication because of their noncompliant, "stiff" lungs. Visceroparietal pleural adhesions also increase the risk of lung puncture. Lung perforation often remains undiagnosed until autopsy with the antemortem chest radiographs having been interpreted as showing the chest tube in place within the thorax [61]. Failure of the chest tube to correct the pneumothorax should signal the possibility of an iatrogenic lung tear [61]. The trocar used to penetrate the chest wall may be more culpable than the tube itself in puncturing the visceral pleura [62]. Within the lung the tube is surrounded by fibrin and compressed hemorrhagic lung tissue [60].

Other complications of chest tube insertion are soft tissue hemorrhage from laceration of an intercostal artery or development of a traumatic arteriovenous fistula between chest wall and lung [62]. In the neonate drainage of

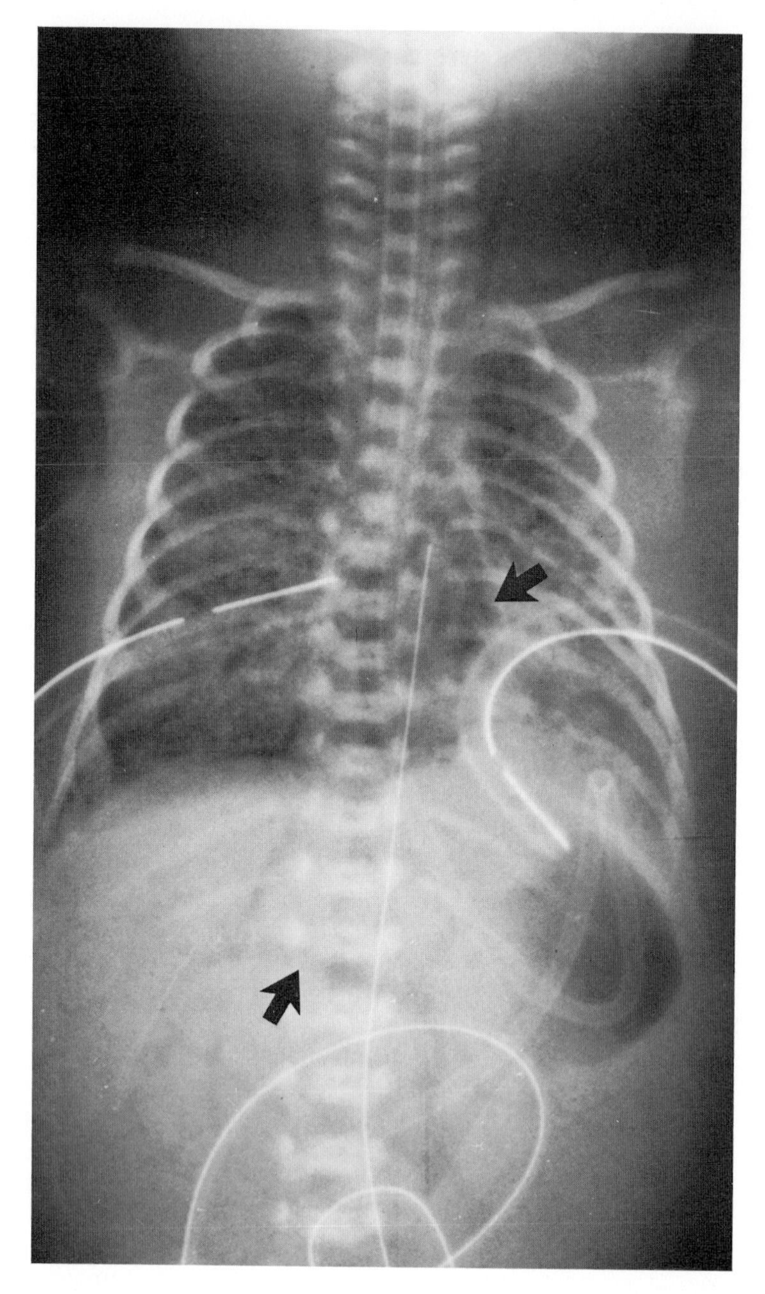

Figure 9 Fatal case of air embolism. Radiograph shows interstitial emphysema and gas filling cardiac chambers (upper arrow) and abdominal blood vessels (lower arrow). (Courtesy of B. Fletcher, Cleveland, Ohio.)

recurrent pneumothorax often requires insertion of several chest tubes. We have seen up to three within a hemithorax. Because of their size they cause significant compression of the lung and limit its expansion.

D. Pulmonary Complications of Parenteral Nutrition

Babies being mechanically ventilated are often maintained for long periods on total intravenous alimentation. Indwelling catheters are themselves a site of infection and a source of pulmonary emboli, perhaps septic ones. A variety of metabolic abnormalities is also associated with alimentation. These include hyperglycemic, nonketotic coma and isosmolar coma, thought to be due to the high amino acid content of protein hydrolysates [63]. Hyperammonemia also is a potentially lethal complication. Up to one-third of neonates receiving total parenteral nutrition show a range of hepatic lesions from intracanalicular bile stasis to severe portal fibrosis [64].

Less well recognized are the pulmonary lesions that affect the newborn receiving intravenous lipid infusions. Dahms and Halpin have reported a series of patients whose small muscular pulmonary arteries were severely narrowed by intimal lipid deposits and fat-laden histiocytes [66]. All were receiving intravenous lipid infusions and had pulmonary hypertension. It is probable that lipid is deposited on the endothelial surface previously damaged by pulmonary hypertension [66]. The lipid vasculopathy in turn exacerbates pulmonary hypertension, contributing to a vicious cycle.

Necrotizing pulmonary vasculitis due to the fungus *Malassezia furfur* has been reported in one patient with BPD receiving intravenous lipid hyperalimentation [67]. *M. furfur,* the causative agent of tinea versicolor and ordinarily a commensal organism of the skin, cannot synthesize medium- and long-chain fatty acids and requires exogenous lipids for metabolism. The arterial intimal lipid deposits seen in infants on intravenous alimentation apparently provide a fertile medium for its growth [67].

V. Pathological Features of Diseases Considered as Differential Diagnosis of the Respiratory Distress Syndrome in the Newborn

Many other congenital and acquired diseases cause respiratory distress in newborns. In some of these disorders, notably streptococcal pneumonia, pulmonary hypoplasia, and cystic adenomatoid malformation, surfactant deficiency with hyaline membrane formation may complicate the clinical course.

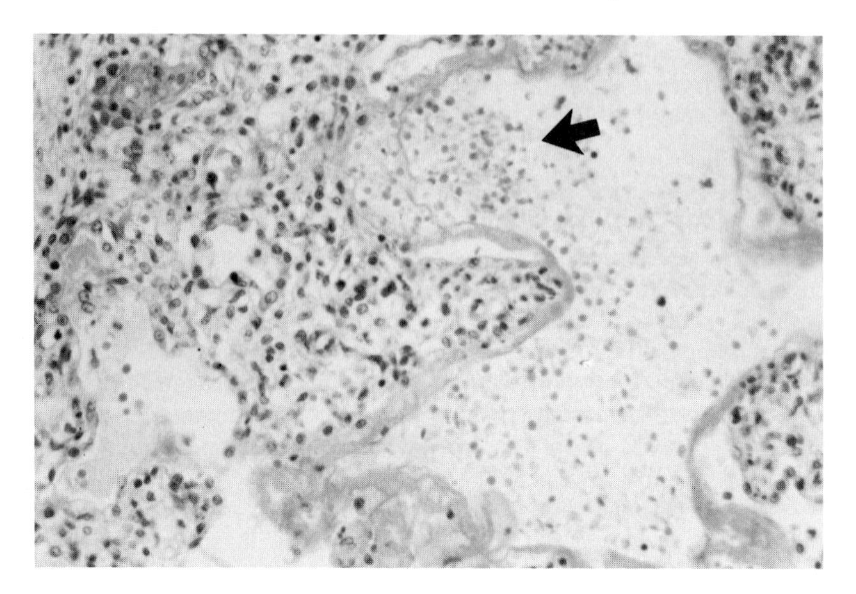

Figure 10 Group B streptococcal infection can easily be mistaken for HMD. It differs from HMD in that peripheral air spaces are also involved and there is little atelectasis. Intra-alveolar exudate (arrow) is seen along with a variable degree of inflammatory cell infiltration. Demonstration of gram-positive streptococci by special strains is necessary to establish the diagnosis. From a newborn weighing 840 g at birth who died 26 hr after birth.

A. Neonatal Pneumonia (Group B Streptococcal)

Pneumonia is the most common serious infection in the newborn period and is found at autopsy in up to 22% of newborns who survive 48 hr or longer [68]. The factors that predispose to neonatal bacterial pneumonia are: (1) prolonged rupture of the membranes, (2) extended labor, and (3) excessive obstetrical manipulations [68]. Group B streptococcal pneumonia is the most common type of bacterial pneumonia seen during this period [68]. When acute in onset it resembles neonatal hyaline membrane disease both clinically and pathologically [69-71]. Histologically, Katzenstein and colleagues noted sparse inflammation with prominent hyaline membranes impregnated with gram-positive cocci [69]. In HMD the membranes are concentrated in the centroacinar areas, while in group B streptococcal infection they are also found at the periphery of the acinus. Ablow et al. reported an interstitial and intraalveolar infiltrate [70]. Lungs affected by streptococcal pneumonia can also be distinguished from those with hyaline membrane disease by the presence of a pleural effusion and minimal atelectasis [69,70].

Other bacteria, particularly *Escherichia coli, Staphylococcus aureus,* or *Pseudomonas aeruginosa,* can cause pneumonias in the neonatal period that can complicate the course of hyaline membrane disease. Pathologically, the hallmark of acute bacterial pneumonia is a fibrinous intra-alveolar exudate (Fig. 10) and an inflammatory cell infiltration of the alveolar wall. Abscess formation is sometimes associated with staphylococcal pneumonia, and necrotizing vasculitis may accompany infection with *Pseudomonas aeruginosa.*

B. Meconium Aspiration

Aspiration of meconium usually occurs in infants who have suffered intra-uterine distress, many of whom are mature or postmature. Microscopically, keratinized squamous cells, meconium bodies, and mucous plugs are impacted in small bronchi and bronchioli [72] (Fig. 11). Infected amniotic fluid also causes an exudate of neutrophils. Distal to the blocked airways, alveoli are hyperinflated,

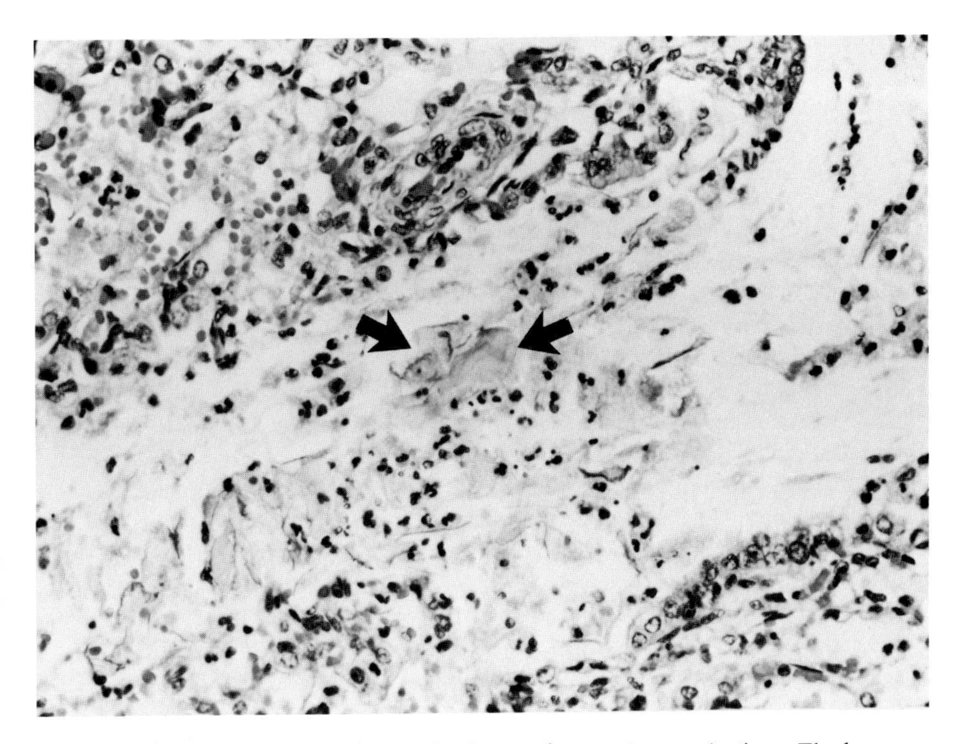

Figure 11 A small airway from a fatal case of meconium aspiration. The lumen contains squamous cells (left arrow), nuclear debris, mucus, and a meconium body (right arrow). A small artery is seen adjacent (Papanicolau stain) (X 250).

and some have ruptured walls. Fatal interstitial emphysema with pneumothorax, pneumomediastinum and air block can occur [72]. A hypercoagulable state is common. Murphy et al., using a quantitative morphometric approach to study the pulmonary vasculature in fatal cases of meconium aspiration, found marked medial hypertrophy of muscular pulmonary arteries and peripheral extension of muscle [73] similar to that seen in patients with persistent pulmonary hypertension of the newborn [74]. These findings in at least some of the patients with meconium aspiration indicate that this perinatal event signals intrauterine maldevelopment perhaps as long as weeks before birth.

C. Pulmonary Hypoplasia

The hypoplastic lung is reduced in size and weight and usually has a decreased number of bronchial branches. To study the anatomical features contributing to the small lung it is necessary to apply quantitative methods to count the number of airways, alveoli, arteries, and veins.

Pulmonary hypoplasia occurs when the available thoracic volume is reduced as in congenital diaphragmatic hernia [75-77]. At birth both lungs are small, especially the ipsilateral one. Following repair of the diaphragm the inflated ipsilateral lung does not immediately fill the hemithorax. Both lungs usually have normal lobation, but often in the ipsilateral lung the lobes are distorted and the bronchi narrowed. The intrasegmental pattern of bronchial branching is disturbed, which is evidence of interference as early as the fifth or sixth week of intrauterine life [78]. Bronchial arrest on the side of the hernia corresponds to an intrauterine development of 10-12 weeks, while that on the contralateral side is 12-14 weeks. This suggests that abdominal organs are in the thorax at least by this stage of development [75].

Microscopically, there is a reduction in the total number of airway branches, particularly small bronchi and bronchioli [75,76]. Reduction in alveolar number also occurs and is more marked on the ipsilateral side. Although alveoli are reduced in size, radial alveolar counts [79,80] (number of alveoli transected by a diagonal between terminal bronchiolus and pleura) are nearly normal, which indicates that the reduction in total alveolar number mainly reflects the reduction in number of bronchioli and, therefore, of acinar units.

Postmortem arteriograms show a reduced number of branches from axial arteries that are characteristically narrow. More medial muscle is present in smaller arteries than in the normal newborn lung, but peripheral extension into acinar vessels is not always seen [76]. The mean arterial medial thickness is slightly higher than normal.

Hypoplastic lungs are capable of catch-up growth following repair of the diaphragmatic defect [81]. By 4 months the radiographic appearance can return to normal. Respiratory function studies, performed on survivors aged

6–19 years, have demonstrated that total lung capacity, vital capacity, and forced expiratory volume are normal [81], whereas blood flow on the side of the hernia is diminished.

Other conditions that limit the thoracic space available to the developing lung, such as phrenic nerve agenesis and diaphragmatic amyoplasia [82], also produce pulmonary hypoplasia and are associated with neonatal respiratory distress.

Chamberlain and colleagues documented pulmonary hypoplasia in babies with severe *Rhesus* isoimmunization [83]. In this series, reduction in airway number was seen in all infants which suggests injury at least by the sixteenth week of intrauterine life. The alveolar abnormality varied from case to case. They suggest that reduction in thoracic volume, which might result from an enlarging liver and spleen, was not the main cause since enlargement of liver and spleen occurs later in the course of the disease [83]. They feel that there may be a hormonal or immune-mediated injury to dividing airway epithelium [83].

Potter has shown that in patients with renal agenesis the lungs are often below normal weight and immature [84]. It seems that this hypoplasia and dysplasia reflects failure of the kidney to produce adequate amounts of proline for use in lung growth [85,86].

D. Wilson-Mikity Syndrome

In 1960 Wilson and Mikity reported a series of premature infants who 1–5 weeks after birth insidiously developed cyanosis and respiratory distress [87]. None of the infants was exposed continually to levels of oxygen of 40% or FI_{O_2} of 0.40 or more, nor did they pass through a phase of RDS or HMD at birth. No infectious cause could be demonstrated. The chest radiographs showed coarse streaky shadows and hyperlucent regions giving a "bubbly" appearance, which is typical of this syndrome. In the original cases the characteristic pathological finding was a regional alveolar inflation, even hyperinflation, with airless compressed zones in between. This appearance of irregular aeration and airlessness of lung is consistent with an uneven maturation of the surfactant system [78]. This suggested that the cause of the radiographic appearance was ventilation of the normal regions and atelectasis of the immature regions. The "disadvantaged" regions might ultimately aerate or persist as scars of condensed lung. If mild recovery of such a condition should occur, its treatment could produce many of the complications described as part of BPD [88]. This term has been used more widely than was justified by this original description. It is appropriate to make a plea here that we return to this more rigid interpretation. In some cases the term has been used to describe any x-ray that shows appearances of hyperlucency with streaky scars.

A similar radiographic picture has been reported as early as day 1 in some premature infants. In one we were able to study personally the lung showed a widespread but focal dysplasia, mixed with regions of more normal lung and ventilation. It is not surprising that the uneven aeration gave a bubbly appearance as described in the original article by Wilson and Mikity [87].

E. Persistent Fetal Circulation

In some neonates the normal postnatal fall in pulmonary artery pressure and pulmonary vascular resistance does not occur. This failure of adaptation cannot be explained by underlying pulmonary or cardiovascular disease. Gersony et al. have termed this disorder *persistent fetal circulation* [89]. Pulmonary hypertension in these patients is often fatal.

Quantitative morphometric studies of the lungs of patients who died with this syndrome have shown a well-developed muscle wall in the alveolar wall arteries that normally at birth are free of muscle [7,20]. The size of arteries and their density and number per unit area of lung, however, are normal. This striking increase in muscle is evidence that a process of vascular remodeling started in utero. The cause or causes of these vascular changes are not known, but it could be sensitivity to some intrauterine stress, abnormal flow in the fetal pulmonary vascular bed, or failure of the mechanisms regulating arterial muscularization and vascular tone [73,74,90]. The degree of extension and hypertrophy of medial smooth muscle in patients with persistent fetal circulation is generally more striking than we have observed in patients with BPD [91].

F. Congenital Lobar Emphysema (Lobar Emphysema of Childhood)

Congenital emphysema, causing respiratory distress in the neonatal period, should not be confused clinically with hyaline membrane disease or BPD in which acquired interstitial or lobar emphysema is present. Radiologically, the pulmonary hyperlucency and mediastinal shift caused by childhood lobar emphysema are distinct from the small lucencies produced by diffuse interstitial emphysema. Acquired lobar emphysema can occur in patients with BPD, but it usually occurs after several weeks of ventilator therapy, and typically involves the right lower lobe, in contrast to congenital lobar emphysema, which has a predilection for the upper lobes.

Lobar emphysema of childhood, if present in the newborn period, represents a disorder of alveolar growth and is of three pathological types: (1) polyalveolar lobe, (2) localized hypoplasia, and (3) bronchial atresia [92]. In the condition known as *polyalveolar lobe* there is a multisegmental increase of normal-sized alveoli localized usually to a few segments. This acinar overgrowth apparently occurs in late intrauterine life. At present, the cause of polyalveolar lobe is unknown, but it may be the result of an imbalance in the regulation of intrauterine growth [93]. It has been associated with abnormal lung fluid retention.

By contrast, in the *localized hypoplasia* form of congenital emphysema, a reduced number of enlarged alveoli is present [94]. Airway number is also reduced, suggesting a defect in lung development beginning before the twelfth week of intrauterine life. In hypoplastic lobar emphysema the total volume of the hyperlucent area may be normal or decreased which is an important diagnostic feature [94].

Bronchial atresia has also been recognized in the neonatal period as a cause of emphysema. Usually, one or two segmental bronchi to the left upper lobe are atretic. Centrally, the bronchus is without communication to the trachea, but distally it branches normally. Alveolar size and number are normal at birth but in those instances in which overinflation via collateral air channels produces air trapping [95] emphysema occurs shortly after birth.

G. Congenital Malformations of the Lung

Pulmonary malformation and dysplasia may present as respiratory distress in the newborn. *Adenomatoid malformation*, a localized unregulated growth of alveolar and bronchiolar tissue, can be either solid or cystic and affect one or more lobes. Three types of this anomaly have been described: solid, large cystic, and small cystic [96,97]. The solid form presents on the chest radiograph as a massive lesion with an accompanying mediastinal shift [96]. Occasionally, cystic adenomatoid malformation is present in edematous premature infants with other congenital anomalies and a history of maternal hydramnios [96,98]. The affected lung may show typical hyaline membrane disease. Some cystic variants are radiolucent on the chest radiograph and are confused with congenital lobar or localized interstitial emphysema. The absence of cartilage in cystic adenomatoid malformation suggests a defect in development before the tenth week of intrauterine life when bronchial cartilage is usually formed [96].

Other dysplastic lesions of the lung have been described as causes of respiratory distress in the neonate. In the patient of Janney et al. a selective retardation in the development of alveolar capillaries was found [99]. Jones has described a malformation in a premature infant similar to cystic adenomatoid malformation of the lung but with excess of mesenchymal tissue [100]. In the cases of pulmonary dysplasia described by Hislop et al. abnormal vascular pathways, ectopic muscle, and air-filled cysts were seen in lungs with either hypoplastic or atretic pulmonary arteries and veins [101].

Finally, congenital pulmonary lymphangiectasia should be mentioned as a lesion which can be difficult to distinguish pathologically from persistent interstitial emphysema, in which air may infiltrate and dilate lymphatic ducts [102].

The presence of hemorrhage and a giant cell reaction to entrapped interstitial gas in interstitial emphysema help to distinguish histologically between these two disorders. Aberrant anomalies of pulmonary venous return are sometimes associated with congenital pulmonary lymphangiectasia.

VI. The Pathology of Bronchopulmonary Dysplasia

Bronchopulmonary dysplasia (BPD) was originally defined by Northway and colleagues as a subacute or chronic fibrosing condition of lung occurring in premature infants following severe hyaline membrane disease [103]. The evolution of this process through the four radiographic stages they described is now rarely observed. More frequently, there is a subtle transition from hyaline membrane disease to BPD [104,105]. The term *bronchopulmonary dysplasia* is now also often applied to the chronic stage of diseases other than HMD (pulmonary surfactant deficiency), such as aspiration or viral pneumonia, both of which resemble BPD both clinically and radiographically [105,106]. This lack of clinical and pathological specificity suggests to some that mechanical ventilation and oxygen toxicity are the key factors in producing the disease [105].

A. Changes in Airways, Alveoli, and Blood Vessels

The morphology of the lung in BPD is the result of a complex interaction of many different factors: the maturity of the lung; the initial cause, severity, evolution, and resolution of the pulmonary abnormality; secondary infection; the effects of therapy [107]; and the extent of postnatal catch-up growth, which may be uneven throughout the lung.

The irregular mottling in the chest radiograph of patients with BPD is produced by the summation of overlying images of hyperaerated and airless pulmonary lobules due either to collapse or to fibrosis. Such lungs are heavy and usually have an increased resting volume. In moderate to severe disease the pleura has the characteristic appearance of a so-called geographical, checkerboard, or fissured look (Fig. 12). The fissures represent the airless or scarred lung. The pathological findings represent a variable admixture of lesions in airways, alveoli, and blood vessels that are conveniently considered separately.

Airways

The damage is more widespread and involves larger airways (as well as the smaller ones) than is typical of RDS. The mildest changes consist of loss of cilia, but as severity increases, epithelial necrosis, hyaline membranes, potentially obstructive abnormal reparative hyperplasia, and squamous metaplasia are all seen in

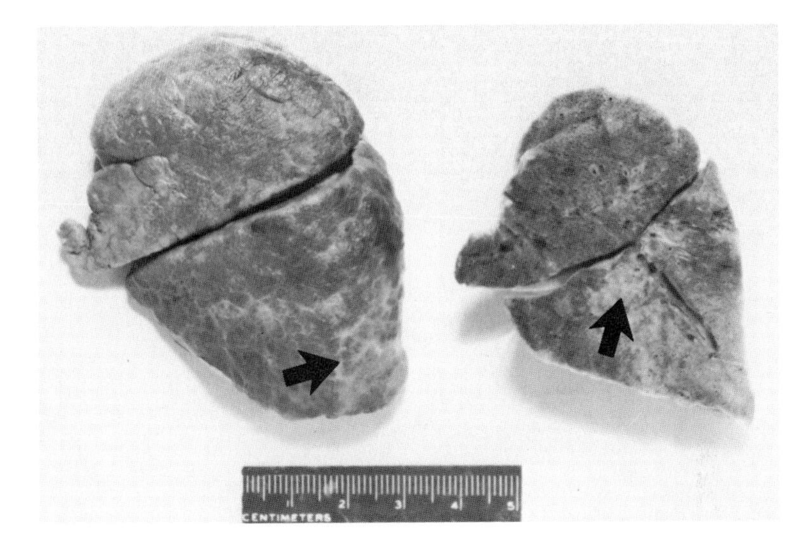

Figure 12 BPD. Macroscopical views of left lung after transbronchial formalin inflation-fixation: On the left the exterior, on the right the cut surface. Indented fissures represent underlying condensation and scarring. The cobblestone appearance seen particularly posteriorly (left arrow) over the lower lobe represents finer scarring and thickening of interlobular connective tissue septa. The cut surface seems solid centrally (right arrow) in the lower lobe and shows irregularity in density and aeration.

the airway epithelium (Fig. 13). Granulation tissue polyps may be found in the terminal airways (Fig. 14). Stasis of mucous or protein exudates in the lumen may progress to organization, which can result in bronchiolitis obliterans [108-115]. Bronchial smooth muscle injury and hyperplasia are common and submucosal fibrosis is occasionally prominent. Goblet cell hyperplasia can also develop.

Alveoli

Patchy hyaline membranes may be seen at any stage of active damage. Chronic interstitial edema, hypercellularity, and irregular hyperplasia of immature type II pneumocytes dominate the picture. Later, fibrosis occurs either as an organization of the interstitial injury or as organization of the alveolar exudate [107]. This may be absorbed into the alveolar wall to cause further thickening, or occasionally fibrous tissue may obliterate the alveolar region, which gives rise to scars that replace a considerable volume of alveoli [108,110].

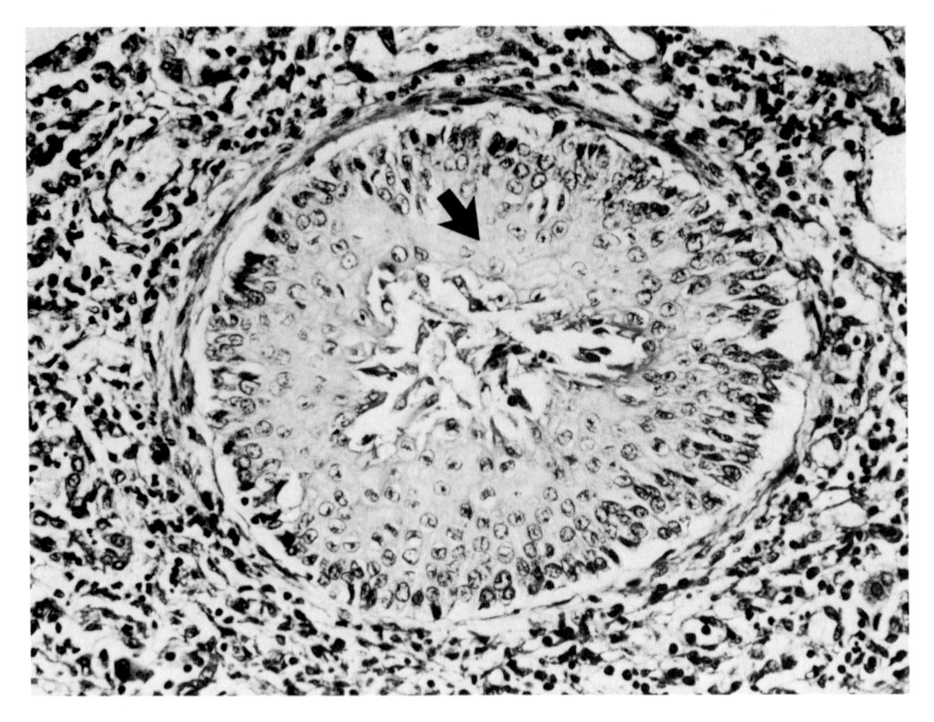

Figure 13 Photomicrograph of a small bronchiolus whose lumen is virtually occluded by hypertrophic epithelium (arrow) that appears squamous. A thin layer of muscle is apparent and heavy infiltration with inflammatory cells is seen (X 160).

Regions of alveolar collapse alternate with scar and regions of emphysema (Figs. 15 and 16). The emphysema which is often especially prominent in the lower lobes results from three processes—hyperinflation, hypoplasia, and regional alveolar destruction [107]. Hyperinflation represents overdistension of a region of lung which may or may not be associated with airway obstruction. Hypoplasia usually reflects interference with alveolar multiplication at an early stage [108]. In one morphometric study of lungs from a patient with prolonged BPD, Sobonya et al. documented a severe reduction in both alveolar number and surface area [116]. Ulceration of an alveolar wall can be part of the process of infection.

Bronchitis, pneumonia, hemorrhage, and interstitial emphysema may punctuate and modify these processes at any time.

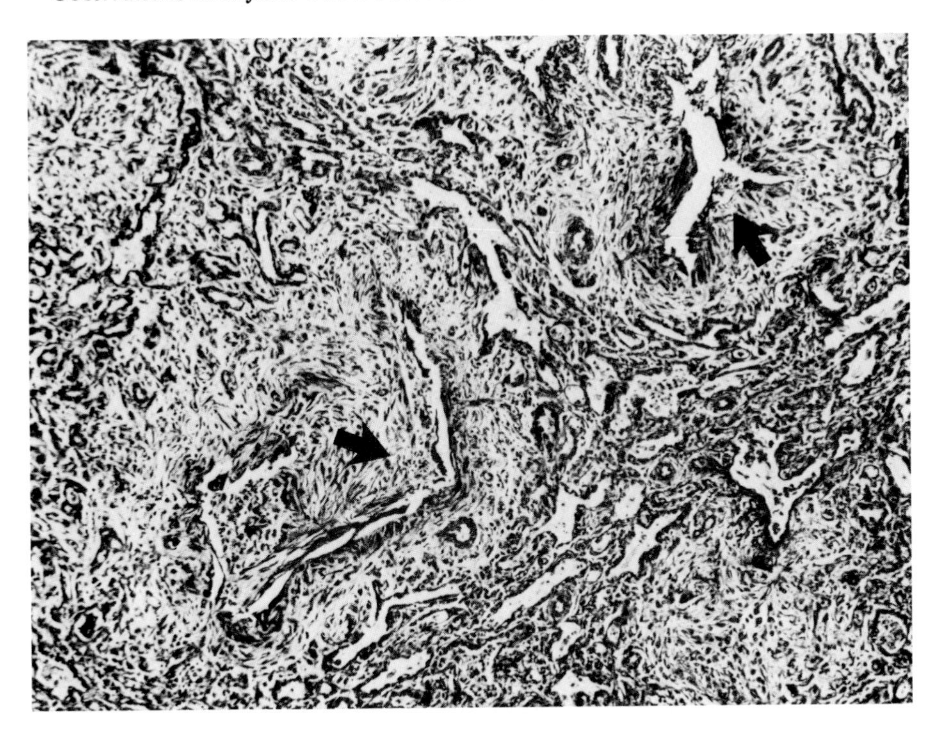

Figure 14 An advanced stage of BPD in which the central region of an acinus is undergoing organization. Granulation tissue polyps (arrows) are seen in terminal airways (X 63).

Blood Vessels

Medial hypertrophy, endothelial hyperplasia, and adventitial fibrosis of the pulmonary arteries have been described [103,109]. Later in the disease there is a reduction in the volume of the capillary and precapillary vascular beds [115]. In our experience, there is considerable variation in the number of capillaries and sometimes regions are seen where there is an increase that can resemble a capillary hemangioma.

A recent quantitative morphometric analysis of the pulmonary vasculature in seven patients with BPD demonstrated both similarities and differences within the group. Postmortem arteriograms indicate branching and lengthening of the axial arteries in BPD similar to controls of like postconceptual age (PCA), but there was considerable variation in arterial diameter, which was normal in

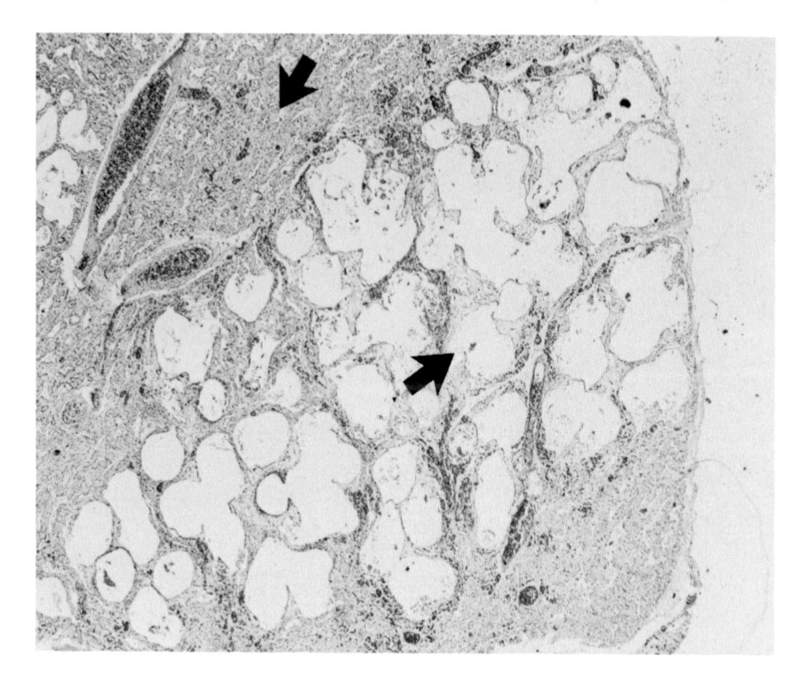

Figure 15 Late BPD. Aerated lung (lower arrow) with alveolar wall fibrosis is seen on the right. This alternates with collapsed alveolar spaces (upper arrow). Radiologically this appears as streaky densities or finely bubbly lung. From an infant born at 7 months' gestational age who died 2 months later after RDS, erythroblastosis fetalis, and BPD.

two, narrowed in three, and dilated either focally or diffusely in two. Two arteriograms are seen in Figure 17a and b. Microscopically, the number of intra-acinar arteries was proportional to PCA. Increase in thickness of the muscular wall was seen in the preacinar arteries, but was less marked than that seen in persistent fetal circulation either of the idiopathic variety or associated with meconium aspiration [73,74]. Muscularization extended abnormally far into the intra-acinar arteries. This suggests that in BPD there is a complex response to vascular injury and attempts at normal adaptation to extrauterine life [91].

In two patients at 38 and 40 weeks PCA the concentration of intra-acinar arteries was increased compared with a term infant, which suggests that patients with BPD have the capacity for an arterial growth spurt and it seems to occur at an earlier PCA. Increased arterial concentration correlated with an increased background haze on postmortem arteriogram [91].

Bronchial arteries are enlarged in patients with BPD, and in our specimens they filled from the pulmonary arteries via bronchopulmonary anastomoses.

The bronchial circulation probably is an important route of collateral blood flow and may play a role in the development of pulmonary hypertension and congestive heart failure. It has recently been suggested that this circulation may play a role in the development of left ventricular hypertrophy, which can occur in patients with BPD [117]. The ductus arteriosus often fails to close in premature infants with hyaline membrane disease, and it often needs to be surgically ligated [118]. In normal infants born at term the ductus usually closes within 24 hr of extrauterine life, but the time of closure in prematurely born infants is less certain. In BPD hypoxia probably contributes a role to the delayed closure [118]. A large left-to-right shunt through the ductus arteriosus worsens pulmonary function by causing left ventricular failure, pulmonary edema, and high-flow pulmonary hypertension.

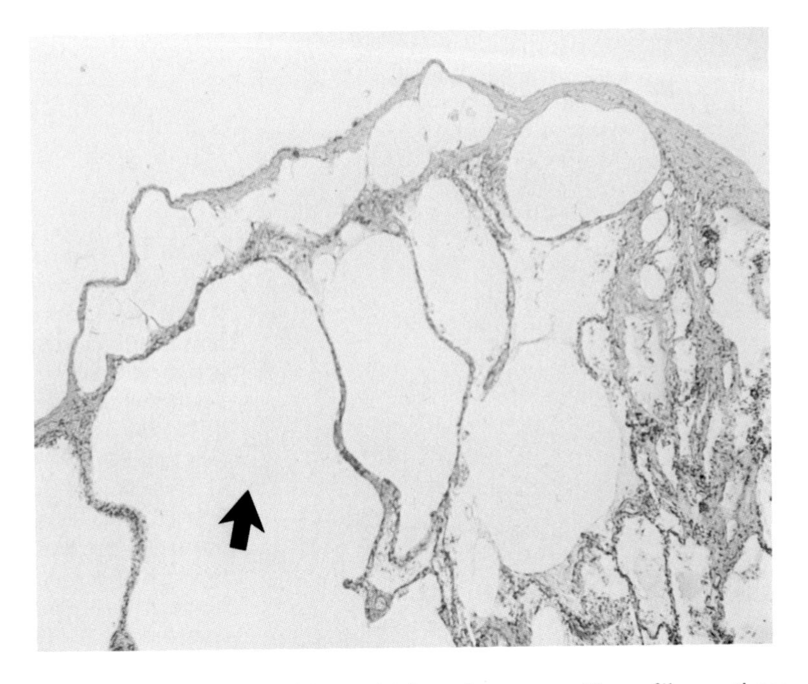

Figure 16 Late BPD. Pleural interstitial emphysema and large fibrous tissue-lined air spaces (arrow) lacking alveolar subdivision. Such changes are often most pronounced in lower lobes and are one reason for overdistension and cystic appearance seen radiologically. From an infant weighing 1000 g at birth who died 7 months later after HMD and BPD.

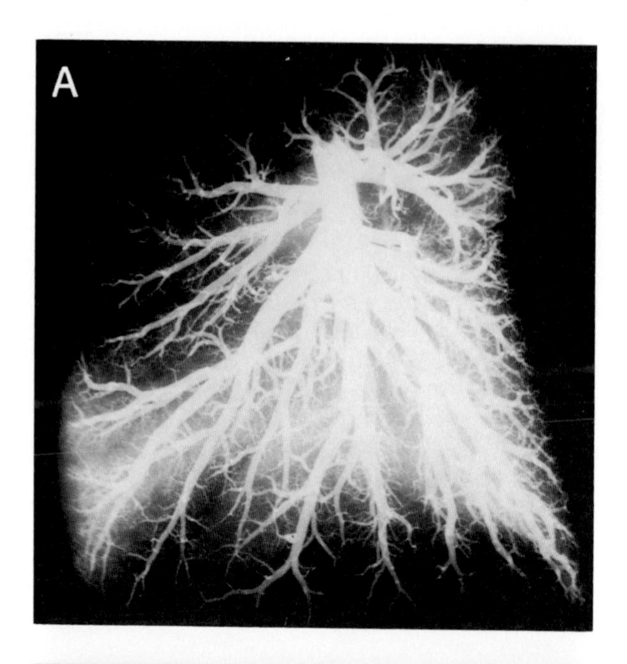

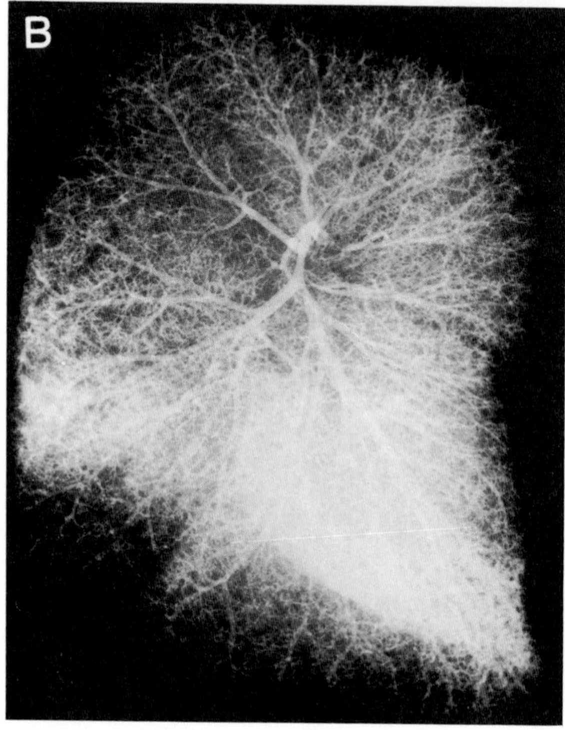

Figure 17 Postmortem arteriograms showing marked variations in central arterial size and peripheral vascular density in two cases of BPD. The postconception age (PCA) of A is 32.5 weeks, and that of B 38.0. Note large central artery size and relative lack of peripheral vascular density in A compared to B. The pattern of A is common in infants who die in the newborn period. The pattern of B is uncommon. Whether this pattern is peculiar to BPD is not known.

B. Right Ventricular Hypertrophy

Right ventricular hypertrophy has been documented both clinically and anatomically in patients with BPD [103,109]. Using the method of Fulton et al. [119], we measured separately the right and left cardiac ventricles of four patients who died with BPD and found rather than a hypertrophied right ventricle a ventricular muscle mass which was smaller than that of fetuses of similar postconceptional age. This suggests that during the early phase of BPD the right ventricle undergoes a regression similar to the survival term infant [91,120]. If lung function progressively deteriorates in those who survive beyond several months, right ventricular hypertrophy develops.

C. Pathogenesis of Vascular Injury in BPD

There is more than one cause of the vascular remodeling seen in BPD and the interaction of these causes is complex. Bronchiolitis is often associated with obliteration and stunted bronchiolar development, as in McLeod's syndrome or unilateral pulmonary hypertransradiancy [121]. The increased muscularization of acinar arteries is probably a response to hypoxia, hyperoxia, and increased flow through the anatomical left to right shunts. It is different from persistence of fetal arterial structure.

Hypoxia

In experimentally induced chronic hypoxia neomuscularization, predominantly of alveolar wall arteries, evolves rapidly by differentiation of normal precursor smooth muscle cells, of the pericyte of nonmuscular arteries, or the intermediate cell of partially muscular arteries [122]. Concomitant endothelial hyperplasia obstructs small vessels, which produces a functional reduction in volume of the lung's peripheral vascular bed. This could lead to an irreversible loss of arterial branches in the alveolar wall.

Left to Right Anatomical Vascular Shunt

In patients with high-flow pulmonary hypertension, as in ventricular septal defects, two types of arteriographic patterns are seen [123,124]. In the first type, characterized by tortuous segmental arteries, the arterial lumen is increased at the hilum and normal or decreased at the periphery, i.e., arteries appear to taper abruptly [123]. Background haze is markedly decreased. Patients having this arteriographic picture had elevated pulmonary artery pressure and resistance at the time of their death, but they also had high pulmonary blood flow and severe congestive heart failure in early infancy. In the second type of arteriographic pattern the internal lumen diameter of the axial arteries is reduced along their length [123]. This is found in infants who had severe elevation in pulmonary vascular resistance from birth, but they were never in congestive heart failure. It is of interest that patients with BPD may show either type of arteriographic pattern [91].

In patients with high-flow pulmonary hypertension, associated with congenital heart disease, the intra-acinar arteries are small in size and few in number. The wall thickness of the muscular preacinar arteries is increased, even above fetal levels, and muscle extends into acinar arteries where it is not normally found in the newborn. The veins are somewhat more muscular than normal [123,124].

Hyperoxia

Increased concentration of oxygen in inspired air, a potent endothelial toxin, probably plays a key role in producing vascular damage in patients with BPD. Oxygen has been linked to a variety of ultrastructural endothelial changes, both in the lungs of humans and experimental animals. Endothelial cell swelling, intracytoplasmic myelin figures, and interstitial edema have all been ascribed to oxygen toxicity [125-127]. Crapo and his colleagues have shown in animals that chronic hyperoxia caused overall loss of endothelial cells as well as large segments of the pulmonary capillary bed [125]. Jones et al. have shown that experimental animals exposed to high F_{IO_2} for 28 days show intimal thickening of intra-acinar arteries, muscular hypertrophy of the normally muscular arteries, and neomuscularization of the nonmuscular segment [128]. There is also dramatic reduction of vascular filling of the postmortem arteriogram due to a reduced concentration of intra-acinar arteries [128]. These changes were only partly reversed when the animals were reacclimated to room air because of irreversible obliterative lesions of the small arteries.

Whether the immature lung responds as the adult to high oxygen is unknown. Although resistance to the effects of oxygen is greater in the newborn than in adult mice [129], it is likely that sustained high F_{IO_2} still results in significant injury.

References

1. E. A. Boyden, Development and growth of the airways. In *Development of the Lung*, vol. 6, *Lung Biology in Health and Disease.* Edited by W. A. Hodson. New York, Marcel Dekker, 1977, p. 3.
2. Hislop, A., and L. Reid, Growth and development of the respiratory system: Anatomical development. In *Scientific Foundations of Paediatrics,* 2nd ed. Edited by J. A. Davis and J. Dobbing. London, Heinemann, 1981, p. 390.

3. Hislop, A., and L. Reid, Formation of the pulmonary vasculature. In *Development of the Lung,* vol. 6. *Lung Biology in Health and Disease.* Edited by W. A. Hodson. New York, Marcel Dekker, 1977, p. 37.
4. Meyrick, B., and L. Reid, Ultrastructure of the alveolar lining and its development. In *Development of the Lung,* vol. 6. *Lung Biology in Health and Disease.* Edited by W. A. Hodson. New York, Marcel Dekker, 1977, p. 87.
5. Bucher, U., and L. Reid, Development of the intrasegmental bronchial tree: The pattern of branching and development of cartilage at various stages of intra-uterine life, *Thorax,* **16**:207 (1961).
6. Hislop, A., and L. Reid, Development of the acinus in the human lung, *Thorax,* **29**:90 (1974).
7. Emery, J. L., and A. Mithal, The number of alveoli in the terminal respiratory unit of man during late intrauterine life and childhood, *Arch. Dis. Childhood,* **35**:544 (1960).
8. Boyden, E. A., and D. H. Tompsett, The changing patterns in the developing lungs of infants, *Acta Anat.,* **61**:164 (1965).
9. Dunnill, M. S., Postnatal growth of the lung, *Thorax,* **17**:329 (1962).
10. Davies, G., and L. Reid, Growth of the alveoli and pulmonary arteries in childhood, *Thorax,* **25**:669 (1970).
11. Hislop, A., and L. Reid, Intrapulmonary arterial development during fetal life – Branching pattern and structure, *J. Anat.,* **113**:35 (1972).
12. Hislop, A., and L. Reid, Pulmonary arterial development during childhood: Branching pattern and structure. *Thorax,* **28**:129 (1973).
13. Elliott, F. M., and L. Reid, Some new facts about the pulmonary artery and its branching pattern, *Clin. Radiol.,* **16**:193 (1965).
14. Reid, L., The pulmonary circulation: Remodelling in growth and disease, *Am. Rev. Respir. Dis.,* **119**:531 (1979).
15. Hislop, A., and L. Reid, Fetal and childhood development of the intrapulmonary veins in man: Branching pattern and structure. *Thorax,* **28**:313 (1973).
16. Rendas, A., M. Branthwaite, S. Lennox, and L. Reid, Response of the pulmonary circulation to acute hypoxia in the growing pig, *J. Appl. Physiol.,* **52**:811 (1982).
17. Krauss, A. N., D. B. Klain, and P. A. M. Auld, Chronic pulmonary insufficiency of prematurity, *Pediatrics,* **55**:55 (1975).
18. Craig, J. M., K. Fenton, and D. Gitlin, Obstructive factors in the pulmonary hyaline membrane syndrome in asphyxia of the newborn, *Pediatrics,* **22**:847 (1958).
19. D'Ablang, G., B. Bernard, I. Zaharon, L. Barton, B. Kaplan, and M. D. Schwinn, Neonatal pulmonary cytology and bronchopulmonary dysplasia, *Acta Cytol.,* **19**:21 (1975).

20. Merritt, T. A., J. M. Puccia, and I. D. Stuard, Cytologic evaluation of pulmonary effluent in neonates with respiratory distress syndrome and bronchopulmonary dysplasia, *Acta Cytol.,* **25**:631 (1981).
21. Chu, J., J. A. Clements, E. Cotton, M. H. Klaus, A. Y. Sweet, M. A. Thomas, and W. H. Tooley, The pulmonary hypoperfusion syndrome, *Pediatrics,* **35**:733 (1965).
22. Lauweryns, J. M., "Hyaline membrane disease" in newborn infants, *Hum. Pathol.,* **1**:175 (1970).
23. Gruenwald, P., The significance of pulmonary hyaline membranes in newborn infants, *J.A.M.A.,* **166**:621 (1958).
24. Buckingham, S., and S. S. Sommers, Pulmonary hyaline membranes, *Am. J. Dis. Child.,* **99**:216 (1960).
25. Gregg, R. H., and J. Bernstein, Pulmonary hyaline membranes and the respiratory distress syndrome, *Am. J. Dis. Child.,* **102**:871 (1961).
26. Gandy, G., W. Jacobson, and D. Gairdner, Hyaline membrane disease. I. Cellular changes, *Arch. Dis. Childhood,* **45**:289 (1970).
27. Finlay-Jones, J. M., J. M. Papadimitriou, and R. A. Barter, Pulmonary hyaline membrane: Light and electron microscopy of the early stage, *J. Pathol.,* **112**:117 (1974).
28. Rendas, A. B., and L. M. Reid, Unpublished data.
29. Johnson, D. E., J. E. Lock, R. P. Elde, and T. R. Thompson, Pulmonary neuroendocrine cells in hyaline membrane disease and bronchopulmonary dysplasia, *Pediatr. Res.,* **16**:446 (1982).
30. Ehrenkranz, R. A., R. C. Ablow, and J. B. Warsham, Prevention of bronchopulmonary dysplasia with vitamin E administration during the acute stages of respiratory distress syndrome, *J. Pediatr.,* **95**:873 (1979).
31. Gitlin, D., and J. M. Craig, The nature of the hyaline membrane in asphyxia of the newborn, *Pediatrics,* **17**:64 (1956).
32. Van Breeman, V. L., H. B. Neustein, and P. D. Bruns, Pulmonary hyaline membranes studied with the electron microscope, *Am. J. Pathol.,* **33**:769 (1957).
33. Larroche, J. C., Developmental Pathology of the Neonates. Amsterdam, *Excerpta Medica,* 1977, p. 3.
34. Morganstern, B., B. Klionsky, and N. Doshi, Yellow hyaline membrane disease, identification of the pigment and bilirubin binding, *Lab. Invest.,* **44**:514 (1981).
35. Blystad, W., B. H. Landing, and C. A. Smith, Pulmonary hyaline membranes in newborn infants, *Pediatrics,* **8**:5 (1951).
36. Esterly, J. R., and E. H. Oppenheimer, Massive pulmonary hemorrhage in the newborn, *J. Pediatr.,* **69**:3 (1966).
37. Phibbs, R. H., P. Johnson, J. A. Kitterman, G. A. Gregory, and W. H. Tooley, Cardiorespiratory status of erythroblastotic infants. I. Relationship

of gestational age, severity of hemolytic disease, and birth asphyxia to idiopathic respiratory distress syndrome and survival, *Pediatrics,* **49**:5 (1972).

38. Sosenko, I. R. S., I. D. Frantz, R. J. Roberts, and B. Meyrick, Morphologic disturbance of lung maturation in fetus of alloxan diabetic rabbits, *Am. Rev. Respir. Dis.,* **122**:687 (1980).
39. Boughton, K., G. Gandy, and D. Gairdner, Hyaline membrane disease. II. Lung lecithin, *Arch. Dis. Child.,* **45**:311 (1970).
40. Boss, J., and J. M. Craig, Reparative phenomena in lungs of neonates with hyaline membranes, *Pediatrics,* **29**:890 (1962).
41. Totten, R. S., and T. J. Moran, Cortisone and atypical pulmonary epithelial hyperplasia, *Am. J. Pathol.,* **38**:575 (1961).
42. Lieberman, J., and F. Kellogg, A deficiency of pulmonary fibrinolysis in hyaline membrane disease, *N. Engl. J. Med.* **262**:999 (1960).
43. Taghizadeh, A., and E. O. R. Reynolds, Pathogenesis of bronchopulmonary dysplasia following hyaline membrane disease, *Am. J. Pathol.,* **82**:241 (1976).
44. Valdes-Dapena, M., Iatrogenic disease in the perinatal period as seen by the pathologist. In *Perinatal Diseases, International Academy of Pathology Monograph.* Edited by R. L. Naeye and J. M. Kissane, Baltimore, Williams & Wilkins, 1981, p. 382.
45. Anderson, K. D., and R. Chandra, Pneumothorax secondary to perforation of segmental bronchi by suction catheters, *J. Pediatr. Surg.,* **11**:687 (1976).
46. Miller, K. E., D. K. Edwards, S. Hilton, D. Collins, F. Lynch, and R. Williams, Acquired lobar emphysema in premature infants with bronchopulmonary dysplasia: An iatrogenic disease?, *Radiology,* **138**:589 (1981).
47. Cooney, D. R., J. A. Menke, and J. E. Allen, "Acquired" lobar emphysema: A complication of respiratory distress in premature infants, *J. Pediatr. Surg.,* **12**:897 (1977).
48. Moylan, F. M. B., and D. C. Shannon, Preferential distribution of lobar emphysema and atelectasis in bronchopulmonary dysplasia, *Pediatrics,* **63**:130 (1979).
49. Kirkpatrick, B. V., A. H. Felman, and D. V. Eitzman, Complications of ventilator therapy in respiratory distress syndrome, recognition and management of acute air leaks, *Am. J. Dis. Child.,* **128**:496 (1974).
50. Macklin, C. C., Transport of air along sheaths of pulmonary blood vessels from alveoli to mediastinum, *Arch. Int. Med.,* **64**:913 (1939).
51. Macklin, M. T., and C. C. Macklin, Malignant interstitial emphysema of the lungs and mediastinum as an important occult complication in many respiratory diseases and other conditions: An interpretation of the clinical literature in the light of laboratory experiment, *Medicine,* **23**:281 (1944).
52. Thibeault, D. W., R. S. Lachman, V. R. Laul, and M. S. Kwong, Pulmonary interstitial emphysema, pneumomediastinum and pneumothorax, occurrence in the newborn infant, *Am. J. Dis. Child.,* **126**:611 (1973).

53. Madansky, D. L., E. E. Lawson, V. Chernick, and H. W. Taeusch, Jr., Pneumothorax and other forms of pulmonary air leak in newborns, *Am. Rev. Resp. Dis.,* **120**:729 (1979).
54. Stocker, J. T., and J. E. Madewell, Persistent interstitial pulmonary emphysema: Another complication of the respiratory distress syndrome, *Pediatrics,* **59**:847 (1977).
55. Leonidas, J. C., I. Bhan, and R. G. K. McCauley, Persistent localized pulmonary interstitial emphysema and lymphangiectasia: A causal relationship?, *Pediatrics,* **64**:165 (1979).
56. Wood, B. P., V. M. Anderson, J. E. Mauk, and T. A. Merritt, Pulmonary lymphatic air: Locating "pulmonary interstitial emphysema" of the premature infant, *Am. J. Roentgenol.,* **138**:809 (1982).
57. Hill, A., J. M. Perlman, and J. J. Volpe, Relationship of pneumothorax to occurrence of intraventricular hemorrhage in the premature newborn, *Pediatrics,* **60**:144 (1982).
58. Oppermann, H. C., L. Wille, M. Obladen, and E. Richter, Systemic air embolism in the respiratory distress syndrome of the newborn, *Pediatr. Radiol.,* **8**:139 (1979).
59. Gregory, G. A., and W. H. Tooley, Gas embolism in hyaline membrane disease, *N. Engl. J. Med.,* **282**:1141 (1970).
60. Moessinger, A. C., J. M. Driscoll, and H. J. Wigger, High incidence of lung perforation by chest tube in neonatal pneumothorax, *J. Pediatr.,* **92**:635 (1978).
61. Wilson, A. J., and H. F. Krous, Lung perforation during chest tube placement in the stiff lung syndrome, *J. Pediatr. Surg.,* **9**:213 (1974).
62. Banagale, R. C., E. W. Outerbridge, and J. V. Aranda, Lung perforation: A complication of chest tube insertion in neonatal pneumothorax, *J. Pediatr.,* **94**:973 (1979).
63. Touloukian, R. J., Isosmolar coma during parenteral alimentation with protein hydrolysate in excess of 4 gm/kg/day, *J. Pediatr.,* **86**:270 (1975).
64. Beale, E. F., R. M. Nelson, R. L. Bucciarelli, W. H. Donnelly, and D. V. Eitzman, Intrahepatic cholestasis associated with parenteral nutrition in premature infants, *Pediatrics,* **64**:342 (1979).
65. Postuma, R., and C. L. Trevenen, Liver disease in infants receiving total parenteral nutrition, *Pediatrics,* **63**:110 (1979).
66. Dahms, B. B., and T. C. Halpin, Jr., Pulmonary arterial lipid deposit in newborn infants receiving intravenous lipid infusion, *J. Pediatr.,* **97**:800 (1980).
67. Redline, R. W., and B. B. Dahms, Malassezia pulmonary vasculitis in an infant on long-term intralipid therapy, *N. Engl. J. Med.,* **305**:1395 (1981).
68. Avery, M., B. Fletcher, and R. G. Williams, The lung and its disorders in the newborn infant. In *The Lung and Its Disorders in the Newborn Infant,* 4th ed. Philadelphia, Saunders, 1981.

69. Katzenstein, A. L., C. Davis, and A. Braude, Pulmonary changes in neonatal sepsis due to group β hemolytic streptococcus: Relation to hyaline membrane disease, *J. Infect. Dis.*, **133**:430 (1976).
70. Ablow, R. C., S. G. Driscoll, E. L. Effman, I. Gross, C. J. Jolles, R. Uauy, and J. B. Warshaw, A comparison of early-onset group B streptococcal neonatal infection and the respiratory distress syndrome of the newborn, *N. Engl. J. Med.*, **294**:65 (1976).
71. Ablow, R. C., I. Gross, E. L. Effman, R. Uauy, and S. Driscoll, The radiographic features of early onset group B streptococcal neonatal sepsis. *Radiology*, **124**:771 (1977).
72. Emery, J. L., Interstitial emphysema, pneumothorax, and "air block" in the newborn, *Lancet*, **i**:405 (1956).
73. Murphy, J. D., M. Rabinovitch, J. D. Goldstein, and L. M. Reid, The structural basis of persistent pulmonary hypertension of the newborn infant, *J. Pediatr.*, **98**:962 (1981).
74. Murphy, J. D., M. Rabinovitch, and L. M. Reid, Pulmonary vascular pathology in fatal neonatal meconium aspiration, *Pediatr. Res.* (Suppl.), **15**:673 (1981).
75. Areechon, W., and L. Reid, Hypoplasia of lung with congenital diaphragmatic hernia, *Br. Med. J.*, **1**:230 (1963).
76. Kitagawa, M., A. Hislop, E. A. Boyden, and L. Reid, Lung hypoplasia in congenital diaphragmatic hernia, a quantitative study of airway, artery and alveolar development, *Br. J. Surg.*, **58**:342 (1971).
77. Hislop, A., and L. Reid, Persistent hypoplasia of the lung after repair of congenital diaphragmatic hernia, *Thorax*, **31**:450 (1976).
78. Hislop, A., and L. Reid, Growth and development of the respiratory system – Anatomical development. In *Scientific Foundation of Paediatrics.* Edited by J. Davis and J. Dobbing. London, Heinemann, 1974, p. 214.
79. Emery, J. L., and A. Mithal, The number of alveoli in the terminal respiratory unit of man during late intrauterine life and childhood, *Arch. Dis. Child.*, **35**:544 (1960).
80. Boyden, E. A., The structure of compressed lungs in congenital diaphragmatic hernia, *Am. J. Anat.*, **134**:497 (1972).
81. Wohl, M. E. B., N. T. Griscom, S. R. Schuster, R. G. Zwerdling, and D. Strieder, Lung growth and function following repair of congenital diaphragmatic hernia, *Pediatr. Res.*, **7**:424 (1973).
82. Goldstein, J. D., and L. M. Reid, Pulmonary hypoplasia resulting from phrenic nerve agenesis and diaphragmatic amyoplasia, *J. Pediatr.*, **97**:282 (1980).
83. Chamberlain, D., A. Hislop, E. Hey, and L. Reid, Pulmonary hypoplasia in babies with severe rhesus isoimmunization: A quantitative study, *J. Pathol.*, **122**:43 (1977).

84. Potter, E., Bilateral absence of ureters and kidneys: A report of 50 cases, *Obstet. Gynec.,* **25**:3 (1965).
85. Hislop, A., E. Hey, and L. Reid, The lungs in congenital bilateral renal agenesis and dysplasia, *Arch. Dis. Child.,* **54**:32 (1979).
86. Clemmons, J. J. W., Embryonic renal injury: A possible factor in fetal malnutrition (abstr.), *Pediatr. Res.,* **11**:404 (1977).
87. Wilson, M. G., and V. G. Mikity, A new form of respiratory disease in premature infants, *Am. J. Dis. Child.,* **99**:489 (1960).
88. Grossman, H., A. R. Levin, P. Winchester, and P. A. M. Auld, Pulmonary hypertension in the Wilson-Mikity syndrome, *Am. J. Roentgenol.,* **114**: 293 (1972).
89. Gersony, W. M., G. V. Duc, and J. C. Sinclair, "P.F.C." syndrome (persistence of the fetal circulation), *Circulation,* **40** (Suppl. III):87 (1969).
90. Haworth, S. G., and L. Reid, Persistent fetal circulation: Newly recognized structural features, *J. Pediatr.,* **88**:614 (1976).
91. Tomashefski, J. F., Jr., H. C. Oppermann, G. F. Vawter, and L. M. Reid, Bronchopulmonary dysplasia: A morphometric study with emphasis on the pulmonary vasculature, *Pediatr. Pathol.,* in press.
92. Reid, L., The lung: Its growth and remodelling in health and disease, *Am. J. Roentgen.,* **129**:777 (1977).
93. Hislop, A., and L. Reid, New pathological findings in emphysema of childhood: 1. Polyalveolar lobe with emphysema, *Thorax,* **25**:682 (1970).
94. Henderson, R., A. Hislop, and L. Reid, New pathological findings in emphysema of childhood. 3. Unilateral congenital emphysema with hypoplasia – And compensatory emphysema of contralateral lung. *Thorax,* **26**:195 (1971).
95. Waddell, J. A., G. Simon, and L. Reid, Bronchial atresia of the left upper lobe, *Thorax,* **20**:214 (1965).
96. Miller, R. K., W. K. Seiber, and E. J. Yunis, Congenital adenomatoid malformation of the lung, a report of 17 cases and review of the literature, *Pathol. Annual,* **15**:387 (1980).
97. Stocker, J. T., J. E. Madewell, and R. M. Drake, Congenital cystic adenomatoid malformation of the lung: Classification and morphologic spectrum, *Hum. Pathol.,* **8**:155 (1977).
98. Bale, P. M., Congenital cystic malformation of the lung, a form of congenital bronchiolar ("adenomatoid") malformation, *Am. J. Clin. Pathol.,* **71**:411 (1979).
99. Janney, C. G., F. B. Askin, and C. Kuhn, III, Congenital alveolar capillary dysplasia – An unusual cause of respiratory distress in the newborn, *Am. J. Clin. Pathol.,* **76**:722 (1981).
100. Jones, C. J., Unusual hamartoma of the lung in a newborn infant, *Arch. Pathol.,* **48**:150 (1949).

101. Hislop, A., M. Sanderson, and L. Reid. Unilateral congenital dysplasia of lung associated with vascular anomalies, *Thorax,* **28**:435 (1973).
102. Norman, J. A., L. R. Walters, and J. T. Reeves, Congenital pulmonary lymphangiectasis, *Am. J. Dis. Child.,* **120**:314 (1970).
103. Northway, W. H., Jr., R. C. Rosan, and D. Y. Porter, Pulmonary disease following respirator therapy of hyaline membrane disease, bronchopulmonary dysplasia. *N. Engl. J. Med.,* **276**:357 (1967).
104. Oppermann, H. C., L. Wille, U. Bleyl, and M. Obladen, Bronchopulmonary dysplasia in premature infants, a radiological and pathological correlation, *Pediatr. Radiol.,* **5**:137 (1977).
105. Edwards, D. K., Radiographic aspects of bronchopulmonary dysplasia, *J. Pediatr.,* **95**:823 (1979).
106. Milner, A. D., Bronchopulmonary dysplasia, *Arch. Dis. Child.,* **55**:661 (1980).
107. Reid, L., Bronchopulmonary dysplasia – Pathology, *J. Pediatr.,* **95**:836 (1979).
108. Taghizadeh, A., and E. O. R. Reynolds, Pathogenesis of bronchopulmonary dysplasia following hyaline membrane disease, *Am. J. Pathol.,* **82**:241 (1976).
109. Bonikos, D. S., K. Bensch, W. H. Northway, Jr., and D. K. Edwards, Bronchopulmonary dysplasia: The pulmonary pathologic sequel of necrotizing bronchiolitis and pulmonary fibrosis, *Hum. Pathol.,* **7**:643 (1976).
110. Anderson, W. R., and M. B. Strickland, Pulmonary complications of oxygen therapy in the neonate, postmortem study of bronchopulmonary dysplasia with emphasis on fibroproliferative obliterative bronchitis and bronchiolitis, *Arch. Pathol.,* **91**:506 (1971).
111. Moylan, F. M. B., and D. C. Shannon, Preferential distribution of lobar emphysema and atelectasis in bronchopulmonary dysplasia, *Pediatrics,* **63**:130 (1979).
112. Miller, K. E., D. K. Edwards, S. Hilton, D. Collins, F. Lynch, and R. Williams, Acquired lobar emphysema in premature infants with bronchopulmonary dysplasia: An iatrogenic disease?, *Radiology,* **138**:589 (1981).
113. Harrod, J. R., P. L'Heureux, O. D. Wangensteen, and C. E. Hunt, Long-term followup of severe respiratory distress syndrome treated with IPPB, *J. Pediatr.,* **84**:277 (1974).
114. Smyth, J. A., E. Tabachnik, W. J. Duncan, B. J. Reilly, and H. Levison, Pulmonary function and bronchial hyperreactivity in long-term survivors of bronchopulmonary dysplasia, *Pediatrics,* **68**:336 (1981).
115. Larroche, J., and C. Nessman, La maladie des membranes hyalines: Evolution, cicatrisation, sequelles etude histologique, *Arch. Fr. Pediatr.,* **28**:113 (1971).

116. Sobonya, R. E., M. M. Logvinoff, L. M. Taussig, and A. Theriault, Morphometric analysis of the lung in prolonged bronchopulmonary dysplasia, *Pediatr. Res.,* **16**:969 (1982).
117. Melnick, G., A. Pickoff, P. L. Ferrer, J. Peyser, E. Bancalari, and H. Galband, Normal pulmonary vascular resistance and left ventricular hypertrophy in young infants with bronchopulmonary dysplasia: An echocardiographic and pathologic study, *Pediatrics,* **66**:589 (1980).
118. Siassi, B., G. C. Emmanouilides, R. J. Cleveland, and F. Hirose, Patent dictus arteriosus complicating prolonged assisted ventilation in respiratory distress syndrome, *J. Pediatr.,* **74**:11 (1969).
119. Fulton, R. M., E. C. Hutchinson, and A. M. Jones, Ventricular weight in cardiac hypertrophy, *Br. Heart J.,* **14**:413 (1952).
120. Keen, E. N., The postnatal development of the human cardiac ventricles, *J. Anat.,* **89**:484 (1955).
121. Reid, L., and G. Simon, Unilateral lung transradiancy, *Thorax,* **17**:230 (1962).
122. Meyrick, B., and L. Reid, The effect of continued hypoxia on rat pulmonary artery circulation, an ultrastructural study, *Lab. Invest.,* **38**:188 (1978).
123. Rabinovitch, M., and L. M. Reid, Quantitative structural analysis of the pulmonary vascular bed in congenital heart defects, *Cardiovasc. Clin.,* **11**:149 (1981).
124. Hislop, A., S. G. Haworth, E. A. Shinebourne, and L. Reid, Quantitative structural analysis of pulmonary vessels in isolated ventricular septal defect in infancy, *Br. Heart J.,* **37**:1014 (1975).
125. Crapo, J. D., M. Peters-Golden, J. Marsh-Salin, and J. S. Shelburne, Pathologic changes in the lungs of oxygen-adapted rats, a morphometric analysis, *Lab. Invest.,* **39**:640 (1978).
126. Gould, V. E., R. Tosco, R. F. Wheelis, and Y. Kapanci, Oxygen pneumonitis in man, ultrastructural observations on the development of the alveolar lesions, *Lab. Invest.,* **26**:499 (1972).
127. Kistler, G. S., P. R. B. Caldwell, and E. R. Weibel, Development of fine structural damage to alveolar and capillary lining cells in oxygen poisoned rat lungs, *J. Cell Biol.,* **32**:605 (1967).
128. Jones, R., W. M. Zapol, and L. Reid, Progressive and regressive structural changes in rat pulmonary arteries during recovery from prolonged hyperoxia, *Am. Rev. Respir. Dis.,* **125**:227 (1982).
129. Bonikos, D. S., K. G. Bensch, and W. H. Northway, Jr., Oxygen toxicity in the newborn, the effect of chronic continuous 100% oxygen exposure on the lungs of newborn mice, *Am. J. Pathol.,* **85**:623 (1976).

130. Dubreuil, G., A. Lacoste, and R. Raymond, Observations sur le développement du poumon humain, *Bull. Histol. Techn. Physiol.,* **13**:235–245 (1936).
131. Loosli, C. G., and E. L. Potter, Pre- and postnatal development of the respiratory portion of the human lung, *Amer. Rev. Resp. Dis.* (Suppl.), **80**:5-23 (1959).
132. Boyden, E. A., Development of the human lung. In *Brennermann's Practice of Pediatrics,* vol. IV. Hagerstown, Maryland, Harper & Row, 1972.

18

Long-Term Consequences of Survivors of Respiratory Distress Syndrome

ROBERT O. FISCH

University of Minneosta Hospitals
Minneapolis, Minnesota

Life is more than survival.

I. Introduction

The long-range outcome of infants who survive respiratory distress syndrome (RDS) is manifested by four important characteristics: (1) RDS is not a single disease entity with a single etiology, but rather it is a consequence of a myriad of complexities associated with prematurity; (2) the etiology, severity, and management of RDS vary from infant to infant; (3) environmental and social factors directly influence the outcome of surviving infants; and (4) the end result of an RDS survivor cannot yet be defined in a cumulative sense from the variety of collected data which reflects vastly different methodologies, aims, and follow-up programs (see Fig. 1).

What is the expected outcome of an RDS survivor? An appreciation for the current literature begins with the realization that this question is too simplistic. The question must be rephrased to include the multifactorial characteristics found throughout the natural history of the disease. Therefore, this chapter will discuss the premature RDS infant in light of methodologies as presented in the literature, mortality and morbidity in regard to separate organ systems, and suggestions for future study designs.

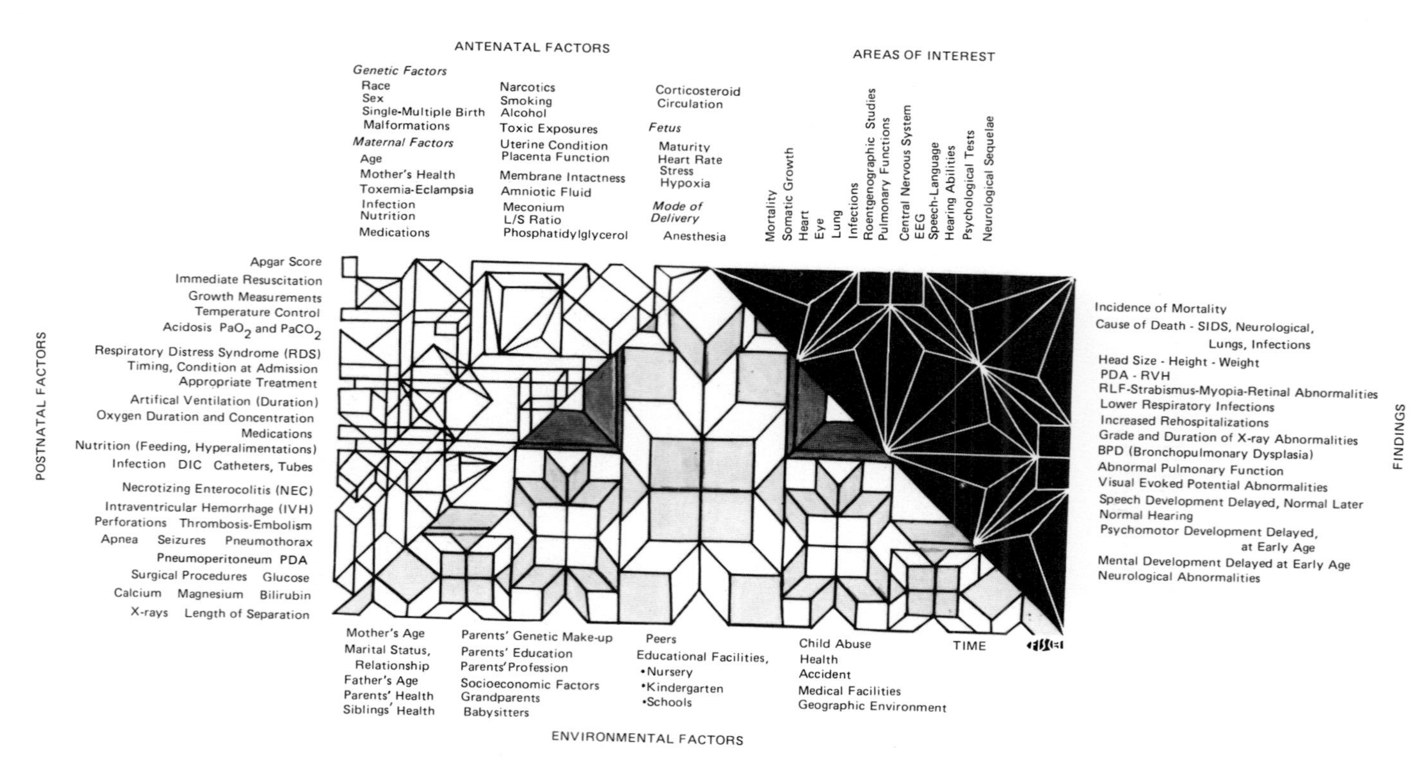

Figure 1 Illustration (in abstract) of the complexity and the importance of inferential multifactorial effects. The upper left triangle represents the infant who finally survives. The lower triangle represents environmental factors. The upper right triangle represents the areas in question as well as the findings about the performances of the infant.

A. Prematurity and RDS

The fetus lives and grows in an optimal environment where rapidly changing needs are efficiently fulfilled throughout the course of its development. The mother adapts physiologically, anatomically, emotionally, and intellectually to her new role as childbearer. The father also gradually becomes a part of the new family unit through direct observation. However, an abrupt, unexpected premature birth throws the infant into a traumatic environment where the essential elements for its survival must be delivered through only partially developed organ systems. The parents of a premature infant inherit the child's complex and confusing problems. Daily explanations of management and complications create enormous and unexpected emotional stresses, while the possible loss of the infant replaces the happy dream of parenthood with the nightmare of the intensive care unit.

Regardless of whether or not the child is premature, the newborn's genetic make-up predetermines its physical, mental, and emotional potentials. The presence or absence of malformations is partly influenced by the mother's age, health, and nutrition. Questions must be asked about maternal health regarding the usage of medications, narcotics, smoking (it was found in one study [1] that the infant's lungs mature more rapidly in a mother who smokes as opposed to one who does not), alcohol, or toxic exposures. Abnormalities in the uterus or placenta – e.g., infectious exposure, lung maturity as assessed by the lecithin-sphingomyelin (L/S) ratio and the presence of phosphatidylglycerol, timing of membrane rupture, presence of meconium or chorioamnionitis, and the usage, dosage, and timing of corticosteroids – are among the many maternal factors which influence the outcome of the newborn.

The status of the fetus prior to birth, its heart rate (decreased heart rate has been shown to be significantly related to the severity of RDS [2]), fetal stress, type of birth and delivery, use of anesthesia, need for obstetrical assistance, Apgar scores (as a predictor of chronic neurological disabilities [3]), condition of the newborn at birth and immediately after, need for resuscitation, birth weight, gestational maturity, and head size are among the determining factors regarding the medical care, the severity of disease, and the management, survival, and prognosis of the RDS infant (see Fig. 1).

What is RDS? RDS is an entity without a comprehensive, simple definition because it is not caused by a single etiological factor [4]. Infants may suffer respiratory distress [5] from pulmonary [6], or nonpulmonary infection or from cardiovascular, metabolic, hemolytic, or central nervous system (CNS) abnormalities [5]. RDS infants are classified by clinical and radiological findings, and an epidemiological reclassification of acute neonatal RDS has been suggested [7]. However, the most commonly accepted condition manifested by RDS is hyaline membrane disease (HMD). The cause of HMD is immaturity – i.e., anatomical, physiological, and biochemical. The clinical and radiological manifestations of HMD as well as its pathophysiology have been well documented [5]. However, in infants with pneumonia, clinical and radiological findings may be indistinguishable from an infant with HMD [6]. Consequently, a variety of conditions may be labeled RDS in a wide range of studies.

B. RDS Infants and Their Survival

Maternal factors influence the severity of RDS. The usage of corticosteroids for the anticipated birth of a premature baby may be influential in reducing mortality and altering morbidity, especially for female and black infants [8,9], although some studies have not documented its usefulness [10]. A quantitative model for HMD can predict the expected course of the disease beyond the first 72 hr of life [11]. The condition of the premature varies in any or all of the following: Apgar score, weight, gestational maturity (these measurements can be used as determinants of neurobehavioral outcomes [12]), intrauterine head growth and head size at birth (which are most important variables affecting later performance [12,13]), sex (females are more likely to survive and are less likely to develop RDS [8,14]), race (blacks are not as susceptible as whites to RDS [10]), and the need for resuscitation.

For many reasons, the interval of time between the onset of symptomatology and appropriate management varies considerably. Temperature control, biochemical consequences of respiratory and metabolic acidosis, appropriate oxygenation, and quality and usage of new respiratory technology are also factors that influence the outcome of the premature infant. In addition, tracheal aspirate for L/S ratio can be used as a predictor for recovery from RDS [15].

The administration of appropriate nutrients or the use of hyperalimentation; intrauterine/iatrogenic infections; complications resulting from treatments (e.g., catheter thrombosis and embolism; nasal, palatal [16], and subglottic [17] abnormalities; scarring from tubes); necrotizing enterocolitis; congenital malformations; surgical procedures; the high incidence of patent ductus arteriosis and consequent abnormal cerebral hemodynamics [18]; the duration of respiratory/oxygen therapy; the severity of the respiratory disease itself; medications; apnea; seizures and/or intraventricular hemorrhage; and the usual problems associated with prematurity (abnormalities in glucose, calcium, and magnesium metabolism) must all be considered in the overall complexity of the premature infant who has RDS (see Fig. 1).

Social and environmental factors also contribute to the ultimate outcome of the RDS infant. The mother's age [19], marital status, and relationship with the father; the genetic potential of the parents; their education, physical and mental health, social and economic status; condition of siblings, grandparents, and peers; additional health problems caused by either the perinatal episode or diseases acquired at a later age; health support; quality of educational facilities (e.g., preschool, kindergarten, elementary); and geographical location all influence the ultimate outcome of the premature infant with RDS. Moreover, the financial burden and emotional stress associated with the care of a chronically ill infant as well as the prolonged separation from the parents during the hospitalizations and bonding difficulties certainly change the environment in which the infant matures. These scenarios predispose to child abuse, especially if the mother is young [19].

In trying to determine a cause-and-effect relationship between neonatal RDS and an observation or measurement made on an infant or child, the time of the measurement is one of the most important factors to be considered. The researcher's ability to detect a cause-and-effect relationship decreases as the infant grows older. The farther away from the perinatal period that one makes the observation or measurement, the more difficult it is to know if RDS was a predisposing cause.

C. Methods Used in the Literature

When presenting a survey of current literature, several points require clarification. First, although numerous papers were reviewed, only about 100 – those which specifically concern RDS infants – have been chosen for presentation.

Second, while many papers concentrated on the outcome of the RDS survivors with respect to a single organ system, other papers presented a more general approach to the picture and evaluated the performances of RDS survivors. Therefore, I have chosen to present articles, not in a certain order, but according to mortality and different morbidities by organs. Consequently, some articles are quoted more than once.

Third, testing quality and aims as well as infant age at the time tests were performed varied greatly among articles and even within a specific article. The quality of the testers as well as the study designs themselves differed considerably from paper to paper. The diagnostic criteria of RDS were not given in certain papers. In many articles, criteria or terminology were different.

Fourth, many of the studies lacked controls and were retrospective, and none of them dealt with the survivors who had the surfactant measured in the amniotic fluid prior to birth as a criterion for RDS. The management of RDS varied from no treatment to the most recent ventilating and additional supports.

Fifth, there are other difficulties with some publications. For example, in a paper stating that 100 RDS infants survived, these infants were followed from 2.5-8.0 years of age. Nine died, 22 were lost for follow-up, 50 had an x-ray, 23 were included in a respiratory function study, and 60 had IQ tests. Therefore, the same article could have different numbers of subjects quoted in different places.

Finally, the consequences from different managements of premature infants are so complex that it is difficult to differentiate the consequences of RDS. Therefore, if something was clearly a consequence of the management (i.e., iatrogenic), then it was excluded from this chapter. For example, a scar on the chest from a chest tube is obviously not the consequence of RDS but of the method of management.

II. Mortality

A. Literature Review

The most severe consequence among RDS survivors is mortality at an early age. Between 1 and 4 years of age the percentage of death was 5.6% of 72 RDS infants, as compared to 0.4% of the control population in a longitudinal study [20,21]. Among 99 infants with HMD requiring artificial ventilation, six (6%) died during the follow-up period, which extended to 5 years of age [22]. Three had neurological deficit (hydrocephalus); one had meningococcemia.

In a study of 20 infants with RDS, one (5%) died at 6 months of age [23]. Among 29 infants with HMD, most of whom were ventilated, two (6.8%) died: one of cardiopulmonary insufficiency at 15 months and one of unknown causes at 3 months [24].

Among 38 RDS infants and 27 non-RDS controls, 11 RDS infants (28%) had bronchopulmonary dysplasia (BPD) and eight (21%) died by the age of 5 months [25]. Two control premature infants (7.4%) died during the first year: one from sudden infant death syndrome (SIDS), the second of pneumococcal pneumonia and sepsis.

Among 20 RDS infants who received continuous positive airway pressure (CPAP), three (15%) died from pulmonary fibrosis, aspiration pneumonia, or hydrocephalus [26]. Among 177 ventilated neonates with HMD, two (1.1%) died in the first year of life from respiratory insufficiency [27]. Among 73 children weighing $<$ 1501 g at birth and requiring mechanical ventilation, two boys died (2.7%), one at 1 month and the other at 13 months of age [28].

In a study of 126 children requiring ventilatory support in the newborn period for respiratory failure, most commonly due to RDS, seven children under 1 year of age died (5.5%) [29]: one of septicemia, one of meningitis, two from BPD, one from total anomalous pulmonary venous return, one from Smith-Lemli-Optiz syndrome, and one of a ruptured stomach from child abuse.

In another study of 148 infants (some ventilated) with birth weights from 501 to 1500 g (40% with RDS), five died (3.4%) [30]: One hydrocephalic child died at 4 months of age with gastroenteritis, one SIDS child at 5 months of age, one at 6 months of age of bronchopneumonia, one at 15 months of age with SIDS, and one at 25 months of age with pulmonary hemosiderosis. Among 136 primarily nonventilated infants with birth weights from 501 to 1500 g, there were two deaths (1.4%) [31] in the follow-up period.

Among 135 prematures assisted with intermittent positive pressure ventilation (IPPV), three died (2.2%) within 6 months of age [32]: One with HMD had findings at autopsy of pneumonia, heart failure, PDA, and BPD; another who had HMD died with SIDS, mild BPD, and signs of encephalomalacia; and the third, who had postasphyxic syndrome at birth, died from aspiration, microcephalus, mild BPD, and subcortical encephalomalacia.

In a study of infants weighing < 1500 g at birth, one (3.8%) died after discharge [33]. Among the eight RDS infants having no BPD, two (25%) died before 4 months of age. Furthermore, a higher rate of SIDS victims was found among infants surviving RDS than among their matched controls in a prospective study [34].

B. Summary

Many researchers have directed their attention to specific problems in their follow-up studies. Although neonatal survival and mortality were mentioned in many reports, not a single article addressed mortality of RDS survivors as its main subject. Frequently, articles either failed to mention RDS survivor mortality or noted that the infants were not available for follow-up study. Moreover, sex was not included in most studies which mentioned mortality. In general, articles pertaining to RDS suggest three things when mentioning the mortality of RDS survivors: (1) SIDS is a common cause of mortality in RDS survivors; (2) severity of lung impairment and neurological complications correlate with a higher incidence of mortality; and (3) it indeed appears that RDS survivors have a higher incidence of mortality, especially with concomitant BPD, than their matched controls during the first 4 years of life and especially during the first year of life. The very limited information available suggests a higher incidence of mortality among male than among female RDS survivors.

III. Somatic Growth

A. Literature Review

Growth measurements of height and weight from three groups of infants with birth weights of < 1500 g were obtained regularly up to 3 years of age [33]. Group A consisted of 26 BPD infants (22 RDS), group B of eight infants with RDS who did not develop BPD. Groups A and B received oxygen therapy for 21 days or longer. Group C consisted of 25 selected infants (10 with RDS) who received oxygen therapy for 5 or fewer days and served as matched controls for the above two groups. At 4 months of age, a significant number of group A fell below the third percentile (in either weight or length) when compared to group C infants ($p < 0.05$). Although the measured length of group A (BPD) infants was less than that in group C infants at 1 year of age, it was not statistically significant. At 24–36 months of age there was no difference between the BPD children and the other groups.

In another study, BPD infants showed weight and height below the third percentile at birth [35]. At 2 years of age weight was at the third to tenth percentile, height at the tenth to twenty-fifth percentile.

In a prospective study, 58 nonventilated RDS survivors were compared with 290 matched and 35,198 unmatched controls regarding height, weight, and occipital-frontal circumference from birth up to 4 years of age [20]. Each group was divided into three subgroups according to birth weight. The RDS survivors and their matched controls attained heights and weights equivalent to those of the unmatched control subjects by 4 years of age. The occipital-frontal circumference was significantly greater in the 4-year-old RDS survivors than in either of the higher birth weight subgroups of the control groups.

With one exception, 47 RDS survivors matched their peers in height, weight, and head circumference when examined between 15 and 24 months of age [36]. Height, weight, and head circumference were compared in 46 preterm RDS, 59 term, and 46 post-term infants up to 1 year of age [37]. The weight and height were significantly less in the preterm RDS group than in the term or post-term infants, probably because of the preterm births and not because of the RDS.

Infants with HMD showed no difference in the three growth parameters at 1 [38] and 4 [39] years of age, whether treated with IV hydrocortisone or not. At 6 years of age, weight and height were below the fiftieth percentile in 89% of ventilated infants and 64% of nonventilated infants [40]. In a long-term follow-up study of HMD infants no relationship was found between birth measurements and eventual size [41]. In a follow-up study [42] of RDS infants treated with CPAP and/or IPPV the mean weight of RDS infants at follow-up was below standard for age, the mean height no different, and the mean head circumference above standard for age. Similarly, normal head circumferences were found at 18 months of age in RDS infants treated with CPAP [43].

Premature infants (some with RDS) were followed up at least to 1 year of age [44]. Weights at 1 year of age tended to remain below the fiftieth percentile, while head circumference was generally above the fiftieth percentile.

Physical growth measurements were done at approximately 12 months of age in infants with birth weights of < 1000 g [45]. These measurements were corrected for gestational age in determining the percentiles. Of the 28 children, 60% had RDS; two-thirds of them were ventilated and one-third were not. At 1 year of age the number of those who were at less than the fifth percentile in length, weight, and head circumference was 14 (50%), 17 (60%), and 11 (39%), respectively. Overall, there was no difference in growth between the ventilated and nonventilated groups.

In another study, mechanically ventilated infants weighing < 1501 g at birth were followed with weight and height measurements to 3 years of age [28]. Fifty-three percent of males and 36% of females had RDS. Growth curves were corrected for gestational age and the children remained slightly below average for weight and height. Growth measurements were recorded in a prospective follow-up study of 184 infants with birth weights between 501 and 1500 g, 40% of whom had RDS [31]. At 3 years of chronological age, 22% of infants were at less than the third percentile in weight and 28% were at less than the third percentile in height. Similar percentiles for weight and height were seen in 28% of infants at 5 years. The head circumference for all infants (except for six hydrocephalic and two microcephalic children) were within the normal range at 3 and 5 years.

At 6 years of age, girls were found to be taller and heavier than boys when their mothers had been treated antenatally with betamethasone, but both groups were in the normal range [46].

B. Summary

Obviously, the findings are not uniform. However, growth studies showed some constant relationships from measurements gathered at birth and on follow-up during the first years of life, when measurements for growth were adjusted according to expected date of confinement (EDC) rather than chronological age. First, most prospective studies with matched controls failed to show any differences between RDS and non-RDS infant growth patterns. Second, infants with BPD might have slow infant growth patterns. Third, the head size of RDS infants appears to be normal or larger than normal after the first year of life. Finally, some studies showed a slowed growth rate for those infants who were small for gestational age, especially those who had been mechanically ventilated.

IV. Effect on Organs

A. Heart

Hypoxia, abnormal vascular resistance, increased pulmonary flow, right-to-left shunting, and vasoconstriction are disease processes that affect long-term cardiac function. In a prospective study, eight (9.4%) HMD infants had a significant patent ductus arteriosus (PDS) [40]. The pathology resolved by 6 months of age in all but one patient; that patient required surgery. In another study of 20 neonates with HMD followed between 1 and 4 years of age (some treated with mechanical ventilation), the EKG was normal in 17 (85%) of the cases and abnormal in three (15%) cases [24]. One infant had an incomplete bundle branch block and two infants had left ventricular hypertrophy (LVH).

Serial EKGs were performed by at least 2 years of age on 16 survivors of severe RDS who had been treated with IPPV [47]. Three of four patients without BPD had normal EKGs, and one had mild RVH. Of the 12 infants with BPD, three (25%) had normal EKGs and two had RVH which progressively improved (one became normal and the other had complete right bundle branch block). The remaining seven patients (58%) had persistent RVH.

Seventy-seven IPPV-treated RDS infants and 60 matched controls were followed between 2.6 and 7.6 years of age [48]. None of the children had clinical or radiological evidence of heart disease. No difference in mean heart volume was found between the two groups. Persistent PDA complicated the clinical course in 45 (15%) of 299 RDS infants presenting over a 3-year period [49]. The incidence of PDA complicating RDS rose with decreasing birth weight and was highest in babies with severe RDS, as judged by the use of assisted ventilation. In infants with birth weights of < 1500 g, PDA occurred as a complication of RDS in 25% of the cases. In RDS survivors, spontaneous closure of the PDA occurred in all except one infant.

Decrease in neonatal heart rate variability (NHRV) was significantly related to the severity of RDS, and the reappearance of NHRV in infants with RDS was associated with good prognosis [2].

HMD was among the perinatal predictors for symptomatic PDA [50]. Preterm infants with PDA demonstrated abnormal cerebral hemodynamics, which returned to normal following the closure of the ductus [18]. The relationship between PDA and brain damage remains to be explained [51].

B. Eye

Oxygen produces detrimental effects on the developing eye, most frequently after high concentrations or prolonged therapeutic duration. Therefore, the incidence of retrolental fibroplasia (RLF) in children with RDS deserves careful attention.

Retrolental Fibroplasia

Among 153 IPPV-treated HMD infants, one had retrolental fibroplasia (0.7%) [32]. No RLF was found among 20 RDS infants with birth weights between 890 and 1570 g who had sustained aortic PO_2 values between 150 mmHg and 300 mmHg [23], nor among any of the 67 HMD infants who were treated with CPAP [52]. Among 74 RDS infants, two had RLF (2.7%) [36].

No RLF was found among 33 neonates with RDS and their 33 matched controls [53]. Follow-up of 76 RDS infants treated with IPPV and 68 matched controls revealed one case of RLF (1.3%) among the RDS group; two had slight cicatricial fibroplasia [54]. Among the controls, one was blind because of RLF (1.4%).

Among 80 ventilated premature infants (60 RDS), RLF occurred in one infant (1.2%) [44]. Thirty-eight infants with a birth weight of < 1000 g, with an RDS-infant subset of 23, were assessed at 1 year of age [45]. Twenty infants received neonatal ventilation. Statistically significant differences were found, with RLF present in 13 (65%) of the ventilated and two (11%) of the nonventilated group.

Among 28 ventilated infants weighing < 1250 g, RLF was diagnosed in 11 infants (39%) in the first 3 months of life [55]. In the RLF group, both birth weight and gestational age were significantly less than in the non-RLF group. Furthermore, a positive blood culture as well as exposure to high O_2 concentrations were significantly higher in the RLF infants than in the non-RLF group. Among 81 children treated with assisted ventilation, one RDS infant (1.2%) had bilateral RLF [56].

Of 161 infants weighing between 501 and 1500 g at birth, ophthalmological assessment was obtained in the nursery and at follow-up examinations [31]. Thirty (18%) had grade I or II RLF; grade III RLF was present in five infants (3.1%); and grade IV or V RLF was found in seven infants (4.3%). Surgery for RLF was done on one infant. No significant perinatal association was found between RDS and RLF.

Other Eye Abnormalities

Forty-seven infants with RDS had ophthalmological examinations between the ages of 15 and 24 months [36]. One child had a scleral crescent in one eye and distortion of the optic disc; three children had squint. Among 22 RDS children, one had strabismus [26]. Among 12 infants with HMD, three had myopia, one had a retinal detachment, one had a retinal traction, one was blind in one eye, and two had resolved stage I retinopathy [55]. Thirty-three RDS and 33 matched control infants had ophthalmological assessment [53]. Squints and refractive errors requiring glasses were found in six RDS children and four controls. Among 19 HMD infants who received CPAP assistance, two had strabismus at ophthalmological follow-up [52]. Among 80 HMD patients treated with artificial ventilation and followed for 2 to 5 years, 11 infants had strabismus [22].

Seventy-six RDS infants treated with IPPV and 68 matched controls were followed [54]. One neonate with RDS had excessive myopia and strabismus amblyopia, and one control suffered from uncomplicated myopia. Furthermore, five RDS infants and four controls presented with uncomplicated squints. Among 161 infants weighing between 501 and 1500 g at birth, vision was severely compromised in association with other problems in four infants (two with unilateral and two with bilateral blindness) [31]. One infant was blind in one eye and severely myopic in the other eye. High myopia was present in nine infants.

Surgery was done for strabismus in eight infants. Severe glaucoma was present in one infant. No correlation was found between neonatal RDS and later development of eye abnormalities. Among 80 children with respiratory insufficiency who were treated with assisted ventilation [56], abnormalities of the eyes were found among one RDS survivor and five others without RDS.

C. Lung

Respiratory Infections

Clinically manifested respiratory infections are a natural consequence in infants who survive RDS. The following articles deal with infants with RDS, of whom some were ventilated and others were not.

The incidence of lower respiratory infection ranged from 5.4% [57] to 19% [58] as well as several percentages in between [24, 36]. The incidence of respiratory symptomatology was much higher among ventilated patients than among nonventilated patients [25]. In another study, the incidence of respiratory infection in childhood was not associated with neonatal respiratory illness, the duration or concentration of the usage of oxygen, or the duration of mechanical ventilation [59]. Rehospitalization of RDS survivors for respiratory symptoms during the first 2 years of life ranged from 5.4% [36] to 20% [59], with other percentages in between [25].

Among all ventilated RDS infants, the ones with BPD subsequently had the most frequent infections [47]. The incidence of severe infections varied from 3.5% [40] to 84% [26], including many percentages in between [22,27,42, 47,52,60]. Some of the symptoms lasted for < 1 year [33], and others for as long as 2-5 years [47]. Although some researchers reported eventual improvement and an absence of chronic symptoms, others reported respiratory problems after 2 years of age, with frequent episodes of pulmonary infections [22].

Control studies of RDS infants who were ventilated reveal that 33% of RDS children < 1 year of age had severe respiratory symptoms, and that between 18 months and 6 years of age, more than half of the 33% remained symptomatic [61]. A matched-control study revealed the incidence of pneumonia or bronchitis to be 48% among infants surviving RDS [48]. The incidence of symptomatology was significantly higher in RDS infants than in the controls. The incidence of upper respiratory infections (URI) was similar for RDS infants and for controls. Episodes of otitis or pneumonia were higher among steroid-treated RDS infants than among controls [39].

Studies of RDS and other premature infants who were ventilated reveal the incidence of lower chest infection to be from 5% [44] to 24% [28], with incidences in between [29,62]. However, among infants who were ventilated for respiratory failure, those with RDS had a higher incidence of infection, and multiple rehospitalization occurred only among the RDS patients [29].

Similarly, neonatal RDS was associated with two-thirds of infections observed at 2 years of age [63]. No differences were found between the rehospitalized and nonrehospitalized RDS patients regarding the total time of oxygen, use of oxygen concentrations over 80%, or time spent on the respirator. The incidence of lower respiratory infection during the second year of life was much higher among infants with BPD whose birth weights were < 1500 g than among infants of similar birth weight with or without RDS alone [28].

In a control study where BPD children were compared with two other non-BPD groups, a significantly higher incidence of respiratory infections was found among the BPD group [33].

Roentgenographic Studies

The early reparative process of hyaline membrane disease in neonates has been reported [64]. The terminology of bronchopulmonary dysplasia by Northway et al. [65] describes those infants who had severe RDS and required respiratory therapy and prolonged oxygen administration at high concentrations. The disease occurs in four stages over a period of 1 month from the acute phase of HMD through the regenerative, transitional, and finally the chronic phases of BPD. All four stages are described clinically, radiologically, and histologically. The disease of BPD is postulated to be the result of a prolonged healing process combined with oxygen toxicity involving mucosal, alveolar, and vascular tissues as evidenced at autopsy. The residual pulmonary consequences of the reparative process in the survivors of ventilated HMD infants were given as the etiological causes of BPD by Shepard et al. [66]. Oxygen detrimentally influenced lung growth by inhibiting DNA synthesis [67]. Since then the roentgenographic findings of RDS survivors have been the topic of many reports.

Studies that include RDS patients [25,27,28,57–59,63,68–70] vary regarding the incidence of residual radiographic changes from 6.2% [25] to 100% [59]. However, the age of the patients at the time of the radiographic studies varied from 1 year to 10 years. In one report, eight of 12 children with RLF but without RDS had abnormal chest roentgenograms, similar to those of the RDS children, in a follow-up study [68]. Meanwhile, another study found no correlation between oxygen therapy and later roentgenographic findings in the children [59]. Another study revealed that 23% of the children who had abnormal chest x-rays were among a nonventilated group [57]. In an opposing study, eight of nine chest x-rays of nonventilated infants were normal between 3 and 13 months of age [25]. In another group of 209 survivors of HMD, 93 nonventilated had no BPD; among the 116 ventilated, 27 infants had BPD and were followed radiologically [69]. Signs of BPD disappeared on long-term radiological follow-up between 3 and 6 months of age in the mild cases and between 18 and 24 months in the severe cases. The incidence of BPD was higher in low birth weight infants (< 1500 g), or those with gestational age of < 32 weeks. The longer an infant is ventilated, the more severe the pulmonary disease. In addition, oxygen use, even at low concentration, demonstrates a similar role in infants presenting with BPD. Chest roentgenogram abnormalities positively correlate with the use of positive pressure ventilation, length of time on the respirator, use of oxygen, and occurrence of chronic symptoms such as pneumonia during the first year of life [27]. Chest roentgenograms do not correlate with negative pressure ventilation or with oxygen concentration. Although more infants survive severe HMD, there has been no increase in the incidence of BPD among survivors within the past 15 years [71].

One hundred and twenty RDS infants were followed radiologically until 4 years of age [72]. The children were grouped according to severity of HMD, mode of artificial ventilation, and duration of oxygen exposure. Of 50 infants with a diagnosis of mild radiological HMD (eight artificially ventilated and 23 subjected to high oxygen exposure) six (12%) had sequelae. Among the 46 cases with a diagnosis of moderate radiological HMD (36 artificially ventilated and 40 subjected to high oxygen exposure), 21 (45%) had sequelae. Of the 24 radiologically severe HMD cases (22 ventilated and all subjected to high oxygen exposure), 21 (88%) had sequelae.

Comparisons were made between RDS children and children receiving intensive care for other causes [73]. The radiographic sequelae of the non-RDS children were much less than those of the RDS group. When high concentrations of oxygen were used for < 3 days in the RDS group, there were no severe sequelae. In moderate HMD cases, children recover completely by about 1 year of age. In severe HMD cases, some children might not be healthy even at 2 years of age. The conclusion was that prematurity, severity of the pulmonary disease, increased concentration of oxygen, and prolongation of oxygen exposure are the major causes of radiographic sequelae.

Studies on ventilated RDS infants who were followed radiologically are plentiful [24,26,40,42,47,52]. The incidence of abnormal x-rays at follow-up varied from 15% [24] to 68% [47], and the age of the follow-up varied from < 1 year up to 6 years. On one hand, there were no statistical correlates reported between the usage of oxygen and subsequent x-ray changes [40]. On the other hand, among 15 BPD infants treated with IPPV, the persistence of abnormal roentgenographic findings was significantly related to the duration of ambient oxygen therapy [47].

Among nine children with BPD, eight (88%) had persistently abnormal chest roentgenograms at 8 years of age [73]. The incidence of BPD among HMD infants treated with IPPV increased over 6 years, from 14% to 28% [32]. Patients with HMD developing BPD had significantly lower gestational ages and birth weights than those without underlying BPD.

In control studies of all ventilated RDS cases, radiological abnormalities were found in 30% of the symptomatic and 6% of the asymptomatic RDS children between 1.5 and 6.0 years of age [61].

In ventilated prematures, some roentgenographic studies have revealed inconsistent results. In a study of 27 survivors, none had abnormal chest x-rays at 1 year of age [44]. In another study of 28 ventilated patients, 11 HMD infants treated wtih negative pressure ventilators had abnormal roentgenograms between 2 and 5 years of age [74]. No conclusion was drawn concerning the administration of oxygen or the use of mechanical ventilation as a major factor in the persistence of roentgenographic abnormalities.

Six infants with various causes for their initial respiratory failure required artificial ventilation for > 6 months [75]. Radiological features resembled those in the chronic phase of BPD. However, only two of the infants in this study had RDS, and only these two received an oxygen concentration > 50%. Therefore, neither the RDS nor the oxygen concentration can be implicated in the BPD-like radiographic picture for the other four infants. Among 38 surviving infants (23 RDS) with birth weights of < 1000 g, chronic BPD was seen in 14 (70%) of the 20 infants who had had prolonged periods of ventilation [45].

Pulmonary Function Studies

Many reports focus on the pulmonary function of RDS survivors. Because the studies employ different technical methodology at different ages and use varied terminology that is understood and appreciated only by those who are highly specialized in lung function and therapy, this section restricts itself primarily to conclusions of the studies rather than to their methodologies.

Among studies where some RDS infants were ventilated, the findings were as follows: In infants who suffered from HMD abnormalities in alveolar-arterial oxygen gradient may exist years after birth [68]. When ventilated and nonventilated RDS infants had respiratory function abnormalities between 5 and 10 years of age it was not possible to establish whether pulmonary disease, high concentration of oxygen, mechanical ventilation, or intubation had been responsible for the abnormalities [57].

During the first months of life functional residual capacity was significantly lower in RDS prematures than in controls [25]. Abnormalities lasted longer in the ventilated than in the nonventilated group. However, only patients with BPD had markedly abnormal blood gasses during the first year of life. By ages 5-10, RDS survivors showed recovery of functional residual capacity and pulmonary function, although minor abnormalities were found in some children. These studies suggest that pulmonary recovery occurs during the first year of life when lung growth is most rapid, and recovery is virtually complete after 5-10 years.

Pulmonary function tests at 7 years of age showed 14% restrictive and 5.5% obstructive abnormalities in ventilated infants. Although those whose pulmonary function tests were normal had had shorter periods of high oxygen concentration, they did not differ significantly from those who had had abnormal pulmonary functions and longer periods of a high oxygen concentration [40].

Studies have been reported involving RDS infants, all of whom were ventilated. In one follow-up study of children between 5 and 10 years of age, 22 severe RDS infants were evaluated. Two had been treated with IPPV and 15 had BPD [47]. Low PaO_2 was found in all BPD and some non-BPD infants at 5 years of age. One-third of all BPD children had normal PaO_2 levels at 10 years of age. At 5 years of age, alveolar-arterial oxygen differences were abnormal, with one exception. No statistical relationship in the follow-ups was found between the abnormalities of pulmonary function and birth weight, gestational age, duration of IPPV, or oxygen therapy. No correlation was found between x-ray and clinical or pulmonary function studies. Between 8 and 48 months, 51% of RDS patients had asymptomatic increased pulmonary resistance [60]. Marginal [26] to normal pulmonary function during the first year of life was found in some studies [52]. However, pulmonary function tests of children with BPD demonstrated airway obstruction and abnormal blood gases at 8 years of age [73]. Bronchial hyperactivity was observed at a mean age of 8.4 years in BPD patients, suggesting that abnormal pulmonary function does not resolve during early childhood, but that abnormalities in fact persist following the completion of lung growth. Seven- and 11-year-old HMD patients still had minimally abnormal pulmonary function studies without a history of exercise intolerance or chronic respiratory symptoms [27]. The presence of chronic respiratory symptoms in infants and the use of mechanical ventilation with subsequent roentgenographic abnormalities at 1 year of age correlated with abnormal pulmonary function tests at 11 years of age.

Several studies included RDS children and controls. A study of children between 1.5 and 6.0 years old revealed not only that there were more statistically significant pulmonary function abnormalities in RDS infants vs. the controls, but also that among RDS infants high concentration of oxygen was an additional etiological factor in lung damage [61]. Data from RDS infants, compared to data from non-RDS preterm and full-term infants, at 6–10 years of age revealed reduced pulmonary gas flow rates in prematurely born children (both with and without RDS), suggesting increased large-airway resistance in both groups of prematurely born infants [76]. Furthermore, additional abnormalities among RDS infants suggested an increase in small airway resistance. Resting BPD infants had significantly higher oxygen consumption than controls, indicating their caloric expenditure was significantly higher [77]. Infants with BPD developed hypercarbia during exercise at 3–5 years of age, while most survivors of

HMD without BPD appear to have normal cardiopulmonary function at this age [78].

Ventilated prematures, including RDS infants, were evaluated with respiratory function studies between 2.5 and 5.5 years of age [79]. They appeared clinically normal and there was no correlation among the conditions requiring ventilation, therapeutic characteristics, or the degree of abnormality in lung function tests.

D. Summary

The incidence of PDA is higher in infants with RDS, but the PDA most often resolves spontaneously. The most serious cardiac complications occur in infants who develop BPD. The abnormal cerebral hemodynamics of infants with RDS suggest intriguing explanations for deficits which do not become manifest until the child is older.

Severe prematurity (< 1000 g birth weight), prolonged use of O_2, severe respiratory disease or sepsis, and mechanical ventilation all contribute to the possibility of a higher incidence of RLF. The etiology of RLF follows a multifactorial pattern with many contributing conditions.

Analytic data from control studies as well as multiple studies fail to suggest that infants with RDS have a higher incidence of other ophthalmological complications.

The clinical problems following the survival of RDS lead to the conclusion that the minor manifestations of URI are more likely for RDS survivors than for control prematures. Hospitalization in the first year of life for high-risk (maternal factors, low birth weight, social factors, etc.) survivors is 9.1% overall, increasing to 38.2% with a decreasing birth weight [80]. Hospitalization is more common in RDS survivors, but most common in those who have later pulmonary complications as a result of prior BPD. Respiratory symptoms will more likely occur in children < 2 years of age because after that lung growth is rapid. The incidence of respiratory disease related to RDS decreases at a later age.

Among the suggested factors responsible for abnormal roentgenograms, the severity of the original HMD (not surprisingly, associated with lower birth weight and gestational age) was frequently mentioned. In addition, the length of mechanical ventilation, oxygen concentration, and duration of oxygen therapy were thought to be iatrogenic causes associated with the radiological findings in some reports. Patients without RDS have considerably less radiological pathology than RDS infants similarly managed during the newborn period. Thus, mechanical ventilatory support is a major cause of the basic residual radiological pathology of HMD, and the iatrogenic disease management is a cause of the residual radiological findings. Clearly, the more mature infant, despite an originally more severe roentgenographic picture, is more likely to recover than the less mature infant with a similar pathology.

Respiratory function studies showed a pattern of disease severity similar to that of radiographic findings. Most of the respiratory functions studies corrèlate with the radiological findings, although not completely. Both the radiological and the respiratory function studies suggest that asymptomatic patients may suffer prolonged functional abnormalities. It also appears that the pulmonary function studies are more sensitive. The abnormalities found by pulmonary function studies persist longer than the clinical or the radiological pathology. Some studies, especially in infants with BPD, showed persistent pulmonary function abnormalities and negate the optimistic view that rapidly growing lungs will eliminate all lung damage [73]. It is not known, however, what complications may arise in survivors of BPD beyond 12 years of age regarding the status of lung function and susceptibility to pulmonary diseases in the future.

Some areas still need to be studied. If males have a higher incidence of RDS at birth, then persistent pulmonary abnormalities would be expected to be found more frequently among males at follow-up. Do males indeed have a more prolonged and troubled course in childhood than females? This question remains open.

V. Effect on Central Nervous System

A. Electroencephalogram

Several researchers have studied RDS as an etiology for hypoxia by making recordings of electroencephalograms (EEGs) and/or visual evoked potentials (VEPs).

In one study, 13 RDS infants, 12 infants suffering from other perinatal syndromes, and 35 controls had serial EEGs [81]. These investigators used VEPs to detect the presence of any abnormalities in the retinocalcarine pathway due to an early anoxic insult in patients who suffered from RDS. Normal VEPs signify normal maturative events in control newborns; whereas the normal response is not obtained after an anoxic insult. Mild RDS infants displayed improved VEP at 6-9 months of age compared to their neonatal recordings. However, in those infants with severe RDS, the improved VEP was not so evident at 9 months of age. In a study of 58 patients (28 RDS and 30 matched controls), normal EEGs were found in 17 RDS infants and 25 controls [53]. Borderline abnormalities were found in seven RDS infants and three controls. Abnormal EEGs occurred in four RDS infants and two controls. Twelve of 24 RDS patients were treated with IV hydrocortisone in the first 24 hr of life [38]. Four abnormal EEG tracings were seen in the steroid-treated children. In the nontreated group, nine were normal and three refused testing. In another steroid-treated RDS study, abnormal EEGs were present with equal frequency in both the treated and the control groups [39]. Among 27 survivors of RDS with assisted ventilation, EEGs were performed on 17 [44]. All recordings were normal for age. Among 80 HMD children treated with artificial ventilation, 33 had an EEG during the neonatal period and a repeated EEG at 2 years of age [22]. Eight normal EEG tracings in premature infants remained normal after 2 years. Twenty-five infants had EEG abnormalities either at initial or at follow-up studies. All 28 RDS survivors who were assisted with constant positive pressure in infancy had normal EEGs at 18 months of age [43]. Among 39 infants who were treated with assisted ventilation because of respiratory insufficiency [56], EEG abnormalities were found among two RDS infants and three others.

B. Speech and Language Development

Does the speech performance of RDS and non-RDS infants differ because of the influence of a prolonged hypoxic episode on the central nervous system at an early point in its development? This question is addressed in several studies.

Among 33 RDS infants and 33 matched controls, speech was tested at 4 years of age [53]. Developmental abnormalities were more frequent in infants with RDS, but the differences were not statistically significant. In a prospective study of 20,137 children, in which speech and language development was determined by complex standardized tests, RDS did not influence performances at 8 years of age, when compared to the control population [82]. The Socio-Economic Index (SEI) was the most significant factor influencing speech and language development.

IPPV-treated RDS infants and matched controls were evaluated between the ages of 2.6 and 7.6 years [54]. The parents of 19 (56%) of 35 RDS survivors reported considerably slower speech development as compared with siblings, while this was reported in only nine (29%) of 31 controls ($p < 0.05$). The average linguistic test score of 37 RDS survivors was lower than that of the controls, but the difference was not significant. Among 51 RDS infants treated with CPAP alone or with CPAP and IPPV, seven had abnormal linguistic performance between 2.5 and 3.5 years of age [42]. Reexamination at age 4-5 showed persistent handicaps among four of the seven children. Three of them had dysphasia. The statistical analysis showed that these children had been more hypoxic at delivery, had been smaller and more premature, and had been hypoxic prior to ventilatory treatment to a greater extent than the control group. There were no differences in speech or language development of 6-year-old children who had RDS as infants, when compared to control children who did not, in a study in which all mothers had been treated antenatally with betamethasone [46].

In a prospective study of 111 selected high-risk newborns, 33 of them had HMD [83]. Speech delay was present at 3 years of age in seven HMD children; however, the incidence was not statistically different from non-HMD infants.

C. Hearing

Whether the hearing capabilities of RDS children vary from those of non-RDS children was the subject of several reports.

Hearing tests performed between 1 and 4 years of age on 33 RDS children and 33 matched controls who had weighed < 2040 g at birth showed one control with hearing loss over 70 dB, but none with hearing loss among the RDS group [53]. In a prospective study in which 20,137 children had audiological evaluation at 8 years of age, the children with RDS did not have a higher incidence of abnormalities compared to the control population [82]. Among 24 RDS infants, 12 of whom were treated with IV cortisone, none of them had hearing loss at 1 year of age [30]. Among 27 RDS infants who received assisted ventilation, two were deaf [44]. A hearing loss > 20 dB was found in nine of 76 (12%) RDS infants treated with IPPV and eight of 68 (12%) matched controls [54]. Eighty HMD infants treated with artificial ventilation were evaluated between 2 and 5 years of age [22]. Seven children had partial hypacusia with bilateral deficit up to 40 dB. Among 67 HMD children treated with CPAP, none had a hearing deficit detected by audiometry between 10 and 14 months of age [52].

D. Psychological Findings

One of the most important questions in the long-term follow-up of RDS infants is whether these children have a higher incidence of abnormalities in later intellectual performance than those infants who did not suffer from RDS. And if they do indeed manifest intellectual impairment, how long will it last?

Studies in Which No Infants Were Ventilated

Sixty patients, including 12 RDS infants, with birth weights between 1500 and 2500 g underwent psychological tests at a mean age of 41 months. The tests revealed that children with higher birth weights and a greater gestational age tended to have higher intelligence [84]. A positive correlation was found between education of parents and intelligence of their children. Similarly, children at a mean age of 4.3 years whose birth weights were < 1500 g displayed a significantly increased incidence of mental retardation compared to normal birth weight infants. Even greater retardation occurred in children with birth weights of < 1250 g and a lower gestational age [85]. The severity and incidence of RDS had an inverse relationship to birth weight, and an increased risk of mental retardation. Socioeconomic standing of the parents and the intellectual performance of the children were positively correlated.

In a prospective study RDS infants whose birth weights were 1501 g and greater had significantly more abnormal performances at 8 months of age with the Bayley Motor Scale than did the controls [86]. The 5- and 20-min Apgar scores were significantly lower and the incidence of resuscitation at birth was significantly higher in the RDS group. Intellectual studies conducted between 1 and 6 years of age in children of < 2040 g birth weight revealed no increased abnormalities among RDS infants [53]. Similar conclusions were derived from studies of RDS and control populations divided into > and < 2000 g birth weight categories studied at 4 years of age [87]. A longitudinal study, which included matched and unmatched controls, revealed that the RDS children with birth weights > 2500 g constituted the only group that at 4 years of age exhibited significantly more psychomotor abnormalities than the control groups [20]. Performances were adversely affected by either low birth weight or low socioeconomic family standing. Comparisons with siblings revealed a fall-off in RDS survivor performance at 8 months of age, but not at 4 years of age. In a study at 1 year of age, where some RDS children received IV cortisone after birth and other RDS children did not, the treated group had significantly lower mental developmental quotient (DQ) [38].

Studies in Which Some Infants Were Ventilated

Among 47 RDS infants followed between 15 and 24 months of age, two (4.2%) had a DQ of < 80 [36]. Among 29 RDS infants with a birth weight < 2000 g, who were evaluated between 1 and 4 years of age, two were mentally retarded [6]. In studies where members of the population were evaluated up to 6 years of age, the DQ showed that those children whose birth weights were < 2000 g ranked significantly below those children whose birth weights were > 2000 g [40,41]. The DQs of children of more highly educated parents were significantly higher. Mechanical ventilation, acidosis, and hypoxia were found to have no effect on DQ. The DQ of RDS children and their siblings was similar. Among 78 RDS children with birth weights < 2000 g, who were tested at 4 years of age, two (3%) had IQs of < 70. Perinatal asphyxia, neonatal acidosis, hypoxia, and hypercapnia did not correlate with cerebral prognosis [88].

Studies in Which All Infants Were Ventilated

In several studies results varied from normal in all RDS infants when tested between 0.5 and 2.5 years of age [26] to a 9% incidence of severe abnormalities at 2-5 years of age [22,29]. RDS infants learned to walk at a significantly later age than their siblings [42]. Among 22 RDS infants (of whom 15 had BPD) tested between 1 and 5 years of age, seven (32%, of whom six were BPD) had abnormal development [47].

Among 76 RDS infants and 68 matched controls tested between 2.6 and 7.6 years of age, walking was delayed significantly among the RDS infants [54]. Five RDS children and one control had an IQ of < 85, although the difference was not significant.

When RDS infants were tested between 1 and 6 years of age RDS per se did not contribute to a higher incidence of impaired development [28,29,44, 56]. No relationship was found between IQs < 85 and the lowest value of PaO_2 or the highest value of $PaCO_2$ [29].

Cognitive development of 6-year-old children who had received mechanical ventilation and whose mothers had been treated antenatally with betamethasone was not different from that of their controls [46].

Among 111 high-risk (e.g., RDS, neurological abnormalities, etc.) newborns followed up to 3 years of age, three RDS children (2.7%) had borderline IQs [83]. Both social and cultural status of the parents seem to play a role in the intellectual performance of infants. In one study of infants with birth weights of < 1000 g, development was assessed at 1 year of age [45]. Within the group of ventilated children there was a correlation between duration of ventilation and low DQ. There was no correlation found between DQ and RDS or the mother's education.

A longitudinal study in which infants of birth weight < 2500 g were studied at early school age revealed that many predictors of abnormal development – such as birth weight, gestational age at birth, early intrauterine insult, social status, and transient neurological abnormalities – were interrelated [90]. Significant correlations were found between school performance and family socioeconomic index. An impairment score – which included family social status, birth weight, gestational age, intrauterine insult, intrauterine growth percentile, postnatal tests, and neurological status at 12 months – was found to have significant relationship to later IQ. In a study where 26 BPD infants were compared to eight similarly treated (> 20 days of oxygen therapy) RDS infants without BPD and to 25 controls (< 6 days of oxygen therapy), including 10 RDS infants [33], a significantly increased mean IQ was found in the two groups without BPD.

E. Neurological Sequelae

The question of the neurological consequences of RDS survivors has been addressed in several articles.

Studies in Which No Infants Were Ventilated

Twelve percent of infants with birth weights < 1500 g displayed neurological abnormalities at 4 years of age, including spastic paraplegia, microcephaly, and quadriplegia [85].

In a longitudinal prospective study where the subjects were divided into birth weight categories of < 1500 g, 1501-2500 g, and > 2500 g, it was found that neurological abnormalities were more frequent during the first year of life in the RDS survivors than in the control subjects in each of the birth weight categories [86]. By 4 years of age, only the group of RDS survivors with birth weights > 2500 g differed significantly from the control group [20]. The incidences of resuscitation, lower Apgar scores at 5 min, and brain abnormalities in the newborn period were significantly higher among the RDS infants than among control subjects in all birth weight categories.

When 33 RDS infants were compared with 33 matched controls at 6 years of age, abnormal neurological findings were present in 16 (48%) of the RDS infants and 11 (33%) of the controls [53]. The differences were not statistically significant. The abnormalities included cerebral palsy and mental retardation. At 4 years of age, RDS infants did not manifest a higher incidence of abnormalities than the controls [87]. A significant negative correlation was found between birth weight and degree of neurological disability. Twelve RDS infants treated with IV cortisone following birth were compared with untreated RDS infants at 1 year of age [38]. Among the treated infants, two (16.6%) were abnormal – one with spastic quadriplegia and one with hypotonia. Among the untreated children, one (8.3%) had spastic diplegia.

Studies in Which Some Infants Were Ventilated

In one study of 47 RDS infants, one (2%) had spastic paraplegia at 2 years of age [36]. Among 29 children evaluated between 1 and 4 years of age who had RDS and a birth weight < 2000 g, four (14%) had major neurological abnormalities [24]. Among 197 RDS children at 1 year of age, three (1.5%) had severe cerebral damage and 14 (7%) had mild cerebral paresis [88]. Mechanical ventilation for more than 14 days increased the risk of cerebral palsy. Very low birth weight and low gestational age increased the risk of abnormal neurological findings only slightly. Perinatal asphyxia, neonatal acidosis, hypoxia, or hypercapnia did not correlate with impaired cerebral prognosis.

No significant reduction was found in the proportion of handicapped, very low birth weight babies (< 1500 g) in the last 15 years in spite of better quality of care [30]. Eighty-eight children with birth weights < 1500 g were followed from 40 weeks up to 55 months of age. Twenty-three percent of them had major neurological abnormalities. Among the 751–1000 g infants, abnormalities were found in 40% [91]. Birth weight and gestational age were significantly lower among the neurologically abnormal infants than among the normal ones. Postnatal factors such as apnea, shock, acidosis, mechanical ventilation for more than 3 days, and moderate to severe RDS were all statistically more common among the neurologically abnormal children. Among children evaluated at 5 years whose birth weight was 501–1500 g, neurological abnormalities were present in 16.8%, and the majority had cerebral palsy [31]. Neurological abnormalities correlated positively with intraventricular hemorrhage, RDS, and the duration of respiratory support. Intraventricular hemorrhage and RDS may be important regarding the underlying risk of neurological problems, but the duration of respiratory support may reflect the severity of the initial state or iatrogenic factors related to the use of mechanical ventilation.

Children followed through school age revealed neurological abnormalities in 60% of those whose birth weights were < 1500 g and 37% of those whose birth weights were between 1501 and 2000 g [88]. A high incidence of postnatal complications was seen in the group suffering intrauterine insult, and this suggested that the postnatal complications were due to existing neurological abnormalities at the time of birth. Social status, intrauterine insult, and transient neonatal neurological abnormalities were predictors of later neurological problems. The handicaps were significantly more frequent in males than in females.

Infants of < 1000 g birth weight studied between 8 and 15 months of age revealed that among 14 ventilated infants, nine (64.2%) had severe handicaps and five (35.7%) were mildly handicapped [45]. Among the 14 control nonventilated infants, one (7.1%) was severely handicapped and three (21%) had mild handicaps.

Among BPD patients, 52% showed neurological abnormalities between 2 and 5 years of age, while only 16% of the non-BPD controls had neurological abnormalities [33]. The abnormalities included spastic diplegia and quadriplegia.

Studies in Which All Infants Were Ventilated

Among 51 RDS infants evaluated between 2.5 and 4.0 years of age, 7.8% had neurological abnormalities [42]. A significant correlation existed among the neurologically abnormal children regarding lower birth weight, lower gestational age, lower Apgar scores, and higher $PaCO_2$ prior to ventilation. Among other studies where follow-up was done between 1 and 7 years of age, the incidence of neurological abnormalities varied from 0% [43] to 40% [91]. The incidence of neurological abnormalities in between was also reported [5,22,28,29,32,44,52, 55,56,58,65,83,92]. Among the neurological abnormalities were hydrocephaly, spastic hemiplegia, diplegia, spastic quadriplegia, and cerebral palsy.

No difference in the incidence of cerebral palsy and hydrocephaly was found among RDS infants than among their matched controls between 2.6 and 7.6 years of age [54]. In several reports the incidence of RDS was higher among the neurologically abnormal children [28,29,32,89]. In one study, major neurological sequelae were closely associated with neonatal seizure and intraventricular hemorrhage and were more common in boys [28]. The severely defective children tended to have longer periods of mechanical ventilation and higher peak bilirubin levels. In another study, birth weight and gestational age of children with severe abnormalities were significantly less than those of children in the remainder of the study [55]. However, no correlation was found among indications for ventilation (RDS, etc.), serum bilirubin, hypernatremia, hypoglycemia, hypocalcemia, or acidemia.

F. Summary

By using the VEP technique, abnormalities were detected in RDS survivors at 9 months of age. In general, the degree of abnormality correlated with the severity of RDS. Other follow-up studies involving EEG measurements in RDS survivors and matched controls failed to demonstrate any consistent abnormalities. Therefore, it seems reasonable to conclude that RDS per se would not produce any persistent EEG abnormalities. However, it likewise seems reasonable to assume that RDS when accompanied by significant hypoxia would result in prolonged (even permanent) EEG changes.

Severe perinatal asphyxia appears to have some untoward effects on early speech development. However, prospective controlled studies at later ages failed to show statistical differences among prematures with or without RDS regarding their speech and language development. Speech and language performances correlated with socioeconomic factors.

In matched control studies, RDS infants did not have a higher incidence of hearing abnormalities.

The psychological performance of RDS infants, especially in terms of motor development, appears to be delayed when compared with their controls and siblings during the first year of life. The differences disappear in later years. The average IQ scores are essentially the same. Socioeconomic and genetic factors are highly influential on later intellectual performance. Small birth weight, lower gestational age, intrauterine growth retardation, and perinatal complications all have an inverse relationship to later intellectual performance, but RDS does not appear to be a significant factor by itself in determining psychological performance.

Neurological abnormalities are higher in RDS survivors than in matched controls of all birth weight groups during the first year of life. The neurological differences were not observed after 4 years of age in matched controls studied. The most recent studies have added further complicating elements—such as

BPD, intraventricular hemorrhage, acidosis, and the introduction of respiratory or oxygen therapy—which appear to correlate with the poor performances of low birth weight infants. The fact that more severely affected RDS infants survive with the newer kinds of respiratory assistance might increase the risk of residual morbidity. Boys appear to have a higher incidence of neurological deficit than girls.

Decreased gestation and low birth weight are very important factors, but above all, the SEI factors (genetic make-up, socioeconomic status, and education of the parents) are most influential in determining performances of both RDS infants and their controls. Natural history again shows clearly that the further away a child is from an RDS episode, the less obvious its "harmful" effects appear to be.

VI. Conclusions

The long-term effects of RDS are still not fully recognized. The reasons for this are fourfold: (1) RDS is a consequence of prematurity and is inseparable from other associated multifactorial perinatal events. (2) Survivors are under the influence of a preset genetic complement and physical environment. (3) RDS infants have such a high mortality rate that it is difficult to analyze many longitudinal studies. (4) The studies of RDS infants that are available have frequently been inappropriately designed.

The results of this survey suggest that RDS survivors have a higher mortality and a higher incidence of lung morbidity, as manifested by increased lower respiratory infections, roentgenographic abnormalities, hospitalizations, and prolonged pulmonary function abnormalities, with males being more severely affected than females. RDS survivors have delayed speech and motor development and a higher incidence of psychoneurological abnormalities at an early age (even with corrected gestation and matched controls), but they do not have similar findings at a later age. The reason for this is unknown.

The birth weight, gestational age at delivery, head size, socioeconomic factors, and perinatal factors (i.e., intraventricular hemorrhage) are better individual predictors for future psychoneurological performance than is RDS itself.

In the future, the incidence and outcomes of RDS will be different because of improving management for prenatal and perinatal care. RDS is currently being managed by a variety of respiratory aids [93-96], and further improvement can be expected. Some complications can now be prevented, and the natural history of BPD is now better elucidated. Newborn tracheal aspirate cytology has been suggested as a potentially useful method for the classification of progressive lung injury in mechanically ventilated RDS patients. This method offers cytological information for predicting and diagnosing BPD [97]. There is a direct relationship between pulmonary barotrauma from pressure ventilation and subsequent development of BPD. The prevention of the latter is associated with a concomitant fall in the employment of the former [98]. Understanding the metabolism of prematures will lead to modified and more appropriate nutritional supportive measures for RDS infants. The use and effectiveness of corticosteroids given antenatally to the mother remains controversial [40,58,99,100]; this is discussed in more detail elsewhere in this book. Follow-up studies suggest no somatic or intellectual disadvantages in children whose mothers received corticosteroids prenatally [46]. However, experimental studies indicate that the use of corticosteroids in pregnant monkeys increases lung volume, suggesting that benefits may result from structural changes rather than from alveolar surfactant production; however, offspring showed serious short-term [101] and long-term [102] side effects. Furthermore, steroid treatment of newborns suggests that immunological alterations may occur [39].

The natural history of RDS remains unclear and, therefore, new approaches toward more appropriate study design are needed.

The relationship between perinatal events and subsequent childhood deficits in physical and mental development remains elusive. Follow-up studies require several years to gather data. During such extensive periods diagnostic criteria and treatment methods are likely to change. Moreover, a myriad of variables and their neurological consequences complicate not only the selection of appropriate control groups but even the criteria for diagnosing the disease itself. However, randomized, double-blind studies, which deny infants updated advances in medical treatment, make some study designs almost impossible, both ethically and practically. Reports indicate that the percentage of deaths among low birth weight prematures who have RDS has fallen. Therefore, questions regarding subsequent morbidity become increasingly important. Some studies deal only with RDS infant survival. There are many mortality rate studies which do indeed give clear results. But life is more than survival.

Personality disorders and organ dysfunctions from multiple intrauterine and extrauterine circumstances call for complex multifaceted studies with properly qualified testers and appropriately applied, well-timed tests.

The greatest difficulty encountered in study design, however, arises because of the number, the complexities, and the interrelations of the problems encountered by the RDS infants, as presented in this chapter (see Fig. 1). To attempt to determine the relationship between only two factors, when many complex variables and interrelated factors mingle beyond the researcher's control, is meaningless. Correlation between two factors cannot be appropriately measured unless the other variables can be controlled [103].

What is the end result? At what age should the study be stopped: after early mortality, after preschool intelligence levels have been reached, after school performance has been assessed, when one begins functioning in a family, or with the end of life itself? Is the small premature who is deprived of maternal support destined to have immunological incompetence at a later age, as manifested by more severe infections or an increased susceptibility to malignancy? These represent a fraction of the questions that so far have not been answered.

Recent years have brought many changes in the management of very low birth weight infants [104]. Higher RDS infant survival rates without increased morbidity are part of the evolution of changing perspectives in premature care [105]. Yet in spite of improved management and survival, a considerable number of very low birth weight infants who survive are neurologically and developmentally handicapped [106]. Neonatologists now routinely attempt to salvage infants at birth weights of < 800 g. The extended limit of salvageability fails to consider the increasing costs, decreasing resources, and additional complications of the undeveloped, immature fetus, as described above. Conflicting opinions in society arise concerning medical management when a healthy fetus can be aborted and the 500-g infant with multiple handicaps is salvaged at any cost.

Newer treatments for managing RDS are not restricted to respirators and instruments. We are now able to influence RDS by giving surfactant directly to the newborn [91,107,108]. Further innovative approaches to managing prematures within an artificial uterine environment are foreseen. Yet no one should forget that the optimal management of the growing fetus is attained in its own intrauterine environment. Are the costs of maintaining an intensive care unit inappropriate? Should we instead use the funds to support obstetrical research and services designed solely to maintain high-risk pregnancies to full term? Regardless of developments and progress in intensive care management and support for the outcome of prematures, the ultimate goal is now, and always should be, to carry the pregnancy to full term.

References

1. Ross, S., and R. L. Naeye, Racial and environmental influences on fetal lung maturation, *Pediatrics.,* **68**:790 (1981).
2. Cabal, L. A., B. Siassi, B. Zanini, J. E. Hodgman, and E. E. Hon, Factors affecting heart rate variability in preterm infants, *Pediatrics,* **65**:50 (1980).
3. Nelson, K. B., and J. H. Ellenberg, Apgar scores as predictors of chronic neurologic disability, *Pediatrics,* **68**:36 (1981).
4. Strang, L. B., Heterogeneity of pathogenetic mechanisms in hyaline membrane disease. In *Surfactant System and Neonatal Lung.* Mead Johnson Symposium on Perinatal and Developmental Medicine, 1978, p. 53.
5. Stahlman, M. T., Acute respiratory disorders in the newborn. In *Neonatology: Pathophysiology and Management of the Newborn.* Edited by G. B. Avery. Philadelphia, Lippincott, 1981, p. 371.

6. Jacob, J., D. Edwards, and L. Gluck, Early-onset sepsis and pneumonia observed as respiratory distress syndrome, *Am. J. Dis. Child.,* **134**:766 (1980).
7. Hjalmarson, O., Epidemiology and classification of acute, neonatal respiratory disorders, *Acta Paediatr. Scand.,* **70**:773 (1981).
8. Papageorgiou, A. N., E. Colle, E. Farri-Kostopoulos, and M. M. Gelfand, Incidence of respiratory distress syndrome following antenatal betamethasone: Role of sex, type of delivery, and prolonged rupture of membranes, *Pediatrics,* **67**:614 (1981).
9. Collaborative Group on Antenatal Steroid Therapy: Effect of antenatal dexamethasone administration on the prevention of respiratory distress syndrome, *Am. J. Obstet. Gynecol.,* **141**:276 (1981).
10. Mead, P. B., Management of the patient with premature rupture of the membranes, *Clin. Perinatol.,* **7**:243 (1980).
11. Rojas, J., R. S. Green, L. Fannon, T. Olsson, D. P. Lindstrom, M. T. Stahlman, and R. B. Cotton, A quantitative model for hyaline membrane disease, *Pediatr. Res.,* **16**:35 (1982).
12. Lipper, E., K. Lee, L. M. Gartner, and B. Grellong, Determinants of neurobehavioral outcome in low-birthweight infants, *Pediatrics,* **67**:502 (1981).
13. Harvey, D., J. Prince, J. Bunton, C. Parkinson, and S. Campbell, Abilities of children who were small-for-gestational-age babies, *Pediatrics,* **69**:296 (1982).
14. Nielsen, H. C., and J. S. Torday, Sex differences in fetal rabbit pulmonary surfactant production, *Pediatr. Res.,* **15**:1245 (1981).
15. Kanto, W. P., R. C. Borer, M. Barr, and D. W. Roloff, Tracheal aspirate lecithin/sphingomyelin ratios as predictors of recovery from respiratory distress syndrome, *J. Pediatr.,* **89**:612 (1976).
16. Duke, P. M., J. D. Coulson, J. I. Santos, and J. D. Johnson, Cleft palate associated with prolonged orotracheal intubation in infancy, *J. Pediatr.,* **89**:990 (1976).
17. Parkin, J. L., M. H. Stevens, and A. L. Jung, Acquired and congenital subglottic stenosis in the infant. *Ann. Otol.,* **85**:573 (1976).
18. Lipman, B., G. A. Serwer, and J. E. Brazy, Abnormal cerebral hemodynamics in preterm infants with patent ductus arteriosus, *Pediatrics,* **69**:778 (1982).
19. Leventhal, J. M., Risk factors for child abuse: Methodologic standards in case-control studies, *Pediatrics,* **68**:684 (1981).
20. Fisch, R. O., M. K. Bilek, L. D. Miller, and R. R. Engel, Physical and mental status at 4 years of age of survivors of respiratory distress syndrome. Follow-up report from the collaborative study, *J. Pediatr.,* **86**:497 (1975).
21. Oleinick, A., Growth and development of survivors of RDS. Letter to the Editor, *J. Pediatr.,* **87**:666 (1975).

22. Cukier, F., C. Amiel-Tison, and A. Minkowski, Hyaline membrane disease in neonates treated with artificial ventilation: Neurological and intellectual sequelae at two to five years of age, *Crit. Care Med.,* **2**:265 (1974).
23. Aranda, J. V., and A. Y. Sweet, Sustained hyperoxemia without cicatricial retrolental fibroplasia, *Pediatrics,* **54**:434 (1974).
24. Goenen, M., J. Ninane, B. Ducoffre, Y. Declerck, D. Claus, G. Ferriere, R. M. Thomas-van-Moerbeke, D. Moulin, R. De Meyer, and J. Tremouroux, Hyaline membrane disease: Prognostic factors and medium-term follow-up, *Eur. J. Pediatr.,* **127**:181 (1978).
25. Bryan, M. H., H. Levison, and P. R. Swyer, Pulmonary function in infants and children following the acute neonatal respiratory distress syndrome, *Bull. Europ. Physiopathol. Respir.,* **9**:1587 (1973).
26. Nilsson, R., and C. J. I. Petersen, Respiratory treatment of neonates with the idiopathic respiratory distress syndrome. II. Follow-up studies, *Ugeskr. Laeger,* **139**:1406 (1977).
27. Stahlman, M., G. Hedvall, D. Lindstrom, and J. Snell, Role of hyaline membrane disease in production of later childhood lung abnormalities, *Pediatrics,* **69**:572 (1982).
28. Fitzhardinge, P. M., K. Pape, M. Arstikaitis, M. Boyle, S. Ashby, A. Rowley, C. Netley, and P. R. Swyer, Mechanical ventilation of infants of less than 1,501 gm birth weight. Health, growth, and neurologic sequelae, *J. Pediatr.,* **88**:531 (1976).
29. Outerbridge, E. W., M. Ramsay, and L. Stern, Developmental follow-up of survivors of neonatal respiratory failure, *Crit. Care Med.,* **2**:23 (1974).
30. Jones, R. A. K., M. Cummins, and P. A. Davies, Infants of very low birthweight. A 15 year analysis, *Lancet,* **i**:1332 (1979).
31. Saigal, S., P. Rosenbaum, B. Stoskopf, and R. Milner, Follow-up of infants 501 to 1,500 gm birth weight delivered to residents of a geographically defined region with perinatal intensive care facilities, *J. Pediatr.,* **100**:606 (1982).
32. Lindroth, M., N. W. Svenningsen, H. Ahlström, and B. Jonson, Evaluation of mechanical ventilation in newborn infants. II. Pulmonary and neurodevelopmental sequelae in relation to original diagnosis, *Acta Paediatr. Scand.,* **69**:151 (1980).
33. Vohr, B. R., E. F. Bell, and W. Oh, Infants with bronchopulmonary dysplasia. Growth pattern and neurologic and developmental outcome, *Am. J. Dis. Child.,* **136**:443 (1982).
34. Naeye, R. L., B. Ladis, and J. S. Drage, Sudden infant death syndrome. A prospective study. *Am. J. Dis. Child.,* **130**:1207 (1976).
35. Markestad, T., and P. M. Fitzhardinge, Growth and development in children recovering from bronchopulmonary dysplasia, *J. Pediatr.,* **98**:597 (1981).

36. Gupta, J. M., G. J. Harrington, and F. C. Hollows, A two year follow-up of infants with respiratory distress syndrome, *Med. J. Aust.,* **1**:819 (1976).
37. Hallock, N., G. Ting, J. Dempsey, C. Dabiri, and H. H. Shuman, A first-year follow-up of high-risk infants: Formulating a cumulative risk index, *Child Devel.,* **49**:119 (1978).
38. Fitzhardinge, P. M., A. Eisen, C. Lejtenyl, K. Metrakos, and M. Ramsay, Sequelae of early steroid administration to the newborn infant, *Pediatrics,* **53**:877 (1974).
39. Gunn, T., E. R. Reece, K. Metrakos, and E. Colle, Depressed T cells following neonatal steroid treatment, *Pediatrics,* **67**:61 (1981).
40. Stahlman, M., G. Hedvall, E. Dolanski, G. Faxelius, H. Burko, and V. Kirk, A six-year follow-up of clinical hyaline membrane disease, *Pediatr. Clin. North Am.,* **20**:433 (1973).
41. Stahlman, M., and V. Kirk, Follow-up studies of infants with hyaline membrane disease. In *Neonatal Intensive Care.* Edited by J. B. Stetson and R. R. Swyer. St. Louis, Green, 1975, p. 487.
42. Kamper, J., and J. Moller, Long-term prognosis of infants with idiopathic respiratory distress syndrome. Follow-up studies in infants surviving after the introduction of continuous positive airway pressure, *Acta Paediatr. Scand.,* **68**:149 (1979).
43. De Miere, R. J. S., C. C. Laiz, A. V. I. Soler, J. M. P. Vinas, and J. I. B. Villalibre, Neurological development of newborn infants with idiopathic respiratory distress syndrome treated with positive pressure, *An. Esp. Pediatr.,* **10**:514 (1977).
44. Brown, J. K., F. Cockburn, J. O. Forfar, R. L. Marshall, and G. W. Stephen, Problems in the management of assisted ventilation in the newborn and follow-up of treated cases, *Br. J. Anaesth.,* **45**(Suppl.):808 (1973).
45. Ruiz, M. P. D., J. A. LeFever, D. O. Hakanson, D. A. Clark, and M. L. Williams, Early development of infants of birth weight less than 1,000 grams with reference to mechanical ventilation in newborn period, *Pediatrics,* **68**:330 (1981).
46. MacArthur, B. A., R. N. Howie, J. A. Dezoete, and J. Elkins, School progress and cognitive development of 6-year-old children whose mothers were treated antenatally with betamethasone, *Pediatrics,* **70**:99 (1982).
47. Harrod, J. R., P. L'Heureux, O. D. Wagensteen, and C. E. Hunt, Long term follow-up of severe respiratory distress syndrome treated with IPPV, *J. Pediatr.,* **84**:277 (1974).
48. Kamper, J., Long term prognosis of infants with severe idiopathic respiratory distress syndrome. II. Cardio-pulmonary outcome, *Acta Paediatr. Scand.,* **67**:71 (1978).

49. Jones, R. W. A., and D. Pickering, Persistent ductus arteriosus complicating the respiratory distress syndrome, *Arch. Dis. Child.,* **52**:274 (1977).
50. Cotton, R. B., D. P. Lindstrom, and M. T. Stahlman, Early prediction of symptomatic patent ductus arteriosus from perinatal risk factors: A discriminant analysis model, *Acta Paedistr. Scand.,* **70**:723 (1981).
51. Bejar, R., T. A. Merritt, R. W. Coen, T. Mannino, and L. Gluck, Pulsatility index, patent ductus arteriosus, and brain damage, *Pediatrics,* **69**:818 (1982).
52. Swenningsen, N. W., B. Jonson, M. Lindroth, and H. Ahlström, Consecutive study of early CPAP-application in hyaline membrane disease, *Eur. J. Pediatr.,* **131**:9 (1979).
53. Robertson, A. M., and J. U. Crichton, Neurological sequelae in children with neonatal respiratory distress. Infants with low birth weight, *Am. J. Dis. Child.,* **117**:271 (1969).
54. Kamper, J., Long term prognosis of infants with severe idiopathic respiratory distress syndrome. I. Neurological and mental outcome, *Acta Paediatr. Scand.,* **67**:61 (1978).
55. Rothberg, A. D., M. J. Maisels, S. Bagnato, J. Murphy, K. Gifford, K. McKinley, E. A. Palmer, and R. C. Vannucci, Outcome for survivors of mechanical ventilation weighing less than 1,250 gm. at birth, *J. Pediatr.,* **98**:106 (1981).
56. Bertelsen, A., B. Bengtsson, B. Rud, and B. Peitersen, Follow-up investigation of children treated with assisted ventilation during the neonatal period, *Ugeskr. Laeger,* **140**:2168 (1978).
57. Lamarre, A., A. L. Linsao, B. J. Reilly, P. R. Swyer, and H. Levison, Residual pulmonary abnormalities in survivors of idiopathic respiratory distress syndrome, *Am. Rev. Respir. Dis.,* **108**:56 (1973).
58. Outerbridge, E. W., and L. Stern, Developmental follow-up of artificially ventilated infants with neonatal respiratory failure. In *Neonatal Intensive Care.* Edited by J. B. Stetson and P. R. Swyer. St. Louis, Green, 1975, p. 471.
59. Outerbridge, E. W., M. B. Nogrady, P. H. Beaudry, and L. Stern, Idiopathic respiratory distress syndrome. Recurrent respiratory illness in survivors, *Am. J. Dis. Child.,* **123**:99 (1972).
60. Bourgeois, J., J. Genoud, J. Cutruge, P. Frappat, and P. Valancogne, Fate of premature infants ventilated for idiopathic respiratory distress, *Pediatrie,* **30**:793 (1975).
61. Benoist, M. R., C. Siguier, R. Jean, J. Fermanian, J. Paupe, and J. Vialatte, Lung function after neonatal respiratory distress syndrome, *Bull. Eur. Physiopathol. Respir.,* **12**:703 (1976).

62. H., Ahlström, Pulmonary mechanics in infants surviving severe neonatal respiratory insufficiency, *Acta Paediatr. Scand.,* **64**:69 (1975).
63. Loc'h, L., J. Lalande, and F. Doyon, Survey on the outcome of newborn infants treated in the pediatric intensive care units, *Arch. Fr. Pediatr.,* **35**:7 (1978).
64. Boss, J. A., and J. M. Craig, Reparative phenomena in lungs of neonates with hyaline membranes, *Pediatrics,* **29**:890 (1962).
65. Northway, W. H., R. C. Rosan, and D. Y. Porter, Pulmonary disease following respiratory therapy of hyaline membrane disease. Bronchopulmonary dysplasia, *N. Engl. J. Med.,* **276**:357 (1967).
66. Shepard, F. M., R. B. Johnston, E. C. Klatte, H. Burko, and M. Stahlman, Residual pulmonary findings in clinical hyaline-membrane disease, *N. Engl. J. Med.,* **279**:1063 (1968).
67. Northway, W. H., L. Rezeau, and K. G. Bensch, Oxygen toxicity in the newborn lung: Reversal of inhibition of DNA synthesis in the mouse, *Pediatrics,* **57**:41 (1976).
68. Westgate, H. D., R. O. Fisch, L. O. Langer, and H. P. Staub, Pulmonary and respiratory function changes in survivors of hyaline membrane disease, *Dis. Chest.,* **55**:465 (1969).
69. Bomsel, F., Pulmonary sequelae of the hyaline membrane disease. Iatrogenic factors? Radiological and anatomical study, *Ann. Radiol.,* **16**:70 (1973).
70. Kanto, W. P., L. P. Kuhns, R. C. Borer, and D. W. Roloff, Failure of serial chest radiographs to predict recovery from respiratory distress syndrome, *Am. J. Obstet. Gynecol.,* **131**:757 (1978).
71. Truog, W. E., J. L. Prueitt, and D. E. Woodrum, Unchanged incidence of bronchopulmonary dysplasia in survivors of hyaline membrane disease, *J. Pediatr.,* **92**:261 (1978).
72. Lalande, J., Pulmonary sequelae of neonatal respiratory distress: Evolution during the first years of life, *Ann. Radiol.,* **16**:74 (1973).
73. Smyth, J. A., E. Tabachnik, W. J. Duncan, B. J. Reilly, and H. Levison, Pulmonary function and bronchial hyperactivity in long-term survivors of bronchopulmonary dysplasia, *Pediatrics,* **68**:336 (1981).
74. Fletcher, B. D., Radiologic findings in mechanically ventilated survivors of neonatal respiratory failure, *Ann. Radiol.,* **16**:78 (1973).
75. Barnes, N. D., D. Hull, W. J. Glover, and A. D. Milner, Effects of prolonged positive pressure ventilation in infancy, *Lancet,* **ii**:630:1096 (1969).
76. Coates, A. L., H. Bergsteinsson, K. Desmond, E. W. Outerbridge, and P. H. Beaudry, Long-term pulmonary sequelae of premature birth with and without idiopathic respiratory distress syndrome, *J. Pediatr.,* **90**:611 (1977).

77. Weinstein, M. R., and W. Oh, Oxygen consumption in infants with bronchopulmonary dysplasia, *J. Pediatr.,* **99**:958 (1981).
78. Heldt, G. P., M. B. McIlroy, T. N. Hansen, and W. H. Tooley, Exercise performance of the survivors of hyaline membrane disease, *J. Pediatr.,* **96**:995 (1980).
79. Borkenstein, J., M. Borkenstein, and H. Rosegger, Pulmonary function studies in long-term survivors with artificial ventilation in the neonatal period, *Acta Paediatr. Scand.,* **69**:159 (1980).
80. McCormick, M. C., S. Shapiro, and B. H. Starfield, Rehospitalization in the first year of life for high-risk survivors. *Pediatrics,* **66**:991 (1980).
81. Gambi, D., P. M. Rossini, G. Albertini, D. Sollazzo, M. G. Torrioli, and G. C. Polidori, Follow-up of visual evoked potential in full-term and preterm control newborns and in subjects who suffered from perinatal respiratory distress, *Electroencephalogr. Clin. Neurophysiol.,* **48**:509 (1980).
82. Fisch, R. O., Overview: Perinatal, medical and growth factors. In *Early Correlates of Speech, Language and Hearing.* Edited by P. J. LaBenz and E. S. LaBenz. Littleton, Massachusetts, PSG Publishing Co., 1980, p. 355.
83. Calame, A., I. Reymond-Goni, M. Maherzi, M. Roulet, C. Marchand, and L. S. Prod'hom, Psychological and neurodevelopmental outcome of high risk newborn infants, *Helv. Paediatr. Acta,* **31**:287 (1976).
84. Bacola, E., F. C. Behrle, L. de Schweinitz, H. C. Miller, and M. Mira, Perinatal and environmental factors in late neurogenic sequelae. II. Infants having birth weights from 1,500 to 2,500 grams, *Am. J. Dis. Child.,* **112**:369 (1966).
85. Bacola, E., F. C. Behrle, L. de Schweinitz, H. C. Miller, and M. Mira, Perinatal and environmental factors in late neurogenic sequelae. I. Infants having birth weights under 1,500 grams, *Am. J. Dis. Child.,* **112**:359 (1966).
86. Fisch, R. O., H. J. Gravem, and R. R. Engel, Neurological status of survivors of neonatal respiratory distress syndrome, *J. Pediatr.,* **73**:395 (1968).
87. Ambrus, C. M., D. H. Weintraub, K. R. Niswander, L. Fischer, J. Fleishman, I. D. J. Bross, and J. L. Ambrus, Evaluation of survivors of respiratory distress syndrome at 4 years of age, *Am. J. Dis. Child.,* **120**:296 (1970).
88. Nars, P. S., L. Schubarth, R. Kinndler, U. Werthemann, and G. Stalder, Systematic follow-up of newborns with idiopathic respiratory distress syndrome. Results in 197 patients born 1971 to 1976, *Helv. Paediatr. Acta,* **36**:389 (1981).
89. Shannon, D. C., R. K. Crone, I. D. Todres, and K. S. Krishnamoorthy, Survival, cost of hospitalization, and prognosis in infants critically ill with respiratory distress syndrome requiring mechanical ventilation, *Crit. Care Med.,* **9**:94 (1981).

90. Drillen, C. M., A. J. M. Thompson, and K. Burgoyne, Low-birthweight children at early school-age: A longitudinal study, *Develop. Med. Child. Neurol.,* **22**:26 (1980).
91. Knobloch, H., A. Malone, P. H. Ellison, F. Stevens, and M. Zdeb, Considerations in evaluating changes in outcome for infants weighing less than 1,501 grams, *Pediatrics,* **69**:285 (1982).
92. Haidvogl, V. M., H. Rosegger, S. Schröfl, and W. D. Müller, The development of infants subjected to aided respiration in the newborn period, *Wein. Klin. Wochenschr.,* **88**:561 (1976).
93. Ballard, R. A., E. N. Kraybill, J. Hernandez, M. L. Renfield, and W. J. Blankenship, Idiopathic respiratory distress syndrome. Treatment with continuous negative-pressure ventilation, *Am. J. Dis. Child.,* **125**:676 (1973).
94. Stewart, A. R., N. N. Finer, R. R. Moriartey, and O. A. Ulan, Neonatal nasotracheal intubation: An evaluation, *Laryngoscope,* **90**:826 (1980).
95. Marchak, B. E., W. K. Thompson, P. Duffty, T. Miyaki, M. H. Bryan, A. C. Bryan, and A. B. Froese, Treatment of RDS by high-frequency oscillatory ventilation: A preliminary report, *J. Pediatr.,* **99**:287 (1981).
96. Alexander, G., T. Gerhardt, and E. Bancalari, Hyaline membrane disease. Comparison of continuous negative pressure and nasal positive airway pressure in its treatment, *Am. J. Dis. Child.,* **133**:1156 (1979).
97. Merritt, T. A., I. D. Stuard, J. Puccia, B. Wood, D. K. Edwards, J. Finkelstein, and D. L. Shapiro, Newborn tracheal aspirate cytology: Classification during respiratory distress syndrome and bronchopulmonary dysplasia, *J. Pediatr.,* **98**:949 (1981).
98. Moylan, F. M. B., A. M. Walker, S. S. Kramer, I. D. Todres, and D. C. Shannon, The relationship of bronchopulmonary dysplasia to the occurrence of alveolar rupture during positive pressure ventilation, *Crit. Care Med.,* **6**:140 (1978).
99. Gluck, L., Administration of corticosteroids to induce maturation of fetal lung, *Am. J. Dis. Child.,* **130**:976 (1976).
100. Ballard, R. A., and P. L. Ballard, Use of prenatal glucocorticoid therapy to prevent respiratory distress syndrome. A supporting view, *Am. J. Dis. Child.,* **130**:982 (1976).
101. Johnson, J. W. C., W. Mitzner, W. T. London, A. E. Palmer, and R. Scott, Betamethasone and the Rhesus fetus: Multisystemic effects, *Am. J. Obstet. Gynecol.,* **133**:677 (1979).
102. Johnson, J. W. C. W. Mitzner, J. C. Beck, W. T. London, D. L. Sly, P. A. Lee, V. A. Khouzami, and R. L. Cavalieri, Long-term effects of betamethasone on fetal development, *Am. J. Obstet. Gynecol.,* **141**:1053 (1981).

103. Weisberg, S., *Applied Linear Regression.* New York, Wiley, 1980.
104. Stewart, A. L., E. O. R. Reynolds, and A. P. Lipscomb, Outcome for infants of very low birthweight: Survey of world literature, *Lancet,* **i**:1038 (1981).
105. Hack, M., A. A. Fanaroff, and I. R. Merkatz, The low-birth-weight infant—Evolution of a changing outlook, *N. Engl. J. Med.*, **301**:1162 (1979).
106. Ment, L. R., D. T. Scott, R. A. Ehrenkranz, S. G. Rothman, C. C. Duncan, and J. W. Warshaw, Neonates of $\leq$ 1,250 grams birth weight: Prospective neurodevelopmental evaluation during the first year post-term, *Pediatrics,* **70**:292 (1982).
107. Notter, R. H., and D. L. Shapiro, Lung surfactant in an era of replacement therapy, *Pediatrics,* **68**:781 (1981).
108. Fujiwara, T., S. Chida, Y. Watabe, H. Maeta, T. Morita, and T. Abe, Artificial surfactant therapy in hyaline-membrane disease, *Lancet,* **i**:8159 (1980).

Part Eight

THE FUTURE

19

Areas of Future Research and Development

GEORGE H. NELSON

Medical College of Georgia
Augusta, Georgia

Regarding early development in utero Ronan O'Rahilly (personal communication) feels that the development of the respiratory system during the embryonic period proper should be reinvestigated in detail in a large series of staged human embryos and the features sorted in ascending order of appearance, thereby allowing a statistical analysis of variations to be made, as well as permitting an appreciation of the detailed relationships to other developing systems.

W. N. Spellacy (personal communication) is of the opinion that one exciting area of future research is in the area of fetal regenerative powers where it is now becoming clear that the removal of a portion of the fetus at an early time period will result in a spontaneous regeneration of that part. It may be that abnormal lung buds may be surgically removed in the future and the fetus will then be able to grow a normal organ. In addition, studies of the maturation process of germinal plate vasculature in the central nervous system of the fetus seem indicated. Clearly, one of our major problems with the premature infant is intraventricular hemorrhage, and if we could predict, prevent, or treat that more effectively in utero, it would have a major impact on infant survival.

With regard to the morphological and biochemical development of fetal lungs, J. M. Johnston, J. M. Snyder, C. R. Mendelson, and J. E. Bleasdale (personal communication) note that the primary emphasis of biochemical investigations has been the elucidation of the molecular mechanism by which the biosyntheses of the glycerophospholipids of surfactant are regulated and integrated. We now have a working hypothesis to explain the integration of the synthesis of the different glycerophospholipids of surfactant. Furthermore, based on the proposed biochemical model, we can now provide a molecular mechanism for the alteration of the glycerophospholipid composition of surfactant that occurs in the fetuses of diabetic mothers. In contrast, limited information is available concerning the origin and function of the proteins that are associated with surfactant. The functions of these proteins, their physiochemical properties, their enzymatic activities, the process by which they may be recycled, and details of their synthesis await future investigations. Johnston et al. also maintain that the precise roles of the various hormones which have been shown to accelerate fetal lung maturation have yet to be established. Contrary to original postulates, the process of acceleration of surfactant biosynthesis may be under the control of several hormones. In addition, the interaction of the type II pneumonocyte with other lung cell types may be involved in the conversion of a less active hormone to the physiologically active form of the hormone. They feel that one of the major voids that we have in the understanding of the process of fetal lung maturation is the biogenesis of lamellar bodies in the type II cell. With the combined efforts of the powerful tools of immunocytochemistry and biochemistry such vital information should be forthcoming in the next few years. The discovery of surfactant and its function and the relationship of the decreased amounts of surfactant to the development of respiratory distress syndrome of the newborn, combined with the increased knowledge that is reviewed in this book, hopefully will provide the impetus for the development of improved therapy for the eradication of neonatal respiratory distress syndrome.

With respect to the use of ultrasound for pregnancy dating, D. L. Levy (personal communication) feels that investigators will continue to report new fetal measurements (some have been reported since he coauthored Chapter 5 of this volume) to correlate with gestational age. Time alone will decide which measurements will survive and which will be abandoned. It seems certain though that as ultrasound technology improves, more accurate measurements will be made and more accurate dating will result. He notes that one development which could slow progress in this area would be public reaction to lay reports regarding the safety vs. the danger of diagnostic ultrasound. The recent report of the NIH task force on the safety of sonography was very positive for its future. However, any adverse reports in the future could retard progress in this area.

Concerning new methods for examination of amniotic fluid for fetal lung maturity evaluation, J. C. McPherson, H. E. Fadel, and G. H. Nelson, (personal communication) feel that three areas are particularly fertile for investigation: (1) the measurement of amniotic fluid phospholipid by attenuated reflection spectroscopy; (2) the measurement of the surfactant protein moiety by radioimmunoassay or enzyme immunoassay; and (3) simple and reliable means of measuring amniotic fluid surface activity.

Morrison (personal communication) perceives that the thyroid hormones may in the future play a larger role as a stimulant of fetal lung maturity. As to other assessments, he believes that in the future we will see less maternal exposure to a variety of prescribed and over-the-counter drugs. As it concerns the development of future tests, he maintains that there will be significant developments in the physiological assessment of the infant to withstand extrauterine life. This is in opposition to the tests currently used, which largely predict, indirectly, the function of one or more systems in a fetus such as lung, renal, or liver maturity. Extensive experience in this area of fetal biophysical functions has already been obtained. This will probably be the area of greatest development in the near future.

R. M. Pitkin (personal communication) feels that a questionable point in patient management is what to do with the patient with premature rupture of the membranes (PROM) near term. The standard approach is to induce labor in these patients who do not go into labor themselves within a reasonable period of time, thinking that infection is the risk to be concerned about. He is currently questioning this approach and is of the opinion that obstetricians may be causing more difficulty by the induction than they are preventing. He believes that a well-controlled study designed to investigate this point would seem to be well worth the effort.

J. F. Evans (personal communication) concludes that consumers will be expecting more from their medical care system than in the recent past. Health care providers will be expected to provide accurate and clear descriptions of their patient's condition, available treatment, and consequences as well as alternatives for care. Maternal transport is a potentially lifesaving mechanism as well as a financial solvency for smaller obstetrical facilities. Evans is of the opinion that maternal transport systems can provide a well-defined, easily accessed mechanism for consultation and transfer. Such a system can also provide needed tertiary support for the infrequent need of expensive equipment and personnel. He feels that in the future the United States can and will support a nationwide system of maternal transport. He is confident that this will result in lower perinatal morbidity and mortality and will in the long run be a cost-saving mechanism.

Concerning premature labor F. Fuchs (personal communication) holds that three things will happen in the next few years: (1) An oxytocin analog which binds to the oxytocin receptor but has no oxytocic properties will be developed. All present tocolytic agents act on several organ systems and, therefore, have side effects; oxytocin only acts on the breast and the uterus, and analogs should not have any side effects on other systems. (2) Combinations of known tocolytic agents will be tested and found superior to single-agent tocolysis because of the different mechanism of action of the various types of agents. (3) Identification of high-risk factors and elimination of risks will spread rapidly and pay off much more than the use of tocolytic drugs. In spite of these developments, preterm birth will remain the most important problem in obstetrics and neonatology for the remaining part of the century.

G. Enhorning (personal communication) is continuing his clinical trial of surfactant instilled prophylactically into the airways of infants born at 29 weeks or earlier and, hence, are at great risk of developing RDS. The surfactant is given prior to the first breath. The study is randomized, and so far they have 66 infants in the trial. Their results were reported at a meeting in Washington, D.C., from November 29 to December 2, 1984. The meeting was organized by Jerold F. Lucey of the University of Vermont in Burlington, who is the editor-in-chief of the journal *Pediatrics.* Lucey invited all investigators involved with clinical trials. Enhorning also believes we are on the threshold of the development of artificial surfactant. The need will probably be enormous because in his opinion treatment of neonatal RDS is only the beginning. Respiratory distress syndrome of the newborn is a fairly clear-cut condition caused mainly by a surfactant deficiency; however, there probably are a number of conditions where surfactant deficiency is also part of the problem, i.e., adult RDS, pneumonia, and possibly asthma.

Considering newborn resuscitation, A. F. Robertson, III and W. P. Kanto, Jr. (personal communication) believe there are several areas that will be interesting for research in the future. The current stress tests, fetal heart rate monitoring, and scalp blood pH determinations are very crude ways of estimating transplacental oxygen delivery. There has to be some better way of measuring this. Perhaps in the future the Doppler technique and computer analysis will be refined to the degree where we can accurately measure placental blood flow and infer oxygen delivery from that. A second area of interest, they feel, is the study of why an asphyxiated baby does not breathe. If this is partially due to endorphins, then obviously the development of more specific endorphin antagonists may be helpful in resuscitation. We need to know much more about brain metabolism in asphyxia. For example, is the damage of asphyxia related to decreased substrate such as glucose or increased product such as lactate? In regard to substrate, what is the capability of the newborn brain for gluconeogenesis? If we knew the correct substrate, the substrate could be replaced immediately in resuscitation. They feel that the future will see the development of the extracorporeal membrane oxygenator. From recent data, it looks as though such an oxygenator will be quite helpful, especially in cases of persistent pulmonary hypertension where the lungs are relatively normal.

G. R. Gutcher and R. H. Perelman (personal communication) believe that the explosive impact of technology on medical care is particularly evident in neonatology. Coupled with an expanding knowledge of fetal and neonatal physiology, the principal effect of this technology is on the increased survival of smaller and smaller infants. However, this improved survival is costly. The technology itself is expensive, while the prolonged hospitalization of these tiny infants imposes additional costs. For the most part, it is not possible for a given family to meet these costs without third-party assistance. Even so, the current system of reimbursement is being stretched to the breaking point. This is and will increasingly provide the impetus to search for better methods of cost containment. Difficult decisions will need to be made. Is the survival of a 500-g infant with some disability cost effective or even desirable? How does one measure cost effectiveness? Who decides? Who pays? Are there means to shorten hospital stays by early discharge? With what criteria? What home-care support systems will be needed? Is early discharge cost effective? When is the preservation of a life too expensive? Who decides? How is the decision made? Furthermore, the expanded technology and protracted hospitalization tend to separate parents from their children in a dehumanizing fashion. This presents an even greater challenge to involve the parents in the care of the infant in the face of the barrier that the technology may physically and psychologically raise. Essentially, the difficult questions ahead reflect the general growing concern in our society with regard to progress. What is it? Gutcher and Perelman believe that there will be a subtle shift in emphasis from what *can* be done to what *should* be done.

A. F. Robertson, III (personal communication) believes that most of the respiratory distress syndromes in newborn infants are related to the following physiological parameters: surfactant synthesis, pulmonary interstitial fluid removal, control of pulmonary arterial resistance, myocardial function, and intrauterine pulmonary growth. Therefore, the future of improved diagnosis and treatment of RDS lies in research having to do with these factors, methods of measuring them, and, ultimately, measures to pharmacologically control them. He looks forward to a better definition of the varying syndromes which we include in the diagnosis of transient tachypnea of the newborn. Some cases are doubtlessly related to the nonremoval of pulmonary interstitial fluid, but in others there may be a myocardial function deficiency. Certainly, it is known that the pulmonary arterial resistance is elevated in some of these babies. If, in infants with transient tachypnea of the newborn, we could define which of these factors is predominant, it would then be possible to treat them more effectively.

In infants with hyaline membrane disease, he hopes for a method of induction of surfactant production which can be used after birth in the infants who already have the disease. Also, there is a need to determine if pharmacological closure of the ductus at birth should be performed in all infants at risk for hyaline membrane disease. Bronchopulmonary dysplasia is the most distressing result of treatment of the respiratory distress syndromes. He is anxious to find out if high-frequency ventilation can be made to work in hyaline membrane disease and if it will circumvent this complication. The meconium aspiration syndrome has decreased in frequency with better obstetrical care at delivery. Since most of the babies who die from this syndrome die as a result of persistent pulmonary hypertension, the next breakthrough would be the development of better pharmacological agents to decrease pulmonary arterial resistance. He believes that the prevention of early-onset streptococcal pneumonia will lie in the immunization of mothers, since the susceptibility of the infant is related to the presence or absence of maternal antibodies. Pulmonary hypoplasia is a diagnostic dilemma. An accurate way to measure pulmonary volume in living infants is needed. Once that is done, the causes of pulmonary hypoplasia and how they relate to intrauterine respiratory activity can be better defined.

G. F. Vawter and L. M. Reid (personal communication) believe that human human autopsy material could be used to explore further the nature of surfactant constituents, including apoprotein. Immunohistochemical and biochemical techniques could be used. Depending on the speed with which tissue is available, lavage, aspirate, biopsy, and even cell or organ culture might be possible. Differences between the various subsets of RDS should be analyzed more carefully—e.g., RDS in the lung of late-gestation infants. The presence of associated hypoplasia should be identified. The reason for the wide range of vascular patterns of early BPD patients should be investigated. In addition, they feel there are three broad questions that should be addressed: What are the mechanisms responsible for the cell necrosis in RDS? What is the nature of adaptation and repair in the premature and immature lung? In late-stage disease what is the injury, response, and repair at all airway levels?

Regarding follow-up studies on RDS infants, R. O. Fisch (personal communication) believes they should be done in a longitudinal prospective fashion, taking other than medical factors into consideration; hence, social and economical factors should also be considered. The only way to really learn the outcome of survivors of RDS is to extend the period of study to the school age and beyond. This is a very necessary endeavor. Follow-up studies should include data not only on infection but also on malignancy. He feels we need to know how these infants will function as adults in a stressful life and if their life expectancy will or will not be shortened.

Comments

Regarding my own thoughts concerning the future, I would like to take this opportunity to close this scientific treatise on a somewhat lighter note. I believe that the incidence of RDS will be shown to be related to the maternal diet. I predict that a team of epidemiologists, obstetricians, and neonatologists will determine that the ingestion of palm oil in the diet of pregnant Nigerian women does result in a lower incidence of RDS in Nigerian newborns. Following this report in the *Journal of the American Medical Association,* controlled studies will be set up in numerous medical centers throughout the United States to determine if the addition of palm oil to the diet of pregnant subjects will accelerate fetal lung maturation and reduce the incidence of RDS in premature births. The obstetrical literature will be flooded with conflicting reports as to the efficacy of this measure. Great debates will take place, and long before the issue is resolved, drug company executives, considering the profitability of a new product, will hold lengthy sessions to determine their course of action. Palm oil, in a variety of brand names, will make its way into the grocery stores alongside cottonseed oil, corn oil, etc. The FDA will rule that palm oil products are approved for human consumption and the race will be on. The first product promoted to obstetricians will be Pulmolac, a palm oil milk shake that will come in three flavors: chocolate, vanilla, and strawberry. Obviously by its name this product will promote pulmonary maturation. Clinical studies with Pulmolac will be initiated. Then the real problem will begin. A second product will be released and it will be called Palmilac. It will look and taste similar to Pulmolac; however, it will contain homogenized, purified palmitic acid. It will be promoted as being "extra strength" on the basis of its higher palmitic acid content. This will result in a pharmacist's nightmare as they attempt to differentiate the "a" from the "u" and the "i" from the "o" on obstetricians' prescriptions. Further complicating the issue will be those prescriptions which really contain a "u" and an "i" and those with an "a" and an "o." What is the poor pharmacist to do?

While in 1984 the likelihood of such a prediction might seem remote at best, stranger things have happened in the field of medicine. Certainly, Sir Alexander Fleming would have seemed wild to predict the antibiotic wars currently taking place among pharmaceutical companies. However, I am convinced that competition is what makes America great, and the Pulmolac–Palmilac conflict to come will be something to see.

AUTHOR INDEX

Italic numbers give the page on which the complete reference is listed.

A

B

C

E

F

G

H

I

J

L

M

N

Q

R

S

T

W

Y

Z

SUBJECT INDEX

D

E

F

G

H

M

N

O

P

R

S

T

U

V

W

6248